Treatment Resistant Depression

Editors

MANISH KUMAR JHA
MADHUKAR H. TRIVEDI

PSYCHIATRIC CLINICS OF NORTH AMERICA

www.psych.theclinics.com

Consulting Editor
HARSH K. TRIVEDI

June 2023 • Volume 46 • Number 2

ELSEVIER

1600 John F. Kennedy Boulevard • Suite 1800 • Philadelphia, Pennsylvania, 19103-2899

http://www.theclinics.com

PSYCHIATRIC CLINICS OF NORTH AMERICA Volume 46, Number 2
June 2023 ISSN 0193-953X, ISBN-13: 978-0-443-18252-5

Editor: Megan Ashdown
Developmental Editor: Malvika Shah

Psychiatric Clinics of North America (ISSN 0193-953X) is published quarterly by Elsevier Inc., 360 Park Avenue South, New York, NY 10010-1710. Months of issue are March, June, September, and December. Business and Editorial Offices: 1600 John F. Kennedy Blvd., Suite 1800, Philadelphia, PA 19103-2899. Periodicals postage paid at New York, NY and additional mailing offices. Subscription prices are $352.00 per year (US individuals), $781.00 per year (US institutions), $100.00 per year (US students/residents), $422.00 per year (Canadian individuals), $519.00 per year (international individuals), $983.00 per year (Canadian & international institutions), and $220.00 per year (international students/residents), $100.00 per year (Canadian & students/residents). Foreign air speed delivery is included in all *Clinics*' subscription prices. All prices are subject to change without notice. **POSTMASTER:** Send address changes to *Psychiatric Clinics of North America*, Elsevier Health Sciences Division, Subscription Customer Service, 3251 Riverport Lane, Maryland Heights, MO 63043. **Customer Service: 1-800-654-2452 (US). From outside the United States, call 1-314-447-8871. Fax: 1-314-447-8029. E-mail: journalscustomerservice-usa@elsevier.com (for print support)** and **journalsonlinesupport-usa@elsevier.com (for online support)**.

Reprints. For copies of 100 or more, of articles in this publication, please contact the Commercial Reprints Department, Elsevier Inc., 360 Park Avenue South, New York, New York 10010-1710. Tel.: 212-633-3874, Fax: 212-633-3820, E-mail: reprints@elsevier.com.

Psychiatric Clinics of North America is covered in *MEDLINE/PubMed (Index Medicus), Current Contents/Social and Behavioral Sciences, Social Science Citation Index, Embase/Excerpta Medica,* and PsycINFO.

Contributors

CONSULTING EDITOR

HARSH K. TRIVEDI, MD, MBA
President and Chief Executive Officer, Sheppard Pratt, Clinical Professor of Psychiatry, University of Maryland School of Medicine, Baltimore, Maryland, USA

EDITORS

MANISH KUMAR JHA, MBBS
Assistant Professor, Department of Psychiatry, Center of Depression Research and Clinical Care, Peter O'Donnell Jr. Brain Institute, The University of Texas Southwestern Medical Center, Dallas, Texas, USA

MADHUKAR H. TRIVEDI, MD
Professor of Psychiatry, Julie K. Hersh Chair for Depression Research and Clinical Care, Betty Jo Hay Distinguished Chair in Mental Health, Department of Psychiatry, Director, Center for Depression Research and Clinical Care, Peter O'Donnell Jr. Brain Institute, The University of Texas Southwestern Medical Center, Dallas, Texas, USA

AUTHORS

HAYLEY ARAMBURU, MHA
Research Study Coordinator, Center for Depression Research and Clinical, Peter O'Donnell Jr. Brain Institute, Department of Psychiatry, The University of Texas Southwestern Medical Center, Dallas, Texas, USA

EMINE RABIA AYVACI, MD
Assistant Professor, Department of Psychiatry, The University of Texas Southwestern Medical Center, Dallas, Texas, USA

KIMBERLYN MARAVET BAIG-WARD, MD, PhD
Psychiatry Research Track Resident Physician, Department of Psychiatry, Center for Depression Research and Clinical Care, The University of Texas Southwestern Medical Center, Dallas, Texas, USA

ANDREA BOSCUTTI, MD
Louis. A. Faillace, MD, Department of Psychiatry and Behavioral Sciences, The University of Texas Health Science Center at Houston, Houston, Texas, USA; Department of Pathophysiology and Transplantation, University of Milan, Milan, Italy

PAOLO CASSANO, MD, PhD
Director of Photobiomodulation, Division of Neuropsychiatry and Neuromodulation, Massachusetts General Hospital, Department of Psychiatry, Harvard Medical School, Boston, Massachusetts, USA

CHERISE R. CHIN FATT, PhD
Assistant Professor of Psychiatry, Center for Depression Research and Clinical Care, UT Southwestern Medical Center, Dallas, Texas, USA

RAYMOND CHO, MD
Baylor College of Medicine, Menninger Department of Psychiatry and Behavioral Sciences, The Menninger Clinic, Houston, Texas, USA

PAUL E. CROARKIN, DO, MS
Professor of Psychiatry, Department of Psychiatry and Psychology, Mayo Clinic, Rochester, Minnesota, USA

AMBER E. DEANE, PhD
Senior Research Scientist, Center for Depression Research and Clinical Care, Peter O'Donnell Jr. Brain Institute, Department of Psychiatry, The University of Texas Southwestern Medical Center, Dallas, Texas, USA

ANNA FEENEY, MD
Clinical Trials Network and Institute, Department of Psychiatry, Massachusetts General Hospital, Harvard Medical School, Boston, Massachusetts, USA

MARIE ANNE GEBARA, MD
Department of Psychiatry, University of Pittsburgh School of Medicine, Pittsburgh, Pennsylvania, USA

MAIA GERSTEN, BS
Division of Neuropsychiatry and Neuromodulation, Massachusetts General Hospital, Boston, Massachusetts, USA

MORA M. GREHL, MA
Department of Psychology and Neuroscience, Temple University, Philadelphia, Pennsylvania, USA

SARA HAMEED, BA
Department of Psychiatry, Depression and Anxiety Center for Discovery and Treatment, Icahn School of Medicine at Mount Sinai, New York, New York, USA

DAN V. IOSIFESCU, MD, MSc
Clinical Research Division, Nathan Kline Institute for Psychiatric Research, Orangeburg, New York, USA; Department of Psychiatry, New York University School of Medicine, New York, New York, USA

AYUSH JAIN
Student, The Shri Ram School, Gurgaon, Haryana, India

MANISH KUMAR JHA, MBBS
Assistant Professor, Department of Psychiatry, Center of Depression Research and Clinical Care, Peter O'Donnell Jr. Brain Institute, The University of Texas Southwestern Medical Center, Dallas, Texas, USA

JULIANA MENDONCA DE FIGUEIREDO, MD
Louis. A. Faillace, MD, Department of Psychiatry and Behavioral Sciences, The University of Texas Health Science Center at Houston, Houston, Texas, USA

SHUBHAM KAMAL, MBBS
Visiting Research Scientist, Department of Psychiatry, Yale School of Medicine, New Haven, Connecticut, USA

ERIC J. LENZE, MD
Department of Psychiatry, Washington University School of Medicine in St. Louis, St Louis, Missouri, USA

SANJAY J. MATHEW, MD
Professor and Vice Chair for Research, Menninger Department of Psychiatry and Behavioral Sciences, Baylor College of Medicine, Michael E. DeBakey VA Medical Center, The Menninger Clinic, Houston, Texas, USA

TARYN L. MAYES, MS
Program Manager, Center for Depression Research and Clinical Care, UT Southwestern Medical Center, Dallas, Texas, USA

KAYLA MARIE MCEACHERN, BS
Division of Neuropsychiatry and Neuromodulation, Massachusetts General Hospital, Boston, Massachusetts, USA

NICHOLAS MURPHY, PhD
Baylor College of Medicine, Menninger Department of Psychiatry and Behavioral Sciences, The Menninger Clinic, Houston, Texas, USA

JAMES W. MURROUGH, MD, PhD
Department of Psychiatry, Depression and Anxiety Center for Discovery and Treatment, Icahn School of Medicine at Mount Sinai, New York, New York, USA

HANADI A. OUGHLI, MD
Department of Psychiatry, Semel Institute for Neuroscience, University of California Los Angeles, Los Angeles, California, USA

BEN JULIAN A. PALANCA, MD, PhD, MSc
Departments of Anesthesiology and Psychiatry, Division of Biology and Biomedical Sciences, Center on Biological Rhythms and Sleep, Neuroimaging Labs Research Center, Washington University School of Medicine in St. Louis, Department of Biomedical Engineering, Washington University in St. Louis, St Louis, Missouri, USA

GEORGE I. PAPAKOSTAS, MD
Clinical Trials Network and Institute, Department of Psychiatry, Massachusetts General Hospital, Harvard Medical School, Boston, Massachusetts, USA

RAJIV RADHAKRISHNAN, MD
Assistant Professor, Departments of Psychiatry, Radiology and Biomedical Imaging, Yale School of Medicine, New Haven, Connecticut, USA

DANA RAZOUQ, MD
Louis. A. Faillace, MD, Department of Psychiatry and Behavioral Sciences, The University of Texas Health Science Center at Houston, Houston, Texas, USA

KARINA RIKHANI, MD
Department of Psychiatry, The University of Texas Southwestern Medical Center, Dallas, Texas, USA

TAYLOR ROGAN, BS
Department of Psychiatry, Yale School of Medicine, New Haven, Connecticut, USA

SUDHAKAR SELVARAJ, MBBS, DPhil (Oxon), FRCPsych
Louis. A. Faillace, MD, Department of Psychiatry and Behavioral Sciences, The University of Texas Health Science Center at Houston, Houston, Texas, USA

SUBHA SUBRAMANIAN, MD
Department of Neurology, Berenson-Allen Center for Noninvasive Brain Stimulation, Department of Psychiatry, Beth Israel Deaconess Medical Center, Harvard Medical School, Boston, Massachusetts, USA

MADHUKAR H. TRIVEDI, MD
Professor of Psychiatry, Julie K. Hersh Chair for Depression Research and Clinical Care, Betty Jo Hay Distinguished Chair in Mental Health, Department of Psychiatry, Director, Center for Depression Research and Clinical Care, Peter O'Donnell Jr. Brain Institute, The University of Texas Southwestern Medical Center, Dallas, Texas, USA

MILI TRIVEDI
Student, Colleyville Heritage High School, Colleyville, Texas, USA

COLLIN VAS, MD
Associate Professor of Psychiatry, The University of Texas Southwestern Medical Center, Dallas, Texas, USA

WILLIANS FERNANDO VIEIRA, PT, MSc, PhD
Division of Neuropsychiatry and Neuromodulation, Massachusetts General Hospital, Department of Psychiatry, Harvard Medical School, Boston, Massachusetts, USA; Department of Anatomy, Institute of Biomedical Sciences (ICB), University of Sao Paulo, Sao Paulo, Brazil

SAMUEL T. WILKINSON, MD
Department of Psychiatry, Yale School of Medicine, New Haven, Connecticut, USA

KUSH YAGNIK
Student, Center for Depression Research and Clinical Care, Peter O'Donnell Jr. Brain Institute, Department of Psychiatry, The University of Texas Southwestern Medical Center, Dallas, Texas, USA

Contents

Major depressive disorder is characterized by depressed mood and/or anhedonia with neurovegetative symptoms and neurocognitive changes affecting an individual's functioning in multiple aspects of life. Treatment outcomes with commonly used antidepressants remain suboptimal. Treatment-resistant depression (TRD) should be considered after inadequate improvement with two or more antidepressant treatments of adequate dose and duration. TRD has been associated with increased disease burden including higher associated costs (both socially and financially) affecting both the individual and society. Additional research is needed to better understand the long-term burden of TRD to both the individual and society.

Measurement-based care (MBC) is the systematic screening and ongoing assessment of symptoms, side effects, and adherence to adjust treatments as needed based on these factors. Studies show MBC leads to improved outcomes for depression and treatment-resistant depression (TRD). In fact, MBC may reduce the chances of developing TRD, as it leads to optimized treatment strategies based on symptom changes and compliance. There are many rating scales available for monitoring depressive symptoms, side effects, and adherence. These rating scales can be used in a variety of clinical settings to help guide treatment decisions, including depression treatment decisions.

Major depressive disorder is a chronic and recurrent illness that affects 20% of adults during their lifetime and is one of the leading causes of suicide in the United States. A systematic measurement-based care approach is the essential first step in the diagnosis and management of treatment-resistant depression (TRD) by promptly identifying individuals with depression and avoiding delays in treatment initiation. As comorbidities may be associated with poorer outcomes to commonly used antidepressants and increase risk of drug-drug interactions, their recognition and treatment is an essential component of management of TRD.

evidence of clinical efficacy, and the clinical aspects of this intervention, including patient evaluation, stimulation parameters selection, and safety considerations. Transcranial direct current stimulation is another neuro-modulation treatment for depression; although promising, the technique is not currently approved for clinical use in the United States. The final section outlines the open challenges and future directions of the field.

Major depressive disorder (MDD) is considered a global crisis. Conventional treatments for MDD consist of pharmacotherapy and psychotherapy, although a significant number of patients with depression respond poorly to conventional treatments and are diagnosed with treatment-resistant depression (TRD). Transcranial photobiomodulation (t-PBM) therapy uses near-infrared light, delivered transcranially, to modulate the brain cortex. The aim of this review was to revisit the antidepressant effects of t-PBM, with a special emphasis on individuals with TRD. A search on PubMed and ClinicalTrials.gov tracked clinical studies using t-PBM for the treatment of patients diagnosed with MDD and TRD.

This article reviews the role of psychotherapy in management of treatment-resistant depression (TRD). Meta-analyses of randomized trials show that psychotherapy has a positive therapeutic benefit in TRD. There is less evidence that one type of psychotherapy approach is superior to another. However, more trials have examined cognitive-based therapies than other forms of psychotherapy. Also reviewed is the potential combination of psychotherapy modalities and medication/somatic therapies as an approach to TRD. There is significant interest in ways that psychotherapy modalities could be combined with medication/somatic therapies to harness a state of enhanced neural plasticity and improve longer-term outcomes in mood disorders.

Major depressive disorder is a substantial public health challenge impacting at least 3 million adolescents annually in the United States. Depressive symptoms do not improve in approximately 30% of adolescents who receive evidence-based treatments. Treatment-resistant depression in adolescents is broadly defined as a depressive disorder that does not respond to a 2-month course of an antidepressant medication at a dose equivalent of 40 mg of fluoxetine daily or 8 to 16 sessions of a cognitive behavioral or interpersonal therapy. This article reviews historical work, recent literature on classification, current evidence-based approaches, and emerging interventional research.

Major depression is common in older adults ($\geq$ 60 years of age), termed late-life depression (LLD). Up to 30% of these patients will have treatment-resistant late-life depression (TRLLD), defined as depression that persists despite two adequate antidepressant trials. TRLLD is challenging for clinicians, given several etiological factors (eg, neurocognitive conditions, medical comorbidities, anxiety, and sleep disruption). Proper assessment and management is critical, as individuals with TRLLD often present in medical settings and suffer from cognitive decline and other marks of accelerated aging. This article serves as an evidence-based guide for medical practitioners who encounter TRLLD in their practice.

Increased awareness of the growing disease burden of treatment resistant depression (TRD), in combination with technological advances in MRI, affords the unique opportunity to research biomarkers that characterize TRD. We provide a narrative review of MRI studies investigating brain features associated with treatment-resistance and treatment outcome in those with TRD. Despite heterogeneity in methods and outcomes, relatively consistent findings include reduced gray matter volume in cortical regions and reduced white matter structural integrity in those with TRD. Alterations in resting state functional connectivity of the default mode network were also found. Larger studies with prospective designs are warranted.

Owing to the link between immune dysfunction and treatment-resistant depression (TRD) and the overwhelming evidence that the immune dysregulation and major depressive disorder (MDD) are associated with each other, using immune profiles to identify the biological distinct subgroup may be the step forward to understanding MDD and TRD. This report aims to briefly review the role of inflammation in the pathophysiology of depression (and TRD in particular), the role of immune dysfunction to guide precision medicine, tools used to understand immune function, and novel statistical techniques.

PSYCHIATRIC CLINICS OF NORTH AMERICA

SERIES OF RELATED INTEREST

Child and Adolescent Psychiatric Clinics of North America
https://www.childpsych.theclinics.com/

Neurologic Clinics
https://www.neurologic.theclinics.com/

Advances in Psychiatry and Behavioral Health
https://www.advancesinpsychiatryandbehavioralhealth.com/

THE CLINICS ARE AVAILABLE ONLINE!
Access your subscription at:
www.theclinics.com

Preface

Treatment-Resistant Depression (TRD): Management Approaches in a Rapidly Evolving Therapeutic Landscape

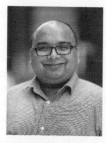
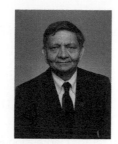

Manish Kumar Jha, MBBS   Madhukar H. Trivedi, MD
Editors

Abbreviations	
TRD	Treatment-Resistant Depression

One in three adults with major depressive disorder may not improve adequately with two or more courses of commonly used antidepressants and may have treatment-resistant depression (TRD). The presence of TRD is associated with impairments in multiple domains of life, higher health care–related expenses, and higher rates of self-harm and all-cause mortality. There is an urgent need to identify individuals with TRD in clinical practice and offer evidence-based treatments to them. With limited benefits of commonly used antidepressants in individuals with TRD, there is also an urgent need to develop novel treatments. This issue of the *Psychiatric Clinics of North America* seeks to address several of these issues starting with a comprehensive overview of TRD, including the public health burden associated with it. Use of measurement-based care is emphasized in this issue, as it can allow for optimizing the use of currently available antidepressants and for early identification of TRD. Currently available treatment options for TRD that are discussed in this issue include the use of medications, such as antidepressants and antipsychotics as well as ketamine and esketamine. Also discussed are neuromodulation approaches, such as repetitive transcranial magnetic stimulation, and psychotherapy treatments, such as cognitive therapy. The current therapeutic landscape of management approaches for TRD is

Psychiatr Clin N Am 46 (2023) xiii–xiv
https://doi.org/10.1016/j.psc.2023.03.014
0193-953X/23/© 2023 Published by Elsevier Inc.

rapidly evolving with the recent approvals by the Food and Drug Administration of intranasal esketamine and cariprazine. This issue takes a deeper dive into several of these promising new treatment approaches, including psychedelics and photobiomodulation. This issue also delves into special considerations associated with TRD in children and adolescents, as well as in the elderly. Readers of this issue will also appreciate the discussion of blood- and brain-based biomarkers that are promising to usher in an era of precision psychiatry for TRD. Together, the reports included in this issue of *Psychiatric Clinics of North America* provide a broad overview of TRD along with the treatment approaches that are currently available as well as those that are on the horizon.

Manish Kumar Jha, MBBS
Center for Depression Research and Clinical Care
Department of Psychiatry
O'Donnell Brain Institute
UT Southwestern Medical Center
5323 Harry Hines Boulevard
Dallas, TX 75390-9119, USA

Madhukar H. Trivedi, MD
Center for Depression Research and Clinical Care
Department of Psychiatry
O'Donnell Brain Institute
UT Southwestern Medical Center
5323 Harry Hines Boulevard
Dallas, TX 75390-9119, USA

E-mail addresses:
Manish.jha@utsouthwestern.edu (M.K. Jha)
Madhukar.Trivedi@utsouthwestern.edu (M.H. Trivedi)

The Individual and Societal Burden of Treatment-Resistant Depression: An Overview

Kimberlyn Maravet Baig-Ward, MD, PhD[a],
Manish Kumar Jha, MBBS[a,b], Madhukar H. Trivedi, MD[a,b],*

KEYWORDS

- Treatment-resistant depression • Depression • Burden of depression
- Major depressive disorder • Quality of life

KEY POINTS

- Depression is a significant cause of disease burden and disability worldwide.
- Depression has a high economic cost for the individual and society.
- Treatment-resistant depression (TRD) lacks a consensus definition and does not have a standard treatment algorithm.
- TRD is associated with protracted burden of disease and is associated with higher treatment costs to the individual and a broader economic impact.
- Consensus definition and additional research on TRD is essential for improved treatment strategies and cost savings.

INTRODUCTION
Depression

Major depressive disorder (MDD) is a heterogenous syndrome that is characterized by depressed mood and/or anhedonia with neurovegetative symptoms and neurocognitive changes experienced nearly every day for a period lasting at least 2 weeks and often associated with significant functional impairments.[1–4] The landmark STAR*D study[5] showed that a third of patients with MDD do not improve adequately with multiple sequential courses of antidepressants, and may have treatment-resistant depression (TRD), a complex condition frequently encountered in those undergoing treatment of MDD.[2] In fact, after inadequate improvement with 2 courses of antidepressants, fewer than 1 in 6 patients with MDD attained remission (ie, no or minimal

[a] Department of Psychiatry, Center for Depression Research and Clinical Care, UT Southwestern Medical Center, 5323 Harry Hines Boulevard, Dallas, TX 75235, USA; [b] O'Donnell Brain Institute, UT Southwestern Medical Center, 6363 Forest Park Road, Dallas, TX 75235, USA
* Corresponding author. Center for Depression Research and Clinical Care, University of Texas Southwestern Medical Center, 5323 Harry Hines Boulevard, Dallas, TX 75235-9086.
E-mail address: madhukar.trivedi@utsouthwestern.edu

Psychiatr Clin N Am 46 (2023) 211–226
https://doi.org/10.1016/j.psc.2023.02.001
0193-953X/23/© 2023 Elsevier Inc. All rights reserved.

symptoms) with a third or fourth medication trial.[5] The presence of TRD further exacerbates the substantial burden associated with MDD. For the patients who do not reach remission after a depressive episode, TRD should be considered. In 2008, the World Health Organization ranked the worldwide burden of disease by cause and listed major depressive disorder as the third highest cause with a prediction that, given the trajectory of the illness, depression could become the number one cause of disease burden worldwide by the year 2030.[1,6] Additionally, a 2017 Lancet report by Vos and colleagues revealed that MDD was the second leading cause of global disability.[7–11] More recently, estimates from the Institute of Health Metrics and Evaluation found that 5% of adults worldwide (estimated to be more than 350 million people by current world population) suffers from depression.[7,12] These sobering indicators highlight the considerable impact of MDD globally and beg the following question: how can we improve our understanding of depression and improve treatments to alleviate suffering and impairment? The answer may, in part, lie in better understanding TRD and the increased individual and societal burden associated with the illness.[1]

EPIDEMIOLOGY

The lifetime risk of experiencing an episode of depression is estimated to be 20% or close to 1 in 5 people.[13,14] MDD can be diagnosed from childhood into older adulthood, with individuals being most likely to experience a first episode of depression between childhood and the fourth decade of life, although it is possible to have later onset.[1] Notably, onset in later years may portend increased treatment difficulty.[1,9,15–18]

Increased prevalence of MDD extends from the 20s through the 30s, with the peak prevalence in adults aged from 18 to 25 years.[19–22] A 2021 report showed that during a 12-month period in the United States, the prevalence of those undergoing medical treatment of MDD was estimated to be 8.9 million adults and of those, 2.8 million were considered to have TRD.[23] Additionally, recent studies have estimated that MDD rapidly increased in prevalence since the onset of the coronavirus disease 2019 (COVID-19) pandemic.[24,25] This increase is alarming and underscores the need for a better understanding of the disease, including the role of biological and social stressors in the disease process, and improved treatments. The recognition of sex as a biological variable and other sociodemographic factors are also important in understanding MDD.[14] Women are nearly twice as likely to have depression compared with men.[26] This so-called gender gap is likely due to an interplay of biopsychosocial factors and is an intriguing area for future cross-disciplinary research.[1,6,15–17,26] When stratified based on other factors, many studies have not shown significant differences in the prevalence of depression based on the income level of an entire country (developed nations versus lower income nations).[1] However, significant differences in prevalence of MDD have been shown based on the socioeconomic status, cultural background, and early life experiences of an individual.[1,27–31]

CAUSE

To treat any disease effectively, basic mechanistic and environmental factors should be understood for the development of novel therapeutic targets. Despite decades of research, there is still much to learn about the functional, molecular, and genetic underpinnings of depression. MDD is a complex disease without a singular cause; rather, the disorder is multifactorial with genetic, epigenetic, biological, environmental, structural, and social factors working together in an intricate network on an individual level making defining treatment targets challenging.[1,32–36] Although strides in the treatment of MDD both pharmacologic and interventional in nature have been made, MDD remains incompletely understood.[1,35,37] Much of the early research on depression was focused on the monoamine neurotransmitter hypothesis for depression and elucidating the role of the hypothalamic-pituitary-adrenal (HPA) axis in depression.[38–40] More recently, studies have shifted to better understand the role of inflammation in depression, environmental stress, genes and epigenetic changes, brain-derived neurotrophic factor, and neurogenesis, as well as structural and functional analyses of the brain, including aberrant neurocircuits, because technological advancements in neuroimaging and other methods (such as EEG) have been made.[1,41–46]

Diagnosis of Major Depressive Disorder

For a diagnosis of MDD by the Diagnostic and Statistical Manual of Mental Disorders fifth edition Text Revision (DSM-5-TR), at least 5 of 9 criteria for depression must be met including the requirement that either depressed mood or anhedonia (lack of interest in things once found enjoyable) is present (criterion A) and represents a departure from the individual's baseline functioning.[4] Briefly, other diagnostic criteria (criterion B) include the following: significant weight loss (or weight gain), insomnia (or hypersomnia), psychomotor retardation (or agitation), reduced energy (or fatigue), feelings of worthlessness (or guilt), poor concentration, and/or recurrent thoughts of suicide or death.[4] Diagnosis also requires that symptoms are not caused by the effects of substance use or other medical condition (criterion C), requires absence of lifetime manic or hypomanic-like episode (criterion D) and require that symptoms are not better explained by a psychotic or schizophrenia spectrum illness, or the like (criterion E).[4] Each of these criteria can be found outlined in greater detail in the DSM-5-TR.[3,4]

VARIATION IN ILLNESS PRESENTATIONS

Given the complexities of the biopsychosocial interactions, presentations of disease can vary from patient to patient. These differences in presentation give way to varying degrees of functional impairment and therefore perception of illness burden by the individual even when overall illness severity seems to be similar.[1,47] To better understand these nuanced differences between experiences, it may be useful to describe episodes of depression using additional specifiers such as those found in the DSM-5-TR and by functional outcomes (such as quality of life, productivity, and the like).[3,48–51] Furthermore, discrete episodes of depression may have other prominent emotions, behaviors, and variations in severity, which can contribute to the overall illness burden experienced at an individual level.[1,3] When present, a description of features of the illness and specifiers describes a more complete clinical picture.[1,14,29,52] Additionally, illness severity is a useful measure that can be accomplished through rating scales such as the Patient Health Questionnaire-9 (PHQ-9), Hamilton Depression Rating Scale, Quick Inventory of Depressive Symptomatology (QIDS), or the like, although clinical judgement still plays a critical role in gauging severity of illness.[28,53]

Anxious distress is the most frequently observed and should not be confused with a comorbid diagnosis of anxiety, which is also frequently occurs in those with MDD.[1] Notably, anxious distress has been linked to a poorer response to commonly used antidepressants (with the exception of ketamine).[54] Other prominent features such as irritability, somatic complaints, and panic are also seen. Irritability is unique among these symptoms because it is considered a criterion symptom of MDD for children and adolescents but not for adults. However, recent studies have shown that presence of irritability (and its related construct of anger attacks) is associated with poorer long-term outcomes (such as persistently elevated suicidal ideation) and that treatment-related changes in irritability can be used to prognostic clinical outcomes including remission and long-term levels of suicidal ideation.[55–58] Although no formal specifier exists for these, it is still important to capture their presence when part of the clinical picture of a depressive episode. Features such as irritability or somatic complaints can be more commonly observed within certain populations.[28,56,57]

Just as variations are observed in the symptoms and presentation of depression, variations in the duration of a single episode of depression have also been observed.[1,59] The average duration for a depressive episode, with treatment, is around 3 to 6 months before remission is reached.[59] However, studies have reported depressive episodes lasting up to 12 months.[1,59] Moreover, other comorbid illnesses can affect the duration and quality of a depressive episode.[1,6,9,60]

Treatment-Resistant Depression

Landmark studies, such as STAR*D, have shown that only around 30% of individuals undergoing "adequate treatment" for MDD will achieve full remission of depression after the first antidepressant trial.[1,5,27,33,37] In fact, most individuals who are treated for MDD either experience a partial response (20%) or no response to the first treatment (50%).[5,27] These treatment partial and nonresponders provide the basis for the concept of TRD.[37,61] TRD should not be confused with a recurrent episode of major depression where the patient previously achieved a period of remission after successful treatment of an episode of depression and experiences another separate and distinct episode of depression. Additionally, it is worth noting that the likelihood of having a recurrent episode of depression increases with increased resistance to treatment.[33,37]

TRD is a complex condition evaluated within the context of MDD.[27,62,63] The concept of treatment resistance is not exclusive to MDD and can also be experienced in bipolar depression and in other psychiatric illnesses.[27,62,63] However, more studies have focused on unipolar depression concerning TRD.[64] To date, no consensus diagnostic criteria with a consistently applied treatment algorithm exists for TRD making the study of TRD difficult.[27,62,63] Given the context of MDD, the cause of TRD is also multifactorial with genetic, epigenetic, biochemical, structural, environmental, and social factors and is not intrinsically resistant to treatment itself despite the current naming convention.[1,27,37] The contribution of each of these factors likely varies from individual to individual adding an additional layer of complexity in understanding the disorder, further convoluting the elucidation of disease mechanisms, and making robust treatment options elusive. The multifaceted cause of TRD and differences in patient presentations with the disorder have made it both diagnostically challenging and difficult when synthesizing the limited evidenced-based findings obtained to date. Furthermore, it has been suggested that TRD could be evaluated along a spectrum rather than by a binary approach (whether a patient has TRD or not).[27] TRD as a spectrum may better represent the diversity of disease seen in practice and myriad of treatment responses observed.

Although the cause of TRD remains enigmatic, certain characteristics, exposures, and comorbid conditions have been identified as risk factors for the development of TRD. Some of the risk factors include the following: comorbid psychiatric illnesses (especially anxiety, substance use disorders, and personality disorders), chronic medical conditions (including pain and inflammatory conditions), and social vulnerabilities (eg, unemployed, divorced, widowed).[65–71] Moreover, extremes of age, severity of illness, and melancholic features have also been shown to be risk factors for TRD.[65–71] Additional risk factors are likely to emerge as more studies are conducted in patients with TRD. Individuals with TRD typically have more comorbidities than those who respond well to treatment and may suggest some degree of biological "loading"; this remains incompletely understood and could be targeted in future research.[66,72,73]

Diagnosis of treatment-resistant depression

The most referenced "criteria" for the diagnosis of TRD require "a minimum of two prior treatment failures and confirmation of prior adequate dose and duration."[27] Despite the morbidity associated with TRD during the last almost 30 years, there is substantial uncertainty among experts or evidence-based guidelines outlining which pharmacologic intervention is preferred and what constitutes an adequate pharmacologic dose or treatment duration to be considered an adequate medication trial. A recent systematic review by Gaynes and colleagues[27] found that out of 185 studies only around 19% applied all components of the most used criteria for TRD. Complicating matters further, there is no consensus whether the adequate medication trial must be for a current episode of depression versus lifetime treatment failures. Furthermore, there was no clear definition for an adequate treatment duration varying from 3 to 12 weeks across the studies analyzed with 4 weeks typically representing the minimum treatment duration.[27] Given the multiple definitions and interpretations of what constitutes treatment resistance and adequate treatment attempts, McAllister-Williams and colleagues proposed the concept of "difficult-to-treat depression" over the naming convention of TRD. The term "difficult-to-treat depression" does not single out any one factor contributing to the continuing burden of illness experienced by the patient and allows for a more patient-centered approach where all treatment modalities are considered.[74]

In 2020, Gaynes and colleagues described screening tools useful in the diagnosis of TRD and assessment of severity of illness. The Antidepressant Treatment History Form stratifies resistance based on prior antidepressant trials with a higher score suggestive of worse patient outcomes and is primarily intended for use in research settings.[27,75] Similarly, the Thase and Rush Staging model and related European Staging model and the Massachusetts General Hospital Staging model also consider the number of antidepressant classes and therapies previously failed by an individual, exposure to a particular treatment (ie, duration), and other treatment strategies considered (such as augmentation), although not every model individually considers each of these factors.[27] Additionally, the Maudsley staging method (MSM) has been shown to predict treatment resistance in 85% of prospective cases studied.[76] This model includes the assessment of baseline characteristics not queried in the other models. The Massachusetts General Hospital Antidepressant Treatment History Questionnaire, a patient self-reported scale, has also been validated and identified around 76% of those with TRD in agreement with the independent examiners in the trial.[77] A newer model, the "Karolinska Institutet (sic) Model" (KIM) as described by Hägg and colleagues,[78] utilizes a precise definition for treatment duration as well as consideration of combination, adjunctive, and electroconvulsive therapy (ECT) treatments.

PSEUDORESISTANCE

If TRD is suspected, it is necessary to ensure all diagnostic possibilities have been considered because symptoms reported are not pathognomonic for depression. Care must be taken to distinguish depression from other psychiatric disorders, including other affective disorders. The psychiatric diagnostic screening questionnaire (PDSQ), as well as the Mini-International Neuropsychiatric Interview (MINI) can be useful tools to screen for other common psychiatric diagnoses.[33,37,79–81] Additionally, medical illnesses may have similar symptomatology (eg, hypothyroidism) and a thorough medical history should be performed.[82] Similarly, pharmacologic effects (substance use or medication side effects) can also mimic symptoms of depression and should be considered.[1] Therefore, treatment nonresponse is not always indicative of TRD, rather, in some instances may indicate an incorrect diagnosis.

When considering reasons for treatment failure, it is also important to verify reported failed medication trials because there could be discrepancies related to recall and medication adherence. Not taking medication correctly can occur for a myriad of reasons including the inability to pay for treatment.[83] In such instances, the patient would not have undergone an adequate trial although they may consider it a failed trial. It is also possible that individuals may inadvertently underestimate how long they were on an earlier medication when discussing past medication trials.

TRACKING TREATMENT OUTCOMES

Impaired function may persist with TRD irrespective of remission of other clinical symptoms.[84,85] Furthermore, the protracted course of illness with TRD makes assessing changes in disease progression challenging. Measurement-based care can be accomplished through a variety of rating scales (detailed in a subsequent section) and should be utilized for tracking treatment outcomes.[1,84,85] Similarly, quality of life measures should be considered when tracking outcomes.[80,85] The selection of which screening instrument is best to use often depends on practice location (ie, acute care setting versus clinic) and purpose (ie, establishment of care with a provider versus research) and time constraints.[28,53,86]

THE BURDEN OF DEPRESSION
Quality of Life

It is well known that depression has a negative impact on an individual's quality of life. However, like the concept of quality of life itself, the subjective degree of burden experienced by an individual with depression has been difficult to quantify; measures such as the global assessment of functioning and quality of life scale are useful in assessing the concept at an individual level.[87] Moreover, the recent COVID-19 pandemic's effect on quality of life has had a profound impact on mental health, the outcomes of which remain to be seen.[88] The determinants of quality of life focus on physical, mental, and social components working together.[89] Per the CDC definition, health-related quality of life is defined as, "an individual's or group's perceived physical and mental health over time."[89]

Those with MDD have a higher risk for cardiovascular events and other chronic medical illnesses.[90–92] Individuals with TRD have been reported to have increased distress and poor overall global functioning.[88,93] A Korean study of depressed individuals by Cho and colleagues[94] found that quality of life varied with age, weight, socioeconomic status, perception of one's own health, level of education, and employment status. Obesity, older age, lower income and education, unemployment, and perception of poor health all correlated with lower quality of life.[94] Similarly, comorbid psychiatric conditions, such as anxiety and substance use disorder, have also been shown to worsen an individual's quality of life.[95] Anxiety is one of the most common co-occurring psychiatric disorders with MDD and has been reported to be diagnosed in almost two-thirds of those with MDD and is often even observed before MDD diagnosis.[96]

Psychosocial Functioning and Productivity

Failing to treat childhood depression often results in a depressed and functionally impaired adult highlighting the "developmental cost" of depression.[28,97] The very nature of depression inhibits psychosocial functioning, causing individuals to have low-energy levels, poor sleep, and limits interpersonal interactions.[1,3] Individuals with depression often face extreme feelings of helplessness, hopelessness, or guilt, further isolating them from engaging with others.[1,3] Findings from a STAR*D secondary analysis showed sad mood and concentration (a subdomain of cognition) to be the most significant psychosocial functional domains affected.[98]

Depression is a significant cause of decreased work productivity as well as activity impairment, which can in part be attributable to the cognitive dysfunction associated with depression.[99] Changes in learning, memory, attention, concentration, and the like can continue even after resolution of the depressive episode.[99] This fact is compounded when decreased work productivity translates into decreased wages and increased unemployment.[1,88,100,101] Areas impacted, such as such as caring for a child or interactions with a partner often have far-reaching consequences to the patient and those who interact with them.[78] Too often these additional aspects of the patient's life are not fully captured in the clinical setting but are important for a holistic evaluation of the patient. Additionally, better understanding the domains affected for that individual will aid in assessing the overall disease burden experienced and will better facilitate connecting individuals with resources most useful for them.

Economic impact

The economic burden of depression is profound both at an individual and societal level. Moreover, studies have shown that TRD is costlier than treatment-responsive MDD due to the protracted duration of an individual episode affecting not only the individual with TRD but also others within their sphere of influence including family, caregivers, and employers.[27,102,103] Furthermore, individuals with TRD are 2 times more likely to endure hospitalization than those with treatment-responsive depression.[27,104] Adding to the economic burden of TRD, hospitalizations of individuals with TRD costs almost 6 times more on average than hospitalizations of individuals with treatment-responsive MDD.[27,105] Ivanova and colleagues[105] reported that TRD nearly doubles the employer-related costs compared with treatment-responsive depression. Those with treatment-responsive depression and commercial insurance spend an estimated US$9,975 after a single medication trial when treated to remission within the first 12 months of starting treatment. However, individuals with TRD who also have commercial insurance incur medical expenses estimated to be US$21,259 in the first 12 months after initiating treatment and undergo 3 or more treatment trials within that period.[106] Given these estimated costs are for those with commercially held insurance, the costs are conceivably much higher for those without insurance. Recent reports have indicated that uninsured individuals are more likely to face treatment barriers and inconsistently engage with the health-care system.[107] Similarly, uninsured individuals are sometimes faced with the burden to afford either medications or food.[83] For these reasons, uninsured individuals often go untreated or undertreated, which has significant implications on the individuals themselves and society overall.[83]

On a national level, reports have estimated the overall annual cost of depression to be around US$326 billion, an increase from the 2010 estimate of US$236 billion.[22] Of the factors considered, the greatest increase observed was due to workplace costs that was accountable for 61% of costs and was increased from 48% estimated in 2010. Moreover, findings from a recent study by Zhdanava and colleagues[23] in US adults undergoing treatment of depression estimated that US$92.7 billion and US$43.8 billion were spent because of MDD and TRD, respectively. Additionally, Zhdanava and colleagues report that the TRD represented US$25.8 billion of the "health care burden," US$8.7 billion of the "unemployment burden," and US$9.3

billion of the "productivity burden" associated with those on medication for the treatment of MDD. From a global perspective, depression and anxiety combined are estimated to cost the global economy around US$1 trillion annually in lost productivity.[108]

The individual and societal burden of suicide

Suicide is a leading cause of death, especially in those aged between the ages of 10 and 34 years.[57,109] Notably, this age range also corresponds with the highest prevalence of depression.[1,22] It is also well established that individuals with depression have a higher risk of suicide and suicide attempts.[1,57] Furthermore, those with TRD have an even higher risk of suicide than those with treatment-responsive depression and should be considered as a distinct outcome in future research studies in this population.[110]

During the last 20 years, the rate of suicide has continued to increase, whereas other major burdens of disease such as cancer and heart disease have declined (**Fig. 1**).[109] Furthermore, individuals who attempt suicide are often seen in the emergency department adding to the overall economic and societal burden of depression.[22] On an individual level, it can be devastating for the loved ones left behind and can create lasting consequences potentially affecting the mental health of the next generation.[111] Failed suicide attempts can also bring a new element of trauma to the already suffering individual.[112]

Lessons learned in improving health outcomes in other medical fields, such as cardiology and cancer, have demonstrated that the identification and utilization of biomarker-guided therapy reduces overall morbidity and mortality for the disease.[113,114] Unfortunately, no validated biomarkers currently exist to guide the treatment of depression.[115] However, cross-disciplinary research approaches seek to elucidate the brain–heart axis, among other promising areas of research.[116] Future research studies to elucidate biomarkers for depression are likely to aid in the

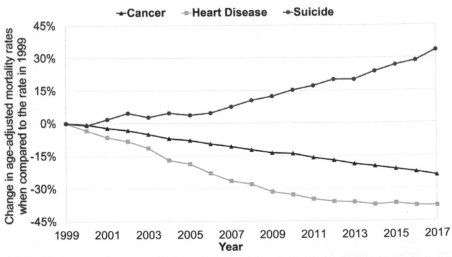

Fig. 1. Change in age-adjusted mortality rate due to suicide in the United States between 1999 and 2017. Age-adjusted mortality rates for suicide, cancer, and heart disease were obtained from the National Center for Health Statistics dataset.[109] The age-adjusted rate in the year 1999 was set as baseline and percent change was calculated for each year. Although rates of cancer and heart disease declined by 24.1% and 38.1%, respectively, the age-adjusted mortality rate of suicide increased by 33.3% between 1999 and 2017.

reduction of suicidality in MDD patients and guide treatments for best outcomes. Other features and measures linked with MDD, such as irritability, should also be considered for future research to better understand this vulnerable population.[57]

DISCUSSION

Barriers to treatment are multifactorial and often mirror the unique biopsychosocial landscape of the individual seeking treatment. The ability to accurately and efficiently stratify need based care is increasingly difficult given the lack of a standardized definition of TRD, the different treatment strategies utilized, the paucity of evidence-based treatment data for TRD, and the significant economic impact both to the individual and society.[27] This treatment conundrum can, in and of itself, act as a barrier to treatment. Moreover, this barrier is often compounded in the pediatric patient population because the therapeutic approach to TRD in these patients is largely based on the adult literature.[27,28] Evidence-based data in the pediatric population are even more limited to the few clinical trials that have been conducted. Treatment of resistant depression in adolescents (TORDIA) trial has been the only large-scale trial to address TRD in the pediatric population.[28,117,118] Of the adult trials that have focused on TRD, the lack of consensus definition of adequate treatment dose and duration has made interpreting findings challenging and limits our ability to compare trials or conduct meta-analyses.[27] However, while the individual and societal burden of depression is immense, especially in cases of TRD, the complexity of the disorder allows for the exciting possibility of personalized therapeutic options in the future.[1,37] Furthermore, improved understanding of TRD can bring about substantial cost savings both for the individual with depression and society overall.

SUMMARY

Given the far-reaching global consequences of depression, governments and other funding institutions must engage in supporting research endeavors to alleviate the burden of depression and better understand this complex illness. A consensus definition and treatment strategy for TRD is essential to help close the knowledge gap that currently exists. More robust research, including randomized clinical trials and meta-analyses, can be performed once this critical illness is better defined leading to better understanding of the illness itself, improved treatment options, and better outcomes for our patients worldwide.

CLINICS CARE POINTS

- Clinicians should be mindful of a patient's prior medication trials for depression. If the patient has already tried 2 different anti-depressants for adequate dose and duration, treatment-resistant depression (TRD) should be considered.

- Screening instruments, such as the Patient Health Questionnaire-9 (PHQ-9), can be utilized in the clinic to track how a patient is responding to treatment.

- Interventional treatment options, such as ECT, as well as clinical trial referral should be considered for TRD patients.

- The "hidden costs" of depression, such as difficulty with interpersonal relationships and economic losses, should be considered in individuals with TRD. Individualized community, therapy, and other resources should be offered, when appropriate.

- If TRD is being considered as a diagnosis, care must be taken to rule out any possible underlying medical or organic causes and other co-morbidities (e.g. hypothyroidism, sleep apnea, etc...).

DECLARATION OF INTERESTS

Dr M.K. Jha has received contract research grants from ACADIA Pharmaceuticals, Neurocrine Bioscience, Navitor/Supernus and Janssen Research & Development, educational grant to serve as Section Editor of the Psychiatry & Behavioral Health Learning Network, consultant fees from Eleusis Therapeutics US, Inc, Janssen Global Services, Janssen Scientific Affairs, Worldwide Clinical Trials/Eliem, and Guidepoint Global, and honoraria from North American Center for Continuing Medical Education, Medscape/WebMD, Clinical Care Options, and Global Medical Education. Dr M.H. Trivedi is or has been an advisor/consultant and received fees from Alkermes Inc, Axsome Therapeutics, Biogen MA Inc., Cerebral Inc., Circular Genomics Inc, Compass Pathfinder Limited, GH Research Limited, Heading Health Inc, Janssen, Legion Health Inc, Merck Sharp & Dohme Corp., Mind Medicine (MindMed) Inc, Merck Sharp & Dhome LLC, Naki Health, Ltd., Neurocrine Biosciences Inc, Noema Pharma AG, Orexo US Inc, Otsuka American Pharmaceutical Inc, Otsuka Canada Pharmaceutical Inc, Otsuka Pharmaceutical Development & Commercialization Inc, Praxis Precision Medicines Inc, SAGE Therapeutics, Sparian Biosciences Inc, Takeda Pharmaceutical Company Ltd, Titan Pharmaceuticals Inc, and WebMD.

REFERENCES

1. Malhi GS, Mann JJ. Depression. Lancet 2018;392(10161):2299–312.
2. Malhi GS, Das P, Mannie Z, et al. Treatment-resistant depression: problematic illness or a problem in our approach? Br J Psychiatry 2019;214(1):1–3.
3. American Psychiatric Association. Diagnostic and statistical manual of mental disorders. 5th edition. Arlington, VA: American Psychiatric Association Publishing; 2013.
4. American Psychiatric Association. Diagnostic and statistical manual of mental disorders: DSM-5-TR. 5th edition, Text revision. ed. Arlington, VA: American Psychiatric Association Publishing; 2022. p. 1050, lxix.
5. Rush AJ, Trivedi MH, Wisniewski SR, et al. Acute and longer-term outcomes in depressed outpatients requiring one or several treatment steps: a STAR*D report. Am J Psychiatry 2006;163(11):1905–17.
6. World Health Organization. The global burden of disease: 2004 update. Geneva: World Health Organization; 2008.
7. Evaluation IoHMa. Global Health Data Exchange (GHDx). Available at: http://ghdx.healthdata.org/gbd-results-tool?params=gbd-api-2019-permalink/d780df fbe8a381b25e1416884959e88b. Accessed June 28, 2022.
8. Vos T, Abajobir AA, Abate KH, et al. Global, regional, and national incidence, prevalence, and years lived with disability for 328 diseases and injuries for 195 countries, 1990–2016: a systematic analysis for the Global Burden of Disease Study 2016. Lancet 2017;390(10100):1211–59.
9. Organization TWH. Depresion and Other Common Mental Disorders: Global Health Estimates. 2017.
10. Friedrich MJ. Depression Is the Leading Cause of Disability Around the World. JAMA 2017;317(15):1517.

11. Disease GBD. Injury I, Prevalence C. Global, regional, and national incidence, prevalence, and years lived with disability for 354 diseases and injuries for 195 countries and territories, 1990-2017: a systematic analysis for the Global Burden of Disease Study 2017. Lancet 2018;392(10159):1789–858.
12. Bank TW. Population, total. The World Bank. Available at: https://data. worldbank.org/indicator/SP.POP.TOTL. Accessed June 28, 2022.
13. Bromet E, Andrade LH, Hwang I, et al. Cross-national epidemiology of DSM-IV major depressive episode. BMC Med 2011;9:90.
14. Hasin DS, Sarvet AL, Meyers JL, et al. Epidemiology of adult DSM-5 major depressive disorder and its specifiers in the United States. JAMA Psychiatr 2018;75(4):336–46.
15. Kessler RC, Bromet EJ. The epidemiology of depression across cultures. Annu Rev Public Health 2013;34:119–38.
16. Hirschfeld RM. The epidemiology of depression and the evolution of treatment. J Clin Psychiatry 2012;73(Suppl 1):5–9.
17. Moffitt TE, Caspi A, Taylor A, et al. How common are common mental disorders? Evidence that lifetime prevalence rates are doubled by prospective versus retrospective ascertainment. Psychol Med 2010;40(6):899–909.
18. Burcusa SL, Iacono WG. Risk for recurrence in depression. Clin Psychol Rev 2007;27(8):959–85.
19. Health NIoM. Major Depression. National Institute of Mental Health. Available at: https://www.nimh.nih.gov/health/statistics/major-depression. Accessed June 28, 2022.
20. Nihalani N, Simionescu M, Dunlop BW. Depression: phenomenology, epidemiology, and pathophysiology. In: Schwartz TL, TPeterson TJ, editors. Depression: treatment strategies and management. CRC Press; 2016. p. 1–22.
21. Kessler RC, Berglund P, Demler O, et al. Lifetime prevalence and age-of-onset distributions of DSM-IV disorders in the National Comorbidity Survey Replication. Arch Gen Psychiatry 2005;62(6):593–602.
22. Greenberg PE, Fournier AA, Sisitsky T, et al. The economic burden of adults with major depressive disorder in the United States (2010 and 2018). Pharmacoeconomics 2021;39(6):653–65.
23. Zhdanava M, Pilon D, Ghelerter I, et al. The Prevalence and National Burden of Treatment-Resistant Depression and Major Depressive Disorder in the United States. J Clin Psychiatry 2021;82(2). https://doi.org/10.4088/JCP.20m13699.
24. Brody DJ, Pratt LA, Hughes JP. Prevalence of depression among adults aged 20 and over: United States, 2013-2016. NCHS Data Brief 2018;(303):1–8.
25. Ettman CK, Cohen GH, Abdalla SM, et al. Persistent depressive symptoms during COVID-19: a national, population-representative, longitudinal study of U.S. adults. Lancet Reg Health Am 2022;5:100091.
26. Kuehner C. Why is depression more common among women than among men? Lancet Psychiatr 2017;4(2):146–58.
27. Gaynes BN, Lux L, Gartlehner G, et al. Defining treatment-resistant depression. Depress Anxiety 2020;37(2):134–45.
28. Dwyer JB, Stringaris A, Brent DA, et al. Annual research review: defining and treating pediatric treatment-resistant depression. J Child Psychol Psychiatry 2020;61(3):312–32.
29. Malhi GS, Outhred T, Hamilton A, et al. Royal Australian and New Zealand College of Psychiatrists clinical practice guidelines for mood disorders: major depression summary. Med J Aust 2018;208(4):175–80.

30. De Aquino J, Londono A, Varvalho AF. An update on the epidemiology of major depressive disorder across cultures. In: Kim Y-K, editor. Understanding depression. Singapore: Springer; 2018. p. 309–15.
31. Heim C, Binder EB. Current research trends in early life stress and depression: review of human studies on sensitive periods, gene-environment interactions, and epigenetics. Exp Neurol 2012;233(1):102–11.
32. Rush AJ, Gullion CM, Basco MR, et al. The Inventory of Depressive Symptomatology (IDS): psychometric properties. Psychol Med 1996;26(3):477–86.
33. Rush AJ, Fava M, Wisniewski SR, et al. Sequenced treatment alternatives to relieve depression (STAR*D): rationale and design. Control Clin Trials 2004; 25(1):119–42.
34. Fabbri C, Corponi F, Souery D, et al. The genetics of treatment-resistant depression: a critical review and future perspectives. Int J Neuropsychopharmacol 2019;22(2):93–104.
35. Rush AJ, Trivedi MH, Stewart JW, et al. Combining medications to enhance depression outcomes (CO-MED): acute and long-term outcomes of a single-blind randomized study. Am J Psychiatry 2011;168(7):689–701.
36. Park C, Rosenblat JD, Brietzke E, et al. Stress, epigenetics and depression: a systematic review. Neurosci Biobehav Rev 2019;102:139–52.
37. Trivedi MH, Rush AJ, Wisniewski SR, et al. Evaluation of outcomes with citalopram for depression using measurement-based care in STAR*D: implications for clinical practice. Am J Psychiatry 2006;163(1):28–40.
38. Hirschfeld RM. History and evolution of the monoamine hypothesis of depression. J Clin Psychiatry 2000;61(Suppl 6):4–6.
39. Pariante CM, Lightman SL. The HPA axis in major depression: classical theories and new developments. Trends Neurosci 2008;31(9):464–8.
40. Segal DS, Kuczenski R, Mandell AJ. Theoretical implications of drug-induced adaptive regulation for a biogenic amine hypothesis of affective disorder. Biol Psychiatry 1974;9(2):147–59.
41. Lohoff FW. Overview of the genetics of major depressive disorder. Curr Psychiatry Rep 2010;12(6):539–46.
42. Risch N, Herrell R, Lehner T, et al. Interaction between the serotonin transporter gene (5-HTTLPR), stressful life events, and risk of depression: a meta-analysis. JAMA 2009;301(23):2462–71.
43. Charney DS, Manji HK. Life stress, genes, and depression: multiple pathways lead to increased risk and new opportunities for intervention. Sci STKE 2004; 2004(225):re5.
44. Stein MB, Campbell-Sills L, Gelernter J. Genetic variation in 5HTTLPR is associated with emotional resilience. Am J Med Genet B Neuropsychiatr Genet 2009; 150B(7):900–6.
45. Polanczyk G, Caspi A, Williams B, et al. Protective effect of CRHR1 gene variants on the development of adult depression following childhood maltreatment: replication and extension. Arch Gen Psychiatry 2009;66(9):978–85.
46. Wang H, Tian X, Wang X, et al. Evolution and emerging trends in depression research from 2004 to 2019: a literature visualization analysis. Front Psychiatry 2021;12:705749.
47. Mitchell AJ, Vaze A, Rao S. Clinical diagnosis of depression in primary care: a meta-analysis. Lancet 2009;374(9690):609–19.
48. Greer TL, Trombello JM, Rethorst CD, et al. Improvements in psychosocial functioning and health-related quality of life following exercise augmentation in

patients with treatment response but nonremitted major depressive disorder: results from the tread study. Depress Anxiety 2016;33(9):870–81.

49. Jha MK, Greer TL, Grannemann BD, et al. Early normalization of Quality of Life predicts later remission in depression: Findings from the CO-MED trial. J Affect Disord 2016;206:17–22.

50. Jha MK, Minhajuddin A, Greer TL, et al. Early improvement in work productivity predicts future clinical course in depressed outpatients: findings from the CO-MED trial. Am J Psychiatry 2016;173(12):1196–204.

51. Jha MK, Teer RB, Minhajuddin A, et al. Daily activity level improvement with antidepressant medications predicts long-term clinical outcomes in outpatients with major depressive disorder. Neuropsychiatr Dis Treat 2017;13:803–13.

52. Malhi GS, Bassett D, Boyce P, et al. Royal Australian and New Zealand College of Psychiatrists clinical practice guidelines for mood disorders. Aust N Z J Psychiatry 2015;49(12):1087–206.

53. Guo T, Xiang YT, Xiao L, et al. Measurement-Based care versus standard care for major depression: a randomized controlled trial with blind raters. Am J Psychiatry 2015;172(10):1004–13.

54. Thase ME, Weisler RH, Manning JS, et al. Utilizing the DSM-5 anxious distress specifier to develop treatment strategies for patients with major depressive disorder. J Clin Psychiatr 2017;78(9):1351–62.

55. Jha MK, Minhajuddin A, South C, et al. Worsening anxiety, irritability, insomnia, or panic predicts poorer antidepressant treatment outcomes: clinical utility and validation of the concise associated symptom tracking (CAST) scale. Int J Neuropsychopharmacol 2018;21(4):325–32.

56. Jha MK, Minhajuddin A, South C, et al. Irritability and its clinical utility in major depressive disorder: prediction of individual-level acute-phase outcomes using early changes in irritability and depression severity. Am J Psychiatr 2019;176(5):358–66.

57. Jha MK, Minhajuddin A, Chin Fatt C, et al. Association between irritability and suicidal ideation in three clinical trials of adults with major depressive disorder. Neuropsychopharmacology 2020;45(13):2147–54.

58. Jha MK, Fava M, Minhajuddin A, et al. Association of anger attacks with suicidal ideation in adults with major depressive disorder: Findings from the EMBARC study. Depress Anxiety 2021;38(1):57–66.

59. Keller MB, Lavori PW, Mueller TI, et al. Time to recovery, chronicity, and levels of psychopathology in major depression. A 5-year prospective follow-up of 431 subjects. Arch Gen Psychiatry 1992;49(10):809–16.

60. Verduijn J, Verhoeven JE, Milaneschi Y, et al. Reconsidering the prognosis of major depressive disorder across diagnostic boundaries: full recovery is the exception rather than the rule. BMC Med 2017;15(1):215.

61. Fava M, Davidson KG. Definition and epidemiology of treatment-resistant depression. Psychiatr Clin North Am 1996;19(2):179–200.

62. Berlim MT, Fleck MP, Turecki G. Current trends in the assessment and somatic treatment of resistant/refractory major depression: an overview. Ann Med 2008;40(2):149–59.

63. Perlis RH, Ostacher MJ, Patel JK, et al. Predictors of recurrence in bipolar disorder: primary outcomes from the Systematic Treatment Enhancement Program for Bipolar Disorder (STEP-BD). Am J Psychiatry 2006;163(2):217–24.

64. Baldessarini RJ, Vazquez GH, Tondo L. Bipolar depression: a major unsolved challenge. Int J Bipolar Disord 2020;8(1):1.

65. Li JM, Zhang Y, Su WJ, et al. Cognitive behavioral therapy for treatment-resistant depression: a systematic review and meta-analysis. Psychiatry Res 2018;268: 243–50.

66. Lahteenvuo M, Taipale H, Tanskanen A, et al. Courses of treatment and risk factors for treatment-resistant depression in Finnish primary and special healthcare: a nationwide cohort study. J Affect Disord 2022;308:236–42.

67. Cepeda MS, Reps J, Ryan P. Finding factors that predict treatment-resistant depression: Results of a cohort study. Depress Anxiety 2018;35(7):668–73.

68. Dome P, Kunovszki P, Takacs P, et al. Clinical characteristics of treatment-resistant depression in adults in Hungary: real-world evidence from a 7-year-long retrospective data analysis. PLoS One 2021;16(1):e0245510.

69. Balestri M, Calati R, Souery D, et al. Socio-demographic and clinical predictors of treatment resistant depression: a prospective European multicenter study. J Affect Disord 2016;189:224–32.

70. Murphy JA, Sarris J, Byrne GJ. A review of the conceptualisation and risk factors associated with treatment-resistant depression. Depress Res Treat 2017;2017: 4176825.

71. Gronemann FH, Jorgensen MB, Nordentoft M, et al. Incidence of, risk factors for, and changes over time in treatment-resistant depression in denmark: a register-based cohort study. J Clin Psychiatry 2018;79(4). https://doi.org/10.4088/JCP. 17m11845.

72. Kornstein SG, Schneider RK. Clinical features of treatment-resistant depression. J Clin Psychiatry 2001;62(Suppl 16):18–25.

73. Huang SS, Chen HH, Wang J, et al. Investigation of early and lifetime clinical features and comorbidities for the risk of developing treatment-resistant depression in a 13-year nationwide cohort study. BMC Psychiatry 2020;20(1):541.

74. McAllister-Williams RH, Arango C, Blier P, et al. The identification, assessment and management of difficult-to-treat depression: an international consensus statement. J Affect Disord 2020;267:264–82.

75. Oquendo MA, Baca-Garcia E, Kartachov A, et al. A computer algorithm for calculating the adequacy of antidepressant treatment in unipolar and bipolar depression. J Clin Psychiatry 2003;64(7):825–33.

76. Fekadu A, Wooderson S, Donaldson C, et al. A multidimensional tool to quantify treatment resistance in depression: the Maudsley staging method. J Clin Psychiatry 2009;70(2):177–84.

77. Chandler GM, Iosifescu DV, Pollack MH, et al. RESEARCH: Validation of the Massachusetts General Hospital Antidepressant Treatment History Questionnaire (ATRQ). CNS Neurosci Ther 2010;16(5):322–5.

78. Hagg D, Brenner P, Reutfors J, et al. A register-based approach to identifying treatment-resistant depression-Comparison with clinical definitions. PLoS One 2020;15(7):e0236434.

79. Sheehan DV, Lecrubier Y, Sheehan KH, et al. The Mini-International Neuropsychiatric Interview (M.I.N.I.): the development and validation of a structured diagnostic psychiatric interview for DSM-IV and ICD-10. J Clin Psychiatry 1998; 59(Suppl 20):22–33 [quiz: 34-57].

80. Perkey H, Sinclair SJ, Blais M, et al. External validity of the psychiatric diagnostic screening questionnaire (PDSQ) in a clinical sample. Psychiatry Res 2018;261:14–20.

81. Zimmerman M, Mattia JI. The psychiatric diagnostic screening questionnaire: development, reliability and validity. Compr Psychiatry 2001;42(3):175–89.

82. Hage MP, Azar ST. The Link between thyroid function and depression. J Thyroid Res 2012;2012:590648.
83. Herman D, Afulani P, Coleman-Jensen A, et al. Food insecurity and cost-related medication underuse among nonelderly adults in a nationally representative sample. Am J Public Health 2015;105(10):e48–59.
84. Trivedi MH, Wisniewski SR, Morris DW, et al. Concise health risk tracking scale: a brief self-report and clinician rating of suicidal risk. J Clin Psychiatry 2011; 72(6):757–64.
85. Trivedi MH, Morris DW, Wisniewski SR, et al. Increase in work productivity of depressed individuals with improvement in depressive symptom severity. Am J Psychiatry 2013;170(6):633–41.
86. Hong RH, Murphy JK, Michalak EE, et al. Implementing measurement-based care for depression: practical solutions for psychiatrists and primary care physicians. Neuropsychiatr Dis Treat 2021;17:79–90.
87. Burckhardt CS, Anderson KL. The Quality of Life Scale (QOLS): reliability, validity, and utilization. Health Qual Life Outcomes 2003;1:60.
88. Proudman D, Greenberg P, Nellesen D. The growing burden of major depressive disorders (MDD): Implications for Researchers and Policy Makers. Pharmacoeconomics 2021;39(6):619–25.
89. Prevention CfDCa. Health Related Quality of Life (HRQOL). Centers for Disease Control and Prevention. Available at: https://www.cdc.gov/hrqol/concept.htm. Accessed June 28, 2022.
90. Dhar AK, Barton DA. Depression and the link with cardiovascular disease. Front Psychiatry 2016;7:33.
91. Seligman F, Nemeroff CB. The interface of depression and cardiovascular disease: therapeutic implications. Ann N Y Acad Sci 2015;1345:25–35.
92. Thom R, Silbersweig DA, Boland RJ. Major depressive disorder in medical illness: a review of assessment, prevalence, and treatment options. Psychosom Med 2019;81(3):246–55.
93. Shah D, Allen L, Zheng W, et al. Economic burden of treatment-resistant depression among adults with chronic non-cancer pain conditions and major depressive disorder in the US. Pharmacoeconomics 2021;39(6):639–51.
94. Cho Y, Lee JK, Kim DH, et al. Factors associated with quality of life in patients with depression: a nationwide population-based study. PLoS One 2019;14(7): e0219455.
95. Thaipisuttikul P, Ittasakul P, Waleeprakhon P, et al. Psychiatric comorbidities in patients with major depressive disorder. Neuropsychiatr Dis Treat 2014;10: 2097–103.
96. Goldberg D, Fawcett J. The importance of anxiety in both major depression and bipolar disorder. Depress Anxiety 2012;29(6):471–8.
97. Dunn V, Goodyer IM. Longitudinal investigation into childhood- and adolescence-onset depression: psychiatric outcome in early adulthood. Br J Psychiatry 2006;188:216–22.
98. Fried EI, Nesse RM. The impact of individual depressive symptoms on impairment of psychosocial functioning. PLoS One 2014;9(2):e90311.
99. Pan Z, Park C, Brietzke E, et al. Cognitive impairment in major depressive disorder. CNS Spectr 2019;24(1):22–9.
100. Trivedi MH, Corey-Lisle PK, Guo Z, et al. Remission, response without remission, and nonresponse in major depressive disorder: impact on functioning. Int Clin Psychopharmacol 2009;24(3):133–8.

101. Mauskopf JA, Simon GE, Kalsekar A, et al. Nonresponse, partial response, and failure to achieve remission: humanistic and cost burden in major depressive disorder. Depress Anxiety 2009;26(1):83–97.

102. Cai Q, Sheehan JJ, Wu B, et al. Descriptive analysis of the economic burden of treatment resistance in a major depressive episode. Curr Med Res Opin 2020; 36(2):329–35.

103. Lerner D, Lavelle TA, Adler D, et al. A population-based survey of the workplace costs for caregivers of persons with treatment-resistant depression compared with other health conditions. J Occup Environ Med 2020;62(9):746–56.

104. Crown WH, Finkelstein S, Berndt ER, et al. The impact of treatment-resistant depression on health care utilization and costs. J Clin Psychiatry 2002;63(11): 963–71.

105. Ivanova JI, Birnbaum HG, Kidolezi Y, et al. Direct and indirect costs of employees with treatment-resistant and non-treatment-resistant major depressive disorder. Curr Med Res Opin 2010;26(10):2475–84.

106. Arnaud A, Suthoff E, Tavares RM, et al. The increasing economic burden with additional steps of pharmacotherapy in major depressive disorder. Pharmacoeconomics 2021;39(6):691–706.

107. Rezaeizadeh A, Sanchez K, Zolfaghari K, et al. Depression screening and treatment among uninsured populations in Primary Care. Int J Clin Health Psychol 2021;21(3):100241.

108. The Lancet Global H. Mental health matters. Lancet Glob Health 2020;8(11): e1352.

109. National Center for Health Statistics. NCHS - Leading Causes of Death: United States. National Center for Health Statistics, Available at: https://data.cdc.gov/NCHS/NCHS-Leading-Causes-of-Death-United-States/bi63-dtpu,   Accessed April 6, 2023.

110. Bergfeld IO, Mantione M, Figee M, et al. Treatment-resistant depression and suicidality. J Affect Disord 2018;235:362–7.

111. de Leo D, Heller T. Social modeling in the transmission of suicidality. Crisis 2008; 29(1):11–9.

112. Stanley IH, Boffa JW, Joiner TE. PTSD from a suicide attempt: phenomenological and diagnostic considerations. Psychiatry. Spring 2019;82(1):57–71.

113. Saijo N. Critical comments for roles of biomarkers in the diagnosis and treatment of cancer. Cancer Treat Rev 2012;38(1):63–7.

114. Sarhene M, Wang Y, Wei J, et al. Biomarkers in heart failure: the past, current and future. Heart Fail Rev 2019;24(6):867–903.

115. Strawbridge R, Young AH, Cleare AJ. Biomarkers for depression: recent insights, current challenges and future prospects. Neuropsychiatr Dis Treat 2017;13:1245–62.

116. Beis D, Zerr I, Martelli F, et al. RNAs in brain and heart diseases. Int J Mol Sci 2020;21(10). https://doi.org/10.3390/ijms21103717.

117. Emslie GJ. Improving outcome in pediatric depression. Am J Psychiatry 2008; 165(1):1–3.

118. Brent D, Emslie G, Clarke G, et al. Switching to another SSRI or to venlafaxine with or without cognitive behavioral therapy for adolescents with SSRI-resistant depression: the TORDIA randomized controlled trial. JAMA 2008; 299(8):901–13.

Improving Identification and Treatment Outcomes of Treatment-Resistant Depression Through Measurement-Based Care

Taryn L. Mayes, MS[a], Amber E. Deane, PhD[a],
Hayley Aramburu, MHA[a], Kush Yagnik[a],
Madhukar H. Trivedi, MD[a],*

KEYWORDS

- Measurement-based care • Treatment-resistant depression • Rating scales
- Improving outcomes

KEY POINTS

- Measurement-based care (MBC) is the systematic use of scales and assessments to measure patient outcomes including assessment of depressive symptoms, side effects, and treatment adherence.
- Critical decision points at regular intervals help determine treatment strategies such as treatment type and dosage.
- MBC improves time to remission in individuals with depression and treatment-resistant depression.
- Barriers to implementing MBC in clinical care include time, resources, training, and challenges with workflow integration.

INTRODUCTION

It is clear that depression leads to significant morbidity and mortality. Depression is a leading cause of global health-related burdens. Although there are effective treatments (described in later sections), many people will not respond to first-line treatments. In fact, although 50% to 65% will respond to treatment, only around 30% to 40% will achieve remission with initial antidepressant monotherapy.[1] Failure to achieve remission contributes to depression relapse, shorter duration between episodes, and increased chronicity.[2]

[a] Center for Depression Research and Clinical, Peter O'Donnell Jr. Brain Institute and the Department of Psychiatry, University of Texas Southwestern Medical Center, 5323 Harry Hines Boulevard, Dallas, Texas, 75390-9119, USA
* Corresponding author. University of Texas Southwestern Medical Center, 5323 Harry Hines Boulevard, Dallas, Texas, 75390-9119.
E-mail address: madhukar.trivedi@utsouthwestern.edu

Psychiatr Clin N Am 46 (2023) 227–245
https://doi.org/10.1016/j.psc.2023.02.002
0193-953X/23/© 2023 Elsevier Inc. All rights reserved.

In an analysis of health care, unemployment, and productivity costs, Zhdanava and colleagues[3] estimated the national economic burden of treatment-resistant depression (TRD) to be $43.8 billion annually. When compared with all adults with medication-treated major depressive disorder (MDD), TRD is disproportionately burdensome. Although the prevalence of TRD is estimated to be 30.9% of US adults with MDD, the national economic burden of TRD is significantly higher and estimated to be 47.2% of the burden of all MDD.[3]

Defining TRD is challenging, as the definitions of outcomes vary across trials. Most clinical trials have used treatment "response" (often defined as a percent improvement on rating scales) as the outcome. However, in the past 2 decades, investigators and clinicians have correctly argued that the goal of treatment should be "remission" (ie, minimal or no symptoms of depression), with emphasis on functional improvements as well as symptom improvements.[4] Several factors may contribute to the lack of improvement with treatment, including inadequate dosing and treatment duration, nonadherence to treatment, and medication side effects. The implementation of measurement-based care (MBC) can address these issues to improve treatment fidelity, which may improve outcomes.

MBC is "systematically using measurement tools to monitor progress and guide treatment choices."[4] In studies examining the effectiveness of MBC, improved patient outcomes are reported.[5] Systematically monitoring patient progress and using that information to continue or modify the treatment strategy in a step-wise fashion can help to address patient concerns about lack of efficacy and tolerability. MBC begins at the very first visit and continues throughout treatment. Although medical illnesses, such as diabetes and heart disease, have long used MBC to guide clinical treatment decisions (eg, hemoglobin A1C and blood pressure), implementation of MBC for psychiatric illnesses in clinical practice has lagged far behind. Owing to the subjective nature of generic and imprecise assessments such as "how are you feeling," global judgments are difficult to quantify and use as a guide for treatment. Although there is clear evidence that global judgments are far less accurate than systematic symptom assessment, adoption of MBC for the treatment of psychiatric illnesses is sparse and infrequent.[6]

In the following review, the authors (1) outline the benefits of MBC to prevent and improve outcomes in TRD; (2) describe how to implement MBC; and (3) discuss future directions to enhance MBC.

BENEFITS OF MEASUREMENT-BASED CARE FOR TREATMENT-RESISTANT DEPRESSION

One key benefit of MBC is demonstrable improvement of depression treatment outcomes, to the degree that MBC may, in fact, prevent TRD. Pence and colleagues[7] estimate that among people reporting lifetime major depressive episodes, the median delay of treatment initiation is about 8 years, significantly increasing the risk of developing new depressive episodes or TRD. Even when depression is identified, only 6% report remission within a 12-month period. Among the earliest trials to illustrate the use of MBC for depression in real-world clinical treatment of depression are the Texas Medication Algorithm Project (TMAP) and Sequenced Treatment Alternatives to Relieve Depressions (STAR*D) trials.[8] Both TMAP and STAR*D were conducted in clinical practice settings and used MBC to guide treatment decisions. TMAP, which used MBC and a treatment algorithm for depression, included 547 adults with MDD. In this trial, 181 participants were treated with the algorithm and MBC and 366 received standard treatment as usual. Treatment with MBC and the algorithm led to greater improvement over usual care within 3 months and continuing through

12 months.[9] One important component of TMAP was the development of critical decision points at weeks 4, 8, and 12, which assisted clinicians in making important decisions about treatment efficacy.[9] This finding supports the incorporation of MBC as an effective strategy to improve treatment outcomes.

STAR*D, the largest depression treatment trial to date, was designed to examine optimal treatment strategies for individuals who were nonresponsive to initial antidepressant treatment. Like TMAP, STAR*D used MBC to assist clinicians in treatment decisions. Remission rates following the first-line treatment with citalopram were around 30%, with similar remission rates with second-line strategies.[10–12] Following the STAR*D and TMAP trials, most American and European guidelines recommend using MBC to guide treatment decisions.[13]

Guo and colleagues prospectively compared MBC versus standard care of MDD in 120 patients over 24 weeks of treatment.[14] Remission rates were significantly higher when clinicians used MBC compared with standard care (73.8% vs 28.8%).[14] More importantly, the time to remission was significantly shorter with MBC than standard care (10.2 weeks vs 19.2 weeks).[14] Narrowing the time to remission window decreases the likelihood of patients developing TRD and increases overall treatment success. It is important to note that patients receiving MBC also received higher doses of their antidepressant treatment, received more treatment adjustments, and were overall more engaged in their treatment process.[14]

In addition to improving initial treatment outcomes (and thereby preventing TRD), the use of MBC will lead to earlier diagnosis of TRD in those patients who are truly resistant to the initial treatment. By diagnosing TRD early in care and adjusting treatments sooner, the length, severity, and consequences from continued depression may lessen or remit entirely. Similarly, because individuals with TRD often receive treatments that are off-label, using MBC to identify response (or lack thereof) more quickly can reduce patient exposure to treatments that are ineffective. For example, McIntyre and colleagues[15] examined 297 adults with TRD to identify a meaningful change threshold in adults being treated with intravenous ketamine. They found a 3.5 change on the Quick Inventory for Depressive Symptomatology (QIDS) was associated with meaningful change.[15] This finding resulted from the use of MBC and could potentially identify ineffective treatment, thus decreasing the likelihood of developing TRD.[15] Similarly, Lee and colleagues[16] examined 139 patients undergoing high-frequency left-sided TMS (HLS-TMS) for MDD. In their study, they found participants that showed less than 20% improvement were unlikely to receive any additional benefit from continued HFL-TMS.[16] However, those who were switched to a different TMS technique (intermittent theta-burst priming of left dorsolateral prefrontal cortex [iTBS]) showed significantly greater improvement by the 30th treatment session.[16] Thus, the ongoing use of measurements to determine treatment effect allows clinicians to make earlier treatment changes (eg, adjusting dose and changing treatments) for improved outcomes.

IMPLEMENTING MEASUREMENT-BASED CARE

Implementing MBC requires the following key components: (1) ongoing measurement of symptoms, side effects, and adherence and (2) critical decision points to determine subsequent treatment strategies.

Ongoing Measurement of Symptoms, Side Effects, and Adherence

Effective MBC includes systematic assessment before and throughout treatment. Yet simply examining depressive symptoms may not be sufficient in guiding treatment decisions. Additional factors, such as side effects and nonadherence to treatment, are important areas to assess in terms of treatment impact. Many assessment measures exist to examine symptom change, side effects, and adherence and include both self-report and clinician-rated rating scales. Although clinical trials have often relied on clinician ratings as the gold standard for outcomes, evidence suggests that there is little difference in depression ratings between clinician and self-report scales.[17,18] Self-report measures may be more easily implemented into busy clinical practices making them an effective, evidence-based option. The authors review a variety of commonly used ratings scales as follows.

Depression Symptom Rating Scales

Table 1 describes commonly used depression severity ratings scales and includes the most widely used treatment response and remission criteria as well as score interpretation when available.

The Patient Health Questionnaire

The Patient Health Questionnaire (PHQ-9) is a widely used nine-item self-report rating scale. The statements are derived from nine criteria symptoms of depression, allowing for the scale to be used to provide initial diagnosis considerations and measure the severity of depression. The questionnaire asks patients to reflect on the last 2 weeks and answer each of the nine statements using the following responses: not at all, several days, more than half of the days, nearly every day on a scale of 0 to 3, respectively.[19] The total possible score ranges from 0 to 27 with results greater than 10 indicating depression. The questionnaire can be self-administered and takes approximately 5 minutes to complete. Owing to the simplicity of the questionnaire, this scale is well suited for use in a general practice setting.

Inventory of Depressive Symptomatology

The Inventory of Depressive Symptomatology (IDS) is a 30-item assessment based on the Diagnostic and Statistical Manual of Mental Disorders, 4th edition (DSM-IV) criteria and associated symptoms for MDD. IDS is available in two different forms, IDS-C (clinician-rated), and IDS-SR (self-report). Each item is scored on a 4-point Likert scale generating a total score of 0 to 84 (only 28 of the 30 items are scored).[20] Internal consistency between the clinician and self-report have been found to be very high.[20] IDS is highly sensitive to change and demonstrates acceptable psychometric properties.[21]

Quick Inventory of Depressive Symptomatology

The QIDS is a 16-item rating scale derived from the IDS. The scale is based on the nine symptoms of depression outlined by the DSM-IV. QIDS is available in two different formats: self-report (QIDS-SR16) and clinician-rated (QIDS-C16). The availability of two formats makes this scale ideal for research purposes.[20] The QIDS-SR16 and QIDS-C16 are generally considered comparable, with studies indicating that the differences between results from the two formats are minimal.[22] Because the differences are minor, QIDS-SR16 is an acceptable substitute for QIDS-C16 and has the advantage of saving time.[22] Each statement is scored based on a 0 to 3 point scale based on the previous week. The total possible score ranges from 0 to 27.[20] Recently, a five-item version of the QIDS was developed (VQIDS), with scores ranging from 0 to 15. The VQIDS is an ideal instrument for large practices or health systems with large patient volumes.

Hamilton Depression Rating Scale

The Hamilton Depression Rating Scale is often referred to as the HAM-D or the HDRS and has several versions, including a 6-item, 7-item, 8-item, 17-item, 21-item. Not only the assessment includes the primary symptoms of depression according to DSM-IV

Table 1
Depression symptom rating scale

Measure	Administration	Assessment Length	Range	Interpretation	Typical Response Criteria	Remission Criteria	References
Depression Symptom Rating Scales							
PHQ-9	Self-report	9 item 5 min	Item score: 0–3 Total score: 0–27	None or minimal: 0–4 Mild: 5–9 Moderate: 10–14 Moderately severe: 15–19 Severe: 20+	≥50% improvement	<5	19
IDS-30	Self-report and clinician versions	Clinician 28-item Self-30-item	Item score 0–3 Total score 0–84	None: 0–13 Mild: 14–25 Moderate: 26–38 Severe: 39–48 Very severe: ≥49	≥50% improvement	≤14	20
QIDS-16	Self-report and clinician versions	16 item 5–7 min	Item score: 0–3 Total score: 0–27	None: 0–5 Mild: 6–10 Moderate: 11–15 Severe 16–20 Very severe: ≥21	≥50% improvement	<5	20
VQIDS-5	Self-report and clinician versions	5 items	Item score: 0–3 Total score: 0–15	None: 0–2 Mild: 3–5 Moderate: 6–8 Severe: 9–12 Very severe: >12	≥50% improvement	≤2	61
HAMD-17	Clinician	17 items 20–30 min	Item score: 0–4 or 0–2 Total score: 0–50	None: 0–7 Mild: 8–16 Moderate: 17–23 Severe: ≥ 24	≥50% improvement	≤7	23,24,62

(continued on next page)

Table 1
(continued)

Measure	Administration	Assessment Length	Range	Interpretation	Typical Response Criteria	Remission Criteria	References
HAMD-6	Clinician	6 items	Item score: 0–4 or 0–2 Total score: 0–22	N/A	≥50% improvement	≤4	24,62,63
MADRS	Clinician	10 item	Item score: 0–6 Total score: 0–60	None: 0–6 Mild: 7–19 Moderate: 20–34 Severe: 35+	≥50% improvement	≤9 Absence of depression: ≤4	25,26,64
BDI-II	Self-report	21 item 10 min	Item score: 0–3 Total Score: 0–63	Minimal: 0–13 Mild: 14–19 Moderate: 20–28 Severe: 29–63	≥50% improvement	≤9	27,65

Abbreviations: BDI-II, beck depression inventory II; HAMD-6, Hamilton Depression Rating Scale-6 item; HAMD-17, Hamilton Depression Rating Scale-17 item; IDS, inventory of depressive symptomatology; MADRS, Montgomery–Asberg depression rating scale; PHQ-9, patient health questionnaire; QIDS, quick IDS; VQIDS, very QIDS.

but also accounts for symptoms of anxiety and drug side effects. The six-item Hamilton Depression Rating Scale (HAM-D-6) is a shorter version of the HAM-D-17 representative of the symptoms of depression according to the DSM-IV.[23] This modified version of the HAM-D has been found to be more sensitive to antidepressant effects than the HAM-D-17. This is possibly due to the exclusion of symptoms such as anxiety and weight gain symptoms.[24] One limitation of the clinician-rated HAM-D is that the accuracy and reliability of this scale depends on the quality of the interviewer,[24] making it less ideal for inexperienced interviewers. The items on the HAM-D include 3-point ranges (0–2) and 5-point ranges (0–4).[23] Cutoff scores are dependent on the version of the HAM-D being used and the interpretation.[24] **Table 1** includes the most commonly used versions (6- and 17-item scales).

Montgomery–Asberg Depression Rating Scale
In 1979, the clinician-administered Montgomery–Asberg Depression Rating Scale (MADRS) was developed to monitor treatment response to antidepression medication.[25] Ten items make up the scale and include apparent sadness, reported sadness, inability to feel, inner tension, suicidal thoughts, lassitude, concentration difficulties, reduced sleep, reduced appetite, and pessimistic thoughts.[26] The items are rated on a seven-point scale ranging from none to severe (0–6, respectively) resulting in a total score of 0 to 60.[25] The MADRS is among one of the most commonly used depression severity measure used in clinical treatment trials behind the HAM-D.[25]

Beck Depression Inventory II
The first Beck Depression Inventory, dating back to 1961, is one of the most well-known depression rating scales and has been revised to create the BDI-IA, BDI-II, and seven-item BDI FastScreen for Medical Patients (BDI-FS).[27] The BDI-II, a 21-item measure of depression severity, is probably the most used version. Each of the 21 items is rated from 0 to 3 with a possible total questionnaire rating of 0 to 63 (higher scores indicating more severe depression).

Special considerations
Many scales such as the BDI and HAM-D have subscales that have been adapted by clinicians and researchers over time to account for varying needs. Although this article covers several depression ratings scales, the above list is not exhaustive. Further scales for consideration include Center for Epidemiologic Studies Depression Scale,[27] Edinburgh Postnatal Depression Scale[28] and age-specific scales such as the Children's Depression Inventory,[29] Children's Depression Rating Scale,[30] and the Geriatric Depression Scale.[27]

Side-effects rating scales
As part of the MBC process, evaluating side effects is essential. One of the primary reasons people with depression discontinue their antidepressant is side effects, often without informing their provider that they have stopped taking the medication.[31,32] Thus, more frequent visits early in treatment or during treatments changes is important for the provider to be able to address side effects through dose reductions, switching to a different medication, or providing short-term interventions to counteract side effects. **Table 2** describes common side-effect rating scales in more detail.

Frequency, Intensity, and Burden of Side-Effects Rating
The Frequency, Intensity, and Burden Side-Effects Rating (FIBSER) was designed to measure the side effects experienced by participants in the STAR*D study. This brief self-report was designed to assist in clinical decision-making. The three-question

Table 2
Side-effect rating and depression adherence scales

Measure	Administration	Assessment Length	References
Side-Effect Rating Scales			
FIBSER	Self-report	3 questions <5 min	33
SAFTEE-GI	Clinician rated	3 questions 5 min	33
SAFTEE-SI	Clinician rated	21 items 15–20 min	33
PRISE	Self-report	32 items 10–15 min	33
Depression Adherence Scales			
AQ	Self-report	2 questions <5 min	32,40
BARS	Clinician rated	3 questions 1 observation < 5 min	41
AAS	Self-report	2–3 min	31,43

Abbreviations: AAS, antidepressant adherence scale; AQ, adherence questionnaire; BARS, brief adherence rating scale; FIBSER, frequency, intensity, and burden of side-effects rating; PRISE, patient-rated inventory of side effects; SAFTEE, systematic assessment for treatment emergent side effects.

assessment is a concise, straight-forward way to measure the frequency, effect, and burden of side effects. The total scores for the FIBSER ranges from 0 to 6, with 0 to 2 being acceptable, 3 to 4 requiring attention, and 5 to 6 being unacceptable (and thus potentially warranting treatment modification). The lack of specificity allows for this assessment to be used in a variety of populations and settings.[33]

Systematic Assessment for Treatment Emergent Side Effects

Sponsored by the National Institute of Mental Health, the Systematic Assessment for Treatment Emergent Side Effects (SAFTEE) was born out of a need for a systematic approach to evaluate side effects in a clinical setting.[34,35] This assessment emphasizes a systematic approach by using preferred terms to eliminate terminology discrepancies between raters and patients.[35] The SAFTEE has two commonly used versions: a shorter general inquiry version (SAFTEE-GI) and a detailed specific inquiry (SAFTEE-SI) assessment.[36] The SAFTEE-GI asks three general questions to elicit adverse events, followed by questions about the pattern, severity, drug relatedness, and action taken, and takes only a few minutes to complete. The SAFTEE-SI elicits information about specific events that are common side effects (eg, headache, nausea, and rash), which is also followed by questions about the pattern, severity, drug relatedness, and action taken. The SAFTEE-SI may take approximately 10 to 15 minutes for each possible symptom to be reviewed. Using the structured SAFTEE-SI in lieu of SAFTEE-GI has the potential benefit of eliciting a response for minor side effects participants might overlook, with the caveat of possible overreporting side effects due to suggestibility.[34]

Patient-Rated Inventory of Side Effects

The Patient-Rated Inventory of Side Effects (PRISE) assessment is used to measure the side effects occurring in nine organ/function domains (gastrointestinal, nervous system, heart, eyes/ears, skin, genital/urinary, sleep, sexual function, and other).[33] Items are scored on a scale of 0 (not present) or 1 (present tolerable) and 2 (present distressing). This assessment was used in the STAR*D study alongside the previously mentioned FIBSER assessment. A study by Winsienwki and colleagues[33] found PRISE to be significantly correlated with FIBSER.

Special considerations

One important consideration for assessing side effects, regardless of the measure selected, is the potential overlap between TRD symptoms and side effects. This is particularly relevant when patients have a worsening of depressive symptoms. For example, fatigue, sleep disturbance, and appetite changes are common side effects, but are also symptoms of depression. If these types of symptoms are not improving or are worsening even after treatment begins, these overlapping symptoms may be mistaken for side effects when they are actually due to worsening illness. It is important for the provider to tease out whether the new or worsening condition is related to side effects (potentially warranting a dose reduction or medication change) or worsening depression (potentially warranting a dose increase or medication change). Assessment of whether other depression symptoms are worsening may provide guidance on the root cause of such overlapping symptoms.

Adherence rating scales

Assessing medication adherence is a vital component to increase the effectiveness of MBC. According to World Healthcare Organization (WHO), nonadherence is precipitated by social, economic, health system, condition-related, therapy-related, and patient-related factors.[37] Treatment adherence is a chronic issue that spans beyond the realm of MDD and impacts virtually all diseases. Improved use of adherence assessments has the potential to improve treatment adherence, which ultimately may improve patient health outcomes. Nonadherence to antidepressant medications and treatment plans contributes to the mounting number of persons deemed to have TRD. According to Lin and colleagues, up to 50% of people treated with antidepressants fail to adhere to their treatment plan.[38] In clinical practice, providers often fail to assess treatment adherence. In clinical trials, traditional methods of measuring medication adherence include pill counts, patient diaries, pharmacy records, urine/blood tests, and electronic monitoring. These methods are not systematic and leave room for error when measuring treatment plan adherence, and some are not feasible in clinical practice.[39] **Table 2** lists several commonly used adherence rating scales.

Adherence Questionnaire

As there is not a gold standard for antidepressant adherence, Warren and colleagues[32] developed the Adherence Questionnaire (AQ) to assess medication adherence of participants in the Combining Medications to Enhance Depression outcomes (CO-MED) study. Unlike other adherence assessments, AQ evaluates missed doses and discontinued doses separately in addition to assessing adherence behavior. The assessment is a two-question self-report that includes a question pertaining to the frequency of missed doses and deviance from the prescribed dosage schedule. This assessment is a behavioral approach and is well suited to identify personal barriers to treatment adherence.[32] AQ (previously called Patient Adherence Questionnaire) was also used in a large program for depression screening and MBC in primary care.[40]

Brief Adherence Rating Scale

Owing to poor adherence of antipsychotic medications in an outpatient setting, Byerly and colleagues[41] developed a four-item assessment called Brief Adherence Rating

Scale (BARS). BARS is a clinician administered assessment composed of three questions and a visual assessment of prescription adherence.[41] Originally designed for use with patients with schizophrenia and schizoaffective disorder, this scale has been used by Low and colleagues[42] to assess the applicability to antidepressant adherence. Results from Byerly and colleagues[37] and Low and colleagues[38] indicate high reliability and validity of the assessment among depressed populations or populations prescribed antidepressants.

Antidepressant Adherence Scale

In 1986, Morisky theorized nonadherence is a multifactor issue influenced by four primary items: forgetfulness, carelessness, discontinuing due to feeling better, and discontinuing due to feeling worse. Morisky created a simple yes/no assessment to measure nonadherence to antihypertensive medication.[43] Guided by Morisky's work, Gabriel and Violato[31] modified the assessment to create the Antidepressant Adherence Scale (AAS). The AAS is a brief questionnaire consisting of four questions designed to identify the source of nonadherence and is scored by continuous numeric responses.[31]

Special considerations

It is important to consider that conventional adherence measures are susceptible to subjectivity. Clear and open communication with the patient is essential to create open dialogue about adherence to treatments in TRD, including educating the patient that nonadherence to the treatment plan may lead to continued depression and ultimately TRD. Objective adherence strategies may also be considered. Pill counts are a common method for assessing adherence. Over the several years, electronic tracking methods have also been used, including pill caps that monitor each time a bottle is opened and pills that have an ingestible imbedded sensor.[44,45]

CRITICAL DECISION POINTS

At the start of treatment of patients diagnosed with depression, regularly scheduled visits are the key to quickly identifying limited depression symptom improvement, troublesome side effects, or nonadherence, all of which may lead to nonresponse, premature discontinuation of treatment, and ultimately TRD. Increased visit frequency early in treatment or following treatment changes also aides in determining whether medication or dosage should be adjusted sooner thus increasing the likelihood of adherence. Visits should be scheduled every 2 weeks for the first 6 weeks, and then every 3 weeks until remission or a change in treatment.[4] Some improvement (at least 25%) is expected within the first 4 weeks of treatment. If patients report less than 25% improvement within that time frame, the treatment may need to be adjusted. For patients showing 25% to 50% improvement during the first 4 weeks of antidepressant treatment, the dose should be optimized to the maximum tolerable dose. For patients showing less than 50% improvement by around 6 to 8 weeks of maximum tolerable dose and the medication adherence is good, a change in antidepressant or augmentation may be considered. In these cases, reevaluation of diagnosis, as well as the consideration of any complicating medical or psychosocial issues, and adherence to treatment is recommended. If the patient is determined to have TRD, changes to the treatment regimen are warranted. Subsequent treatment strategies are described in later sections.

Increased frequency of visits during medication initiation, dose adjustments, or switching medications can be challenging in a busy clinical practice. Given this is a key component to improve treatment outcomes, it is essential for clinicians to educate their patients about the importance of these visits, as well as to establish workflows to accommodate increased visit frequency.

NAVIGATING THE MEASUREMENT-BASED CARE COURSE AHEAD

Although MBC leads to more effective treatment outcomes and can prevent or reduce the effects of TRD, further enhancement of MBC may improve prognostication. Here, the authors review two areas of interest: measurement of functional outcomes, other depression-related symptom outcomes, and implementation of MBC in primary care and health care systems.

Functional Outcomes

Functional outcomes encompass day-to-day living functioning, and these outcomes are equally or more important than symptom reduction to individuals suffering from depression.[46] A functional outcome differs from clinical outcomes in that it focuses on day-to-day functioning of an individual rather than symptom remission.[47] Clinicians may use functional outcome measurements to assess the impact of disease on daily life and social functioning. Different aspects that factor into functional outcomes include work attendance, productivity, quality of life, well-being, and suicidal risk.

When completing an assessment, screening for background information that includes lifestyle information such as demographics, work life, home life, and family life are vital. Susceptibility to many disorders can be influenced by lifestyles and genetic factors. Conducting a thorough evaluation that evaluates symptoms in both the home and work context assists clinicians in identifying potential barriers and sources of support for patients. Using systematic measurements to evaluate functional improvements also enables providers and patients to explore other components of improvement even in the absence of significant changes in symptoms. Below the authors examine several rating scales that examine factors associated with depression that are not simply symptom focused, but address functioning and wellness.

THE WORLD HEALTHCARE ORGANIZATION WELL-BEING INDEX

The World Healthcare Organization Well-Being Index (WHO-5), developed in 1998, is a generic, unidimensional assessment designed to measure well-being regardless of a specific diagnosis.[48] Topp and colleagues suggest that WHO-5 is well suited for clinical practices and research settings due to the simplicity and validity of the assessment. Like other WHO scales, the assessment has been widely translated and is used globally.[48]

WHO Quality of Life Brief Version (WHOQOL-BREF)

WHOQOL-BREF is a globally used questionnaire that includes four domains of quality of life: environmental, social, physical, and psychological.[49] Developed by the World Health Organization, this scale is both validate and reliable for use across cultures. This is also available in multiple languages.[49]

Work Productivity and Activity Impairment Questionnaire

The Work Productivity and Activity Impairment Questionnaire (WPAI) is a brief self-report questionnaire that has been adapted by multiple medical fields to measure the impact of health problems on productivity and nonwork related activities.[50] Beck and colleagues[50] examined the relationship between PHQ-9 scores and WPAI scores and found a significant relationship between the severity of depression and the impact of depression on participants' work productivity. In other words, depression impacts productivity which supports the assertion that mental illness impacts society at both the macrolevel and microlevel.

The Remission from Depression Questionnaire

Remission from Depression Questionnaire (RDQ) is a unique measure in that the primary focus of the questionnaire is to evaluate patients' perception of remission rather than symptom resolution. Previous studies that explored the validity of measuring symptom reduction to determine remission have found that patient perception to be a more adequate measure of remission.[51] This is important because the goal for providers should be relevant to patient goals of improvement which extend beyond the textbook definition of remission. The RDQ covers domains determined to be important by patients including ability to cope, positive mental health, impact of functionality, life satisfaction, symptoms of depression, anxiety and irritability, and sense of well-being.[51] Although this measure takes a more patient-centered approach, it is subjective and should be used in conjunction with other MBC scales.

Work and Social Adjustment Scale

The Work and Social Adjustment Scale is a five-item self-report used to measure functional impairment. Items are scored from 0 to 8, with 0 indicating no impairment and 8 indicating very severe impairment.[52] Total scores greater than 20 indicate moderately sever psychopathology, whereas scores ranging between 10 and 20 indicate significant functional impairment.[52]

Other Depression-Related Outcomes

Concise Health Risk Tracking Scale

The Concise Health Risk Tracking (CHRT) Scale was designed to measure suicidal ideation (SI) in a research setting.[53] The assessment focuses not only on suicidal behaviors but also factors associated with suicidal risk, such as pessimism, helplessness, lack of social support, and despair. Each item is measured on a five-point Likert scale. Several versions of the CHRT self-report are available, all of which have demonstrated reliability and validity among adults and adolescents with depression, bipolar disorder, and substance use disorders.[53,54] The CHRT also has a clinician-rated behavioral module that includes the Columbia Classification Algorithm for Suicide Assessment suicidal behavior categories.

Concise Associated Symptoms Tracking

The Concise Associated Symptoms Tracking (CAST) is a self-report measure based on the warning the FDA added to antidepressants in 2005. This 17-item measure examines the five signs of activation syndrome: irritability, anxiety, mania, insomnia, and panic. The CAST is a 17-item scale with each item rated on a five-point scale of strongly disagree to strongly agree. The simplicity of the assessment makes it easy to administer and interpret making it a cost-effective option.[55]

Further investigation of functional outcomes and depression severity are critical to bridging the gap between symptom remission and functional outcome. Armed with this knowledge, providers can leverage MBC to better treat depression with functional outcomes in mind.

Altman Self-Rating Mania Scale

Some individuals with depression may experience manic or hypomanic symptoms either as part of a bipolar disorder or as a result of medication-induced mania/hypomania. Thus, providers may choose to monitor these symptoms. The Altman Self-Rating Mania Scale is a commonly used five-item self-report rating scale that takes about 5 minutes to complete. The scale has strong psychometric properties.[56]

Pain Frequency, Intensity, and Burden Scale

Pain is often associated with depression and can impact functioning and treatment outcomes. The Pain Frequency, Intensity, and Burden Scale is brief four-item self-report developed to examine frequency, intensity, and burden of pain. Items are rated on a 0 to 8 Likert scale. This brief scale has been determined to have consistent reliability and validity.[57]

Implementing measurement-based care in primary care and health care systems

Although MBC is considered best practice when treating depression, implementation by primary care providers and health systems has been slow. There are several factors that influence the slow uptake; they include the lack of training medical providers receive for mental and behavioral health care as well as difficulty in integrating depression screening and treatment within the clinic workflow. However, the principles and foundations of MBC are universal for most medical conditions, depression care should be no different. Importantly, patients with chronic conditions such as diabetes and cardiovascular disease and other illness are at greater risk not only for depression but also for TRD. Conversely, people diagnosed with depression likely have other co-occurring health conditions resulting in worse overall health outcomes. Poor mental health outcomes for patients lead to significant economic burdens for health systems and society, and people with depression and related mood disorders are high health care resource users. Thus, failing to address mental health is costly for both patients and health systems alike. Integrating screening and treatment for depression in health care settings is a key next step for MBC.

A common misconception that depression care is too complex for those outside the field of psychiatry persists. However, just as primary care doctors do not need to have extensive training in cardiology to treat high blood pressure, primary care doctors do not need extensive training in psychiatry to treat depression. Despite evidence that suggests using an MBC model to treat depression is effective and efficient for primary care providers, many practitioners are reluctant to implement MBC to guide treatment and choose to refer patients out for specialty care, such as a psychiatrists, psychologists, or therapists for mental health services. This is particularly true when treating general mental distress, and even more so with TRD. As psychiatry prioritizes identification of more severe mental illnesses (eg, schizophrenia, bipolar disorder), this practice creates a bottleneck for patients who struggle to gain access to clinicians due to a lack of specialty providers, lengthy wait times, and delayed treatment. The use of MBC and treatment algorithms provide easy solutions for primary care providers to treat depression. Even for TRD, algorithms and decision support applications provide primary care providers the tools they need to be able to continue to treat within the primary care home for at least one to two additional treatment trials before referring out to a psychiatrist.

Another strategy to assist with TRD cases is the collaborative care model, which involves collaborating with a mental health provider (psychiatrist or therapist) within primary care clinics or health systems. By incorporating a collaborative care model to address mental health care and behavioral needs of patients, providers may be more agile and better able to provide cost saving treatments as opposed to expensive emergency care and hospitalizations during a mental health crisis. Collaborative care also frees up valuable time for providers by training support staff to administer screening tools before the provider–patient encounter. By using validated tools and systematic screening and monitoring, providers are armed with knowledge prior entering the patient room and can engage in more informed, concise discussions. More importantly, identifying the most effective treatment of a particular patient quickly reduces the pain and suffering of patients and their families. Thus, when primary care providers and health systems adopt universal depression screening, patients with mild to moderate depression are identified early and can begin treatments that are cost-effective and more readily available than through advanced specialty psychiatric care.

Large scale efforts in Texas have demonstrated the feasibility of implementing MBC in real-world clinics. In 2014, the Center for Depression Research and Clinical Care at the University of Texas Southwestern Medical Center developed a comprehensive program (VitalSign[6]) to help community health organizations, primary care, specialty care, and pediatric practices routinely screen patients for depression, accurately diagnose and manage patients who screen positive, and provide MBC to those needing treatment for depression.[58] Providers receive training in depression diagnosis and MBC, and the VitalSign6 application provides decision support tools to assist with treatment decisions based on symptom change, side effects, and adherence. Since 2014, over 80,000 patients have been screened, with approximately 20% screening positive for depression. Remarkably, roughly 35% of those receiving treatment for depression reach remission,[59,60] which is significantly greater than the 6% remission rate for the national average.[7]

The second project to implement MBC on a large scale focused on youth. The Texas Youth Depression and Suicide Research Network (TX-YDSRN) was developed in 2020 to leverage the expertise and clinical and research capabilities of 12 Texas health-related universities to improve identification and treatment for youth and young adults (ages 8–20 years) with depression and suicidal thoughts or behaviors. The objective of the first research study was to develop a Network Participant Registry to characterize systems and interventions to examine statewide population health outcomes, particularly as they relate to depression and suicide. Data collected include mood symptoms, SI and behavior, associated comorbidities, treatment history, services use, and social determinants of health. In addition, providers deliver MBC within the clinics and complete data forms documenting treatments. We are well into our second year of building the Texas Youth Depression and Suicide Research Network, with approximately 40 clinics across the state involved in the project. To date, over 1100 youth have been enrolled, and over 6200 visits have been completed. Even more striking, 83% of youth have provided data at five or more visits.

DISCUSSION

MBC is demonstrated to improve outcomes for individuals suffering from depression and may reduce incidence of apparent TRD by identifying factors associated with nonresponse, such as underdosing, intolerable side effects, and nonadherence. When treating depression, it is important to not only evaluate symptom changes but to also assess side effects and adherence to treatment. Functional outcomes are important to assess, as patients are often as much or more concerned with functional outcomes as symptom reduction. These strategies may reduce the overall incidence of TRD, but more importantly will lead to faster and more robust improvements in individuals suffering from TRD. A variety of rating scales to assess symptoms, side effects, and adherence are available as self-reports or clinician-rated measures, and self-report measures may reduce the challenges of time and resources, leading to easier integration into clinic workflows. Using these scales at critical decision points throughout treatment will improve patient outcomes, including those with TRD. There are challenges to implementing MBC, including time, resources, training, and establishing workflow processes; however, the benefits of improving outcomes for individuals suffering from TRD warrant addressing each provider's or clinic's identified barriers.

CLINICS CARE POINTS

- Measuring symptoms, adherence, and adverse effects throughout treatment leads to improved outcomes.
- Many rating scales are available as self-report or clinician-rated measures to assess symptoms, adherence, and adverse events.
- Using measurement-based care during the treatment of depression may reduce the chance of developing treatment resistant depression by making treatment modifications as needed.

DISCLOSURE

Dr M.H. Trivedi is or has been an advisor/consultant and received fees from: Alkermes Inc, Axsome Therapeutics, Biogen MA Inc, Cerebral Inc, Circular Genomics Inc, Compass Pathfinder Limited, GH Research Limited, Heading Health Inc, Janssen, Legion Health Inc, Merck Sharp & Dohme Corp, Mind Medicine (MindMed) Inc, Merck Sharp & Dhome LLC, Naki Health, Ltd, Neurocrine Biosciences Inc, Noema Pharma AG, Orexo US Inc, Otsuka American Pharmaceutical Inc, Otsuka Canada Pharmaceutical Inc, Otsuka Pharmaceutical Development & Commercialization Inc, Praxis Precision Medicines Inc, SAGE Therapeutics, Sparian Biosciences Inc, Takeda Pharmaceutical Company Ltd, Titan Pharmaceuticals Inc, and WebMD. Ms T.L. Mayes, Dr A.E. Deane, Ms H. Aramburu, and Mr K. Yagnik have nothing to disclose.

REFERENCES

1. Henssler J, Kurschus M, Franklin J, et al. Trajectories of acute antidepressant efficacy: how long to wait for response? A systematic review and meta-analysis of long-term, placebo-controlled acute treatment trials. J Clin Psychiatry 2018;79(3). https://doi.org/10.4088/JCP.17r11470.
2. Mendlewicz J. Towards achieving remission in the treatment of depression. Dialogues Clin Neurosci 2008;10(4):371–5.
3. Zhdanava M, Pilon D, Ghelerter I, et al. The prevalence and national burden of treatment-resistant depression and major depressive disorder in the United States. J Clin Psychiatry 2021;(2):82. https://doi.org/10.4088/JCP.20m13699.
4. Trivedi MH. Tools and strategies for ongoing assessment of depression: a measurement-based approach to remission. J Clin Psychiatry 2009;70(Suppl 6):26–31.
5. Fortney JC, Unutzer J, Wrenn G, et al. A tipping point for measurement-based care. Psychiatr Serv 2017;68(2):179–88.
6. Biggs MM, Shores-Wilson K, Rush AJ, et al. A comparison of alternative assessments of depressive symptom severity: a pilot study. Psychiatry Res 20 2000; 96(3):269–79.
7. Pence BW, O'Donnell JK, Gaynes BN. The depression treatment cascade in primary care: a public health perspective. Curr Psychiatry Rep 2012;14(4):328–35.

8. Trivedi MH, Daly EJ. Measurement-based care for refractory depression: a clinical decision support model for clinical research and practice. Drug Alcohol Depend 2007;88(Suppl 2):S61–71.

9. Trivedi MH, Rush AJ, Crismon ML, et al. Clinical results for patients with major depressive disorder in the Texas Medication Algorithm Project. Arch Gen Psychiatry 2004;61(7):669–80.

10. Rush AJ, Trivedi MH, Wisniewski SR, et al. Bupropion-SR, sertraline, or venlafaxine-XR after failure of SSRIs for depression. N Engl J Med 2006; 354(12):1231–42.

11. Trivedi MH, Fava M, Wisniewski SR, et al. Medication augmentation after the failure of SSRIs for depression. N Engl J Med 2006;354(12):1243–52.

12. Trivedi MH, Rush AJ, Wisniewski SR, et al. Evaluation of outcomes with citalopram for depression using measurement-based care in STAR*D: implications for clinical practice. Am J Psychiatry 2006;163(1):28–40.

13. Gelenberg AJ. A review of the current guidelines for depression treatment. J Clin Psychiatry 2010;71(7):e15.

14. Guo T, Xiang YT, Xiao L, et al. Measurement-based care versus standard care for major depression: a randomized controlled trial with blind raters. Am J Psychiatry 2015;172(10):1004–13.

15. McIntyre RS, Lipsitz O, Lui LMW, et al. The meaningful change threshold as measured by the 16-item quick inventory of depressive symptomatology in adults with treatment-resistant major depressive and bipolar disorder receiving intravenous ketamine. J Affect Disord 2021;294:592–6.

16. Lee JC, Wilson AC, Corlier J, et al. Strategies for augmentation of high-frequency left-sided repetitive transcranial magnetic stimulation treatment of major depressive disorder. J Affect Disord 2020;277:964–9.

17. Rush AJ, Carmody TJ, Ibrahim HM, et al. Comparison of self-report and clinician ratings on two inventories of depressive symptomatology. Psychiatr Serv 2006; 57(6):829–37.

18. Hershenberg R, McDonald WM, Crowell A, et al. Concordance between clinician-rated and patient reported outcome measures of depressive symptoms in treatment resistant depression. J Affect Disord 2020;266:22–9.

19. Kroenke K, Spitzer RL, Williams JB. The PHQ-9: validity of a brief depression severity measure. J Gen Intern Med 2001;16(9):606–13.

20. Rush AJ, Trivedi MH, Ibrahim HM, et al. The 16-item Quick Inventory of Depressive Symptomatology (QIDS), clinician rating (QIDS-C), and self-report (QIDS-SR): a psychometric evaluation in patients with chronic major depression. Biol Psychiatry 2003;54(5):573–83.

21. Trivedi MH, Rush AJ, Ibrahim HM, et al. The Inventory of Depressive Symptomatology, Clinician Rating (IDS-C) and Self-Report (IDS-SR), and the Quick Inventory of Depressive Symptomatology, Clinician Rating (QIDS-C) and Self-Report (QIDS-SR) in public sector patients with mood disorders: a psychometric evaluation. Psychol Med 2004;34(1):73–82.

22. Bernstein IH, Rush AJ, Carmody TJ, et al. Clinical vs. self-report versions of the quick inventory of depressive symptomatology in a public sector sample. J Psychiatr Res 2007;41(3–4):239–46.

23. Ma S, Yang J, Yang B, et al. The Patient Health Questionnaire-9 vs. the Hamilton Rating Scale for Depression in assessing major depressive disorder. Front Psychiatry 2021;12:747139.

24. Carrozzino D, Patierno C, Fava GA, et al. The Hamilton Rating Scales for Depression: a critical review of clinimetric properties of different versions. Psychother Psychosom 2020;89(3):133–50.

25. Quilty LC, Robinson JJ, Rolland JP, et al. The structure of the Montgomery-Asberg depression rating scale over the course of treatment for depression. Int J Methods Psychiatr Res 2013;22(3):175–84.

26. Montgomery SA, Asberg M. A new depression scale designed to be sensitive to change. Br J Psychiatry 1979;134:382–9.

27. Smarr KL, Keefer AL. Measures of depression and depressive symptoms: Beck Depression Inventory-II (BDI-II), Center for Epidemiologic Studies Depression Scale (CES-D), Geriatric Depression Scale (GDS), Hospital Anxiety and Depression Scale (HADS), and Patient Health Questionnaire-9 (PHQ-9). Arthritis Care Res (Hoboken) 2011;63(Suppl 11):S454–66.

28. Gibson J, McKenzie-McHarg K, Shakespeare J, et al. A systematic review of studies validating the Edinburgh Postnatal Depression Scale in antepartum and postpartum women. Acta Psychiatr Scand 2009;119(5):350–64.

29. Smucker MR, Craighead WE, Craighead LW, et al. Normative and reliability data for the Children's Depression Inventory. J Abnorm Child Psychol 1986;14(1): 25–39.

30. Poznanski EO, Grossman JA, Buchsbaum Y, et al. Preliminary Studies of the Reliability and Validity of the Children's Depression Rating Scale. J Am Acad Child Psychiatry 1984;23(2):191–7.

31. Gabriel A, Violato C. Knowledge of and attitudes towards depression and adherence to treatment: the Antidepressant Adherence Scale (AAS). J Affect Disord 2010;126(3):388–94.

32. Warden D, Trivedi MH, Carmody T, et al. Adherence to antidepressant combinations and monotherapy for major depressive disorder: a CO-MED report of measurement-based care. J Psychiatr Practice® 2014;20(2):118–32.

33. Wisniewski SR, Rush AJ, Balasubramani GK, et al. Self-rated global measure of the frequency, intensity, and burden of side effects. J Psychiatr Pract 2006; 12(2):71–9.

34. Jacobson AF, Goldstein BJ, Dominguez RA, et al. Interrater agreement and intraclass reliability measures of SAFTEE in psychopharmacologic clinical trials. Psychopharmacol Bull 1986;22(2):382–8.

35. Levine J, Schooler NR. SAFTEE: a technique for the systematic assessment of side effects in clinical trials. Psychopharmacol Bull 1986;22(2):343–81.

36. Vanderkooy JD, Kennedy SH, Bagby RM. Antidepressant side effects in depression patients treated in a naturalistic setting: a study of bupropion, moclobemide, paroxetine, sertraline, and venlafaxine. Can J Psychiatry 2002;47(2):174–80.

37. Chaudri NA. Adherence to Long-term Therapies Evidence for Action. Ann Saudi Med 2004;24(3):221–2.

38. Lin J, Szukis H, Sheehan JJ, et al. Economic burden of treatment-resistant depression among patients hospitalized for major depressive disorder in the United States. Psychiatr Res Clin Pract 2019;1(2):68–76.

39. Nakonezny PA, Hughes CW, Mayes TL, et al. A comparison of various methods of measuring antidepressant medication adherence among children and adolescents with major depressive disorder in a 12-week open trial of fluoxetine. J Child Adolesc Psychopharmacol 2010;20(5):431–9.

40. Dela Cruz AM, Walker R, Pipes R, et al. Creation of an algorithm for clinical decision support for treatment of opioid use disorder with buprenorphine in primary care. Addict Sci Clin Pract 2021;16(1):12.

41. Byerly MJ, Nakonezny PA, Rush AJ. The Brief Adherence Rating Scale (BARS) validated against electronic monitoring in assessing the antipsychotic medication adherence of outpatients with schizophrenia and schizoaffective disorder. Schizophr Res 2008;100(1–3):60–9.

42. Low PT, Ng CG, Kadir MS, et al. Reminder through mobile messaging application improves outpatient attendance and medication adherence among patients with depression: An open-label randomised controlled trial. Med J Malaysia Sep 2021; 76(5):617–23.

43. Morisky DE, Green LW, Levine DM. Concurrent and predictive validity of a self-reported measure of medication adherence. Med Care 1986;67–74.

44. Rosen MI, Rigsby MO, Salahi JT, et al. Electronic monitoring and counseling to improve medication adherence. Behav Res Ther Apr 2004;42(4):409–22.

45. Alipour A, Gabrielson S, Patel PB. Ingestible Sensors and Medication Adherence: Focus on Use in Serious Mental Illness. Pharmacy (Basel) 2020;8(2). https://doi.org/10.3390/pharmacy8020103.

46. Zimmerman M, McGlinchey JB, Posternak MA, et al. How should remission from depression be defined? The depressed patient's perspective. Am J Psychiatry 2006;163(1):148–50.

47. Remington G. Functional Outcome. In: Stolerman IP, editor. Encyclopedia of Psychopharmacology. Springer Berlin Heidelberg; 2010. p. 546–7.

48. Topp CW, Østergaard SD, Søndergaard S, et al. The WHO-5 Well-Being Index: a systematic review of the literature. Psychother Psychosom 2015;84(3):167–76.

49. Lex H, Ginsburg Y, Sitzmann AF, et al. Quality of life across domains among individuals with treatment-resistant depression. J Affect Disord 2019;243:401–7.

50. Beck A, Crain AL, Solberg LI, et al. Severity of depression and magnitude of productivity loss. Ann Fam Med 2011;9(4):305–11.

51. Zimmerman M, Martinez JH, Attiullah N, et al. A new type of scale for determining remission from depression: The Remission from Depression Questionnaire. J Psychiatr Res 2013;47(1):78–82.

52. Mundt JC, Marks IM, Shear MK, et al. The Work and Social Adjustment Scale: a simple measure of impairment in functioning. Br J Psychiatry 2002;180(5):461–4.

53. Trivedi MH, Wisniewski SR, Morris DW, et al. Concise Health Risk Tracking scale: a brief self-report and clinician rating of suicidal risk. J Clin Psychiatry Jun 2011; 72(6):757–64.

54. Ostacher MJ, Nierenberg AA, Rabideau D, et al. A clinical measure of suicidal ideation, suicidal behavior, and associated symptoms in bipolar disorder: Psychometric properties of the Concise Health Risk Tracking Self-Report (CHRT-SR). J Psychiatr Res 2015;71:126–33.

55. Trivedi MH, Wisniewski SR, Morris DW, et al. Concise Associated Symptoms Tracking scale: a brief self-report and clinician rating of symptoms associated with suicidality. J Clin Psychiatry 2011;72(6):765–74.

56. Altman EG, Hedeker D, Peterson JL, et al. The Altman Self-Rating Mania Scale. Biol Psychiatry 1997;42(10):948–55.

57. dela Cruz AM, Bernstein IH, Greer TL, et al. Self-rated measure of pain frequency, intensity, and burden: psychometric properties of a new instrument for the assessment of pain. J Psychiatr Res 2014;59:155–60.

58. Trivedi MH, Jha MK, Kahalnik F, et al. VitalSign(6): A Primary Care First (PCP-First) Model for Universal Screening and Measurement-Based Care for Depression. Pharmaceuticals (Basel) 2019;12(2). https://doi.org/10.3390/ph12020071.

59. Jha MK, Grannemann BD, Trombello JM, et al. A Structured Approach to Detecting and Treating Depression in Primary Care: VitalSign6 Project. Ann Fam Med 2019;17(4):326–35.
60. Wang MZ, Jha MK, Minhajuddin A, et al. A primary care first (PCP-first) model to screen and treat depression: A VitalSign(6) report from a second cohort of 32,106 patients. Gen Hosp Psychiatry 2022;74:1–8.
61. Rush AJ, Madia ND, Carmody T, et al. Psychometric and Clinical Evaluation of the Clinician (VQIDS-C(5)) and Self-Report (VQIDS-SR(5)) Versions of the Very Quick Inventory of Depressive Symptoms. Neuropsychiatr Dis Treat 2022;18:289–302.
62. Hamilton M. A rating scale for depression. J Neurol Neurosurg Psychiatry 1960; 23:56–62.
63. Kyle PR, Lemming OM, Timmerby N, et al. The Validity of the Different Versions of the Hamilton Depression Scale in Separating Remission Rates of Placebo and Antidepressants in Clinical Trials of Major Depression. J Clin Psychopharmacol 2016;36(5):453–6.
64. Zimmerman M, Posternak MA, Chelminski I. Defining remission on the Montgomery-Asberg depression rating scale. J Clin Psychiatry 2004;65(2): 163–8.
65. Reeves GM, Rohan KJ, Langenberg P, et al. Calibration of response and remission cut-points on the Beck Depression Inventory-Second Edition for monitoring seasonal affective disorder treatment outcomes. J Affect Disord 2012;138(1–2): 123–7.

Approach to Diagnosis and Management of Treatment-Resistant Depression

Karina Rikhani, MD[a], Collin Vas, MD[a],
Manish Kumar Jha, MBBS[a,b],*

KEYWORDS

- Treatment-resistant depression • Diagnosis and treatment
- Management approaches • Structured assessment

KEY POINTS

- Treatment-resistant depression (TRD) should be considered in patients with major depressive disorder (MDD) who have inadequate improvement with 2 or more courses of antidepressant of adequate dose and duration.
- Measurement-based care approach of using rating scales at each visit helps in prompt identification and diagnosis of TRD.
- Differential diagnoses including other psychiatric disorders such as bipolar depression and medical conditions such as untreated hypothyroidism and obstructive sleep apnea should be considered.
- Presence of comorbidities such as anxiety disorder and substance use disorder is associated with more treatment-refractory course and should be systematically assessed.
- Management approaches for TRD include use of another medication to augment current antidepressant, switch to another antidepressant, or the use of a TRD-specific treatment (such as intranasal esketamine or electroconvulsive therapy).

INTRODUCTION

Major depressive disorder (MDD) is a chronic and recurrent illness that affects 20% of adults in the United States during their lifetime (Hasin and colleagues, JAMA Psychiatry). Disability associated with MDD has increased greater than 53% in last 2 decades and is now the second leading cause of disability.[1] Depression is also one of the leading causes of suicide. In fact, age-adjusted mortality rates due to suicide have continued to increase over the past 2 decades, even as age-adjusted mortality rates

[a] Department of Psychiatry, University of Texas Southwestern Medical Center, 5323 Harry Hines Boulevard, Dallas, TX 75390-9119, USA; [b] Peter O'Donnell Jr. Brain Institute, University of Texas Southwestern Medical Center, 5323 Harry Hines Boulevard, Dallas, TX 75390-9119, USA
* Corresponding author. University of Texas Southwestern Medical Center, 5323 Harry Hines Boulevard, Dallas, TX 75390-9119.
E-mail address: manish.jha@utsouthwestern.edu

Psychiatr Clin N Am 46 (2023) 247–259
https://doi.org/10.1016/j.psc.2023.02.011
0193-953X/23/© 2023 Elsevier Inc. All rights reserved.

psych.theclinics.com

due to other causes, such as cancer and heart disease, have steadily declined.[2] Based on data from the National Center for Health Statistics, and with the age-adjusted mortality rate in the year 1999 set as baseline, mortality rates due to cancer and heart disease have declined by 24.1% and 38.1%, respectively, between 1999 and 2017, whereas the mortality rate due to suicide has increased by 33.3% in the same period.[2] These declines in heart disease– and cancer-related mortality rates reflect successes in screening, preventative approaches, and development of treatments that are based on a deeper understanding of the underlying biological mechanisms.

Adoption of the United States Preventive Services Task Force recommendation of universal screening for depression may help in promptly identifying individuals suffering from depressive symptoms. Because of shortage of behavioral health services, most of the burden of screening, diagnosis, treatment, and follow-up of depression is usually thrust onto other medical providers. Unfortunately, half of the patients with MDD who are seen in medical settings will not be recognized as suffering from depression.[3,4] For those actually treated with antidepressants, only 1 out of 5 patients will receive adequate dosing.[5,6] A primary care provider (PCP) first approach that empowers PCPs to effectively manage depression in their patients may be instrumental in leveraging advanced health information technology tool. This approach allows for universal screening that is followed by diagnostic assessment in those who screen positive and selection and implementation of treatment.[7] Prior studies in real-world community practices have demonstrated the feasibility of this approach.[8,9] A team-based approach that leverages this model, as shown in **Fig. 1**, may be an essential first step in the diagnosis and management of treatment-resistant depression (TRD) by prompt identification of individuals with depression and avoiding unnecessary delays in the onset of care.

APPROACH TO IDENTIFICATION OF TREATMENT-RESISTANT DEPRESSION

TRD is most commonly defined as an inadequate treatment response following at least 2 consecutive antidepressant trials of adequate dose, duration, and treatment adherence among patients suffering from unipolar depressive disorders.[10] A measurement-based care approach that incorporates systematic assessment of symptom severity, tolerability, and adherence is therefore critical in maximizing treatment effectiveness (thereby preventing the onset of TRD) and in promptly identifying those who have not improved even after treatment optimization.[11] When evaluating patients who did not respond to antidepressant treatment, the clinician should verify that the primary diagnosis is correct and determine the presence of psychiatric or medical comorbidities that could affect the treatment response. Thoroughly evaluating risk factors for treatment resistance can help the clinician in choosing the best strategies for their patients with TRD.[12]

DIFFERENTIAL DIAGNOSIS OF TREATMENT-RESISTANT DEPRESSION

The first question to consider when evaluating response to antidepressant treatment is whether the primary diagnosis of MDD is correct. Instead of having TRD in the context of MDD, the patient may have previously received treatment for an incorrect diagnosis.[13] Therefore, it is important to differentiate unipolar depression from other conditions that have the same or very similar symptoms such as bipolar disorder, chronic medical condition, and obstructive sleep apnea (OSA).

Bipolar Disorder

Bipolar depressive episodes can be difficult to distinguish from MDD. The evidence suggests that there is an average delay of 10 years between initial symptoms and

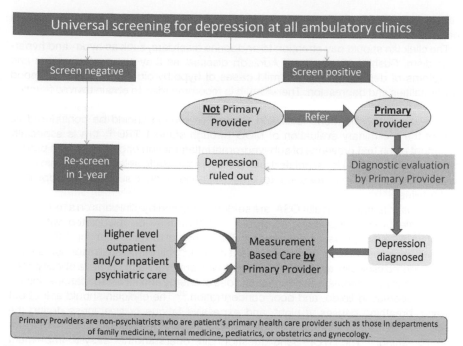

Fig. 1. A primary care provider–first approach of team-based screening and management of depression in health care settings.

diagnosis of bipolar disorder[14,15] and higher rates of undiagnosed bipolar disorder in treatment-resistant versus nonresistant depression.[16,17]

Unipolar and bipolar depression share similar clinical presentations, often making the differential diagnosis challenging. Unclear history of manic or hypomanic episodes leads to the misdiagnosis of bipolar disorder as unipolar depression.[18] Obtaining key information from the patient's medical history as well as information from the patient's family members may be very helpful to identify bipolar disorder.[12] The Mood Disorders Questionnaire[19] and the Hypomania/Mania Symptom Checklist[20] are available for the clinician in the differential diagnosis of bipolar versus unipolar depression.[18]

Chronic Medical Conditions

A variety of medical conditions need to be considered before making the diagnosis of TRD, as they can mimic symptoms of depression. Untreated or inadequately treated hypothyroidism should be considered as a differential diagnosis in patients with depression, and levels of thyroid hormones should be checked if presence of TRD is suspected. Multiple other medical conditions such as fibromyalgia, chronic fatigue syndrome, irritable bowel syndrome, and vitamin deficiencies are often associated with depressive symptoms and may be considered in the workup of patients with depression, as treatment of these conditions may result in significant improvement in depression symptoms.[21,22] Common medications used for management of medical conditions, including opiate analgesics and calcium channel blockers, may be associated with either causing or exacerbating depression.[23] Additional medications implicated for their role in causing or exacerbating depression include the systematic use of corticosteroids,[23] the interleukins, and interferons.[24,25] A careful history from the patient may be helpful in revealing a pattern of worsening depressive symptoms with initiation or changes in the dosage of these medications.

The clinician should pay attention to endocrine disorders, such as hypo- and hyperthyroidism, Cushing disease, and Addison disease, as they can produce signs and symptoms of depression.[26] Even mild cases of hypothyroid state can cause mood abnormalities and depression. Therefore, it is recommended to obtain thyroid function tests for patients with atypical or TRD.[27] Kirstein and colleagues suggested that a thyroid-stimulating hormone level and C-reactive protein should be considered as part of the preliminary evaluation of MDD through stage 1 TRD[28]; this is especially important given that presence of subsyndromal inflammation or obesity (which predisposes to inflammation) is associated with poorer response to selective serotonin reuptake inhibitors and may respond to other first-line agents such as bupropion or nortriptyline.[29–32]

Sleep disorders, in particular OSA, are seldom assessed by clinicians on a regular basis in patients with depressive disorders, but they may be associated with poor response to antidepressant treatment.[33] Even though assessment for OSA is not routinely recommended for the management of TRD,[34] this differential diagnosis should be considered clinically, especially in patients who are overweight or have obesity,[35] as it shares many symptoms with depression: loss of energy and increased fatigue, loss of interest, decreased libido, and poor concentration.[36] The clinician should ask about snoring, breathing pauses at night, and excessive fatigue or sleepiness during the day.[35] The Berlin Questionnaire is developed for use in the primary care setting for OSA screening.[37] The STOP-Bang questionnaire offers another easy-to-implement and practical approach to screen for OSA in clinical practice.[38] Other medical conditions that should be considered include diabetes, hypertension, and hypercholesterolemia, which are associated with higher rates of treatment resistance.[39] Chronic pain conditions are also associated with greater severity and longer duration of depressive symptoms and tend to show a lower response rate to antidepressant treatment.[40] Therefore, workup for TRD should include systematic assessment to identify potential medical illnesses that may resemble symptoms of depression or make it less likely for commonly used antidepressants to work effectively.

COMORBIDITIES

Recognition of comorbidities is essential because of its clear impact on the clinical severity of MDD and as risk factor for development of TRD. Individuals with comorbid conditions follow a more chronic and treatment-resistant course than those with only one depressive disorder.[41–43] They are more likely to have more severe depressive symptoms, decreased responsiveness to antidepressant treatment, and greater susceptibility to side effects.[28] Therefore, comprehensive management of comorbidities is essential to reduce the overall symptom burden in patients with depression.[44]

Substance Use Disorders

Substance use disorders are often comorbid with MDD, especially alcohol use disorder, and is associated with more severe depression symptoms, lower functioning, increased suicidality, a harder-to-treat depression, and a lower likelihood of remission.[45] The course of each of these problems seems to be complicated by the other.[46] A study with fluoxetine at the Depression Research Program of the Clinical Psychopharmacology Unit at the Massachusetts General Hospital found that even moderate alcohol consumption correlated with poorer response to the antidepressant treatment. This relationship remained significant even after adjusting for the severity of depression at baseline.[47]

Anxiety Disorders

Anxiety disorders are highly comorbid with depression, and rates of cooccurrence are greater than with any other psychiatric disorder.[48,49] Patients with MDD and comorbid anxiety have more severe depression symptoms and increased risk for suicide than patients without comorbid anxiety.[50] They tend to have a slower response to medication and an incomplete remission of symptoms.[28] Patients with depression with mixed states involving panic attacks have the poorest outcomes and are most likely to be chronically depressed.[51] Therefore, the clinical evaluation of TRD must include screening for anxiety symptoms and disorders.[28]

Personality Disorders

It is estimated that 1 in 2 patients with MDD may have comorbid personality disorders.[28] Presence of personality disorders is often associated with an earlier age of onset of depression and has a positive relationship with the degree of treatment resistance.[28,52,53] The evidence indicates that depressed patients with comorbid personality disorders are less responsive to the treatment with antidepressant medications compared with patients with no history of personality disorders and have a worse prognosis for long-term outcomes.[53,54]

However, chronic depressive symptoms may alter the presentation of personality traits to an extent that a valid personality assessment is almost impossible. Fava and colleagues reported that 44% of patients with depression and borderline personality disorder no longer met the criteria for the personality disorder after 8 weeks of treatment with fluoxetine. Therefore, it is very important to not prematurely diagnose personality disorders in patients with depression.[28,55]

Other Comorbidities

Medical conditions such as irritable bowel syndrome, fibromyalgia, migraine, atypical facial pain, premenstrual dysphoric disorder, and chronic fatigue syndrome are often associated with depressive symptoms. They are important diagnoses to consider in the evaluation of TRD, as they go often underrecognized and undertreated by most clinicians. When the associated depression is treated with a psychotropic drug, there is usually an improvement in the somatic symptoms as well. This observation suggests a common etiologic step in these disorders that are addressed by the antidepressant.[56]

STRUCTURED ASSESSMENT FOR TREATMENT-RESISTANT DISORDER

Structured assessments are reliable and valid instruments to verify the accurate diagnosis of TRD. Standardized rating scales are used to assess depression severity and determine treatment response. The response to antidepressant treatment is usually classified into 4 categories: nonresponse (patients who have no clinically meaningful response to treatment), partial response (a greater than 25% but less than 50% decrease in depression assessment scale scores), treatment response (defined as a 50% or greater decrease in scores), and remission (absence of depressive symptoms or the presence of minimal residual symptoms).[57]

The Massachusetts General Hospital Antidepressant Treatment History Questionnaire (MGH-ATRQ) is a clinician-rated scale used to determine treatment resistance in MDD. The MGH-ATRQ examines the patient's antidepressant treatment history and usually defines 8 weeks on an adequate dose (such as a dose approved by

Food and Drug Administration [FDA]) of antidepressant medication as an adequate duration of treatment. It also provides specific criteria for adequate dosage for each antidepressant trial and the degree of symptomatic improvement obtained with each trial. Research studies have shown good validity of this measure; in a previous study, no subjects deemed treatment resistant by the MGH-ATRQ were found to be nonresistant by the clinician.[58]

Another clinician-rated scale, the Antidepressant Treatment History Form (ATHF), offers the advantage of incorporating clinical judgment in the assessment of treatment resistance,[59] and it is one of the most commonly used instrument to evaluate the adequacy of prior antidepressant treatment.[60] The ATHF was developed to organize information from various sources about the treatment history of patients with major depression and to rate the antidepressant potency of medication trials or other somatic treatments that a patient may have received in the current or previous episodes.[59] This instrument has separate criteria for unipolar and bipolar major depressive (MDE), as well as psychotic and nonpsychotic MDE.[61] The ATHF uses a 5-point scale to rate each antidepressant trial and requires clinical judgment regarding adherence and clinical outcome. Patients are not considered as resistant to a treatment if they did not receive it due to nonadherence.[62,63]

MANAGEMENT APPROACHES FOR TREATMENT-RESISTANT DISORDER

Approaches for management of TRD include augmenting antidepressant with nonantidepressant medication, combining antidepressant therapies, and switching therapies.[64,65] Several effective FDA-approved treatments and commonly used off-label treatment strategies are available to clinicians for use in treating their patients with TRD. The goal of treatment is to attain remission, to reduce the risk of relapse,[66,67] and to improve psychosocial functioning.[68] To address each individual patient's priorities, clinicians should use a shared decision-making approach for treatment selection.[60] These medications have been discussed in other reports within this issue of the Clinics and are referred to in this article briefly.

Augmentation and Combination Approach

Several second-generation antipsychotics, such as aripiprazole, brexpiprazole, cariprazine, and quetiapine extended release, are approved as augmentation agents, that is, they can be considered for management of TRD. The olanzapine-fluoxetine combination was the first medication combination to be specifically approved for TRD. These medications may have a decreased risk of extrapyramidal effect as compared with first-generation antipsychotics but have other side effects including metabolic dysfunction and weight gain.[70] A report by Vas and colleagues in the current issue of the Clinics discusses in detail the FDA-approved second-generation antipsychotics.

Other effective strategies include augmentation with lithium and liothyronine (T3) to the effectiveness of antidepressant medications.[69] Lithium is also effective for relapse prevention and reduction of long-term risk of suicide. Medications that can be used in off-label fashion include pramipexole and lamotrigine[71] as well as combinations of antidepressants including bupropion, mirtazapine, or tricyclic antidepressants.[69]

Switching to an Alternative Antidepressant

Studies of insurance databases suggest that clinicians often use an alternative antidepressant after inadequate improvement with 2 sequential courses of treatment. In the

Sequenced Treatment Alternatives to Relieve Depression (STAR*D) study, the participants who required 3 treatment steps had a depression remission rate of 13.7%. Participants who required more antidepressant trials tended to have greater depressive illness burden and more concurrent psychiatric and general medical disorders.[72] Therefore, evidence supporting the use of alternative antidepressant in management of TRD is limited. Alternative antidepressants may be considered if prior course of antidepressant trials were limited due to side effects, resulting in inadequate dose and duration. Because of the potential side effects and risk of hypertensive crises, monoamine oxidase inhibitors are usually considered in clinical practice only after multiple first-line antidepressants and other augmentation strategies have been proved to be ineffective.

Treatment-Resistant Depression–Specific Interventions

Ketamine and esketamine

Ketamine seems to be effective for the treatment and reduction of suicidal ideation in patients with TRD in several randomized blinded and open-label studies.[73–75] The antisuicidal ideation effect is seen with both single and repeat dosing.[76] Esketamine is an FDA-approved treatment of TRD and of major depression with suicidal ideation and behavior[77] when used in conjunction with an oral antidepressant. The intranasal formulation allows the medication to bypass the first-pass metabolism in liver and improves bioavailability and has a quick onset of antidepressant effects.[78] Intranasal esketamine was studied in several trials before regulatory approval, and the meta-analysis of the efficacy reported significant improvement in depression symptoms.[79,80] Current approval of esketamine is in conjunction with another antidepressant but ongoing studies are evaluating it as monotherapy. Ketamine has been used as a monotherapy in research studies, often administered intravenously at 0.5 mg/kg infusion over 40 minutes. This issue of the *Clinics* includes detailed information on these rapid-acting antidepressants.

Neuromodulation interventions

Neuromodulation techniques such as transcranial magnetic stimulation (TMS), electroconvulsive therapy (ECT), and vagus nerve stimulation (VNS) may be used either alone or in combination with antidepressants for management of TRD. TMS is a noninvasive brain stimulation technique approved by the US FDA for TRD if pharmacotherapy trials fail.[81] Treatment with repetitive transcranial magnetic stimulation (rTMS) was found to be safe and effective in pregnant patients and elderly patients in whom treatment options are limited because of a possible risk of adverse reactions and negative child development outcomes.[82] Intermittent theta-burst stimulation (iTBS), an FDA-approved form of rTMS, produces equivalent antidepressant responses[83,84] with shorter session duration (3 minutes with iTBS).[85]

ECT is an alternative approach for management of TRD. The American Psychiatry Association guidelines suggest ECT as a first-line option for patients with psychotic symptoms or with a positive response to psychotherapy in the past. This method can be used for more severe, incapacitating forms of TRD, especially where there is a need for an early response because of the risk of harm to self.[81] Studies suggest that ECT has a response rate of 50% to 70% in patients with TRD.[86] Pharmacotherapy should not be stopped when initiating ECT, as maintenance of antidepressant therapy reduces relapses after course of ECT treatment.[87]

The VNS is FDA approved as adjunctive therapy for patients with TRD with 4 prior antidepressant treatment failures.[86] VNS has been shown to exhibit antidepressant and antisuicidal effects and improve quality of life of patients with TRD.[88] Side effects related to VNS often limit its use. As VNS is a neuromodulatory intervention that involves surgical attachment of an electrode to the vagus nerve, it carries risks associated with any surgical intervention[89] and may cause damage to the vagus nerve or result in alteration of voice and hoarseness.[90] Because VNS requires months to demonstrate clinical efficacy, this treatment method should not be used in acutely suicidal patients.[91]

SUMMARY

One in three patients with MDD, an often chronic and recurrent condition that affects 1 in 5 adults in the United States, may have TRD. A team-based approach that brings together primary care providers and psychiatric providers may be an essential first step in the diagnosis and management of TRD by prompt identification of individuals with depression and avoiding unnecessary delays in the onset of care. A measurement-based care approach that incorporates systematic assessment of symptom severity, tolerability, and adherence is critical in maximizing treatment effectiveness and thereby preventing the onset of TRD. With the approval of new treatments, such as intranasal esketamine, and others that are in the pipeline, clinicians may have more tools to work with their patients with TRD.

CLINICS CARE POINTS

- Measurement-based care approach aids in early identification of treatment-resistant depression (TRD).
- Consider using structured assessments to verify drug dose, duration, and degree of improvement when evaluating individuals for TRD.
- Use of TRD-specific interventions should be considered when TRD is present.

DISCLOSURE

Dr M.K. Jha has received contract research grants from Acadia Pharmaceuticals, Neurocrine Bioscience, Navitor/Supernus, and Janssen Research & Development; educational grant to serve as Section Editor of the Psychiatry & Behavioral Health Learning Network; consultant fees from Eleusis Therapeutics US, Inc, Janssen Global Services, Janssen Scientific Affairs, Worldwide Clinical Trials/Eliem and Inversargo, Boehringer Ingelheim, and Guidepoint Global; and honoraria from North American Center for Continuing Medical Education, Medscape/WebMD, Clinical Care Options, and Global Medical Education. Drs K. Rikhani and C. Vas have nothing to disclose.

ACKNOWLEDGMENTS

Dr M.K. Jha is supported by a career development award from National Institute of Mental Health (MH126202), the O'Donnell Clinical Neuroscience Scholar Award from UT Southwestern Medical Center, and the resources from the Center for Depression Research and Clinical Care (CDRC) at UT Southwestern Medical Center.

REFERENCES

1. Vos T, Barber RM, Bell B, et al. Global, regional, and national incidence, prevalence, and years lived with disability for 301 acute and chronic diseases and

injuries in 188 countries, 1990–2013: a systematic analysis for the Global Burden of Disease Study. Lancet 2013;386(9995):743–800.

2. NCHS. National Center for Health Statistics. Leading Causes of Death: United States. 2020. Available at: https://data.cdc.gov/NCHS/NCHS-Leading-Causes-of-Death-United-States/bi63-dtpu. 2020. Accessed on 26 September 2021.

3. Pignone M.P., Gaynes B.N., Rushton J.L., et al., Screening for depression in adults: a summary of the evidence for the US Preventive Services Task Force, Annals of internal medicine, 136 (10), 2002,765–776.

4. Coyne JC, Schwenk TL, Fechner-Bates S. Nondetection of depression by primary care physicians reconsidered. Gen Hosp Psychiatr 1995;17(1):3–12.

5. Kessler RC, Berglund P, Demler O, et al. The Epidemiology of Major Depressive Disorder. JAMA, J Am Med Assoc 2003;289(23):3095–105.

6. Young AS, Klap R, Sherbourne CD, et al. The quality of care for depressive and anxiety disorders in the United States. Arch Gen Psychiatr 2001;58(1):55–61.

7. Trivedi MH, Jha MK, Kahalnik F, et al. VitalSign[6]: A Primary Care First (PCP-First) Model for Universal Screening and Measurement-Based Care for Depression. Pharmaceuticals 2019;12(2):71.

8. Jha MK, Grannemann BD, Trombello JM, et al. A Structured Approach to Detecting and Treating Depression in Primary Care: VitalSign6 Project. Ann Fam Med 2019;17(4):326–35.

9. Wang MZ, Jha MK, Minhajuddin A, et al. A primary care first (PCP-first) model to screen and treat depression: A VitalSign[6] report from a second cohort of 32,106 patients. Gen Hosp Psychiatr 2022;74:1–8.

10. Souery D, Papakostas GI, Trivedi MH. Treatment-resistant depression. J Clin Psychiatr 2006;67:16.

11. Trivedi MH, Rush AJ, Wisniewski SR, et al, STAR*D Study Team. Evaluation of outcomes with citalopram for depression using measurement-based care in STAR*D: implications for clinical practice. Am J Psychiatr 2006;163(1):28–40.

12. Gaynes BN. Identifying difficult-to-treat depression: differential diagnosis, subtypes, and comorbidities. J Clin Psychiatr 2009;70(suppl 6):8452.

13. Fava M. Diagnosis and definition of treatment-resistant depression. Biol Psychiatr 2003;53(8):649–59.

14. Lish JD, Dime-Meenan S, Whybrow PC, et al. The National Depressive and Manic-depressive Association (DMDA) survey of bipolar members. J Affect Disord 1994;31(4):281–94.

15. Baldessarini RJ, Tondo L, Baethge CJ, et al. Effects of treatment latency on response to maintenance treatment in manic-depressive disorders. Bipolar Disord 2007;9(4):386–93.

16. Perugi G, Pacchiarotti I, Mainardi C, et al. Patterns of response to antidepressants in major depressive disorder: Drug resistance or worsening of depression are associated with a bipolar diathesis. Eur Neuropsychopharmacol 2019;29(7): 825–34.

17. Sharma V, Khan M, Smith A. A closer look at treatment resistant depression: is it due to a bipolar diathesis? J Affect Disord 2005;84(2–3):251–7.

18. Trivedi MH. *Depression*. New York, NY: Oxford University Press; 2020.

19. Hirschfeld RMA, Williams JBW, Spitzer RL, et al. Development and validation of a screening instrument for bipolar spectrum disorder: the Mood Disorder Questionnaire. Am J Psychiatr 2000;157(11):1873–5.

20. Angst J, Adolfsson R, Benazzi F, et al. The HCL-32: towards a self-assessment tool for hypomanic symptoms in outpatients. J Affect Disord 2005;88(2):217–33.

21. Phillip S. A Clinically Relevant Guide to the Differential Diagnosis of Depression. J Nerv Ment Dis 1985;173(4):199–211.
22. Gruber AJ, Hudson JI, Pope HG. The management of treatment-resistant depression in disorders on the interface of psychiatry and medicine. Psychiatr Clin North Am 1996;19:351–69.
23. Patten SB, Lavorato DH. Medication use and major depressive syndrome in a community population. Compr Psychiatry 2001;42(2):124–31.
24. Wilson DR, Warise L. Cytokines and their role in depression. Perspect Psychiatr Care 2008;44(4):285–9.
25. Van De Putte DE, Fischer K, Posthouwer D, et al. Occurrence, course and risk factors of depression during antiviral treatment for chronic hepatitis C in patients with inherited bleeding disorders: a prospective study. Haemophilia 2009;15(2):544–51.
26. Wolkowitz OM, Rothschild AJ. Psychoneuroendocrinology: the scientific basis of clinical practice. Arlington, VA: American Psychiatric Pub; 2008.
27. Gold MS, Pottash ALC, Extein IRL. Hypothyroidism and depression: evidence from complete thyroid function evaluation. JAMA 1981;245(19):1919–22.
28. Kornstein SG, Schneider RK. Clinical features of treatment-resistant depression. J Clin Psychiatr 2001;62:18–25.
29. Jha MK, Wakhlu S, Dronamraju N, et al. Validating pre-treatment body mass index as moderator of antidepressant treatment outcomes: Findings from CO-MED trial. J Affect Disord 2018;234:34–7.
30. Jha MK, Minhajuddin A, Chin-Fatt C, et al. Sex differences in the association of baseline c-reactive protein (CRP) and acute-phase treatment outcomes in major depressive disorder: Findings from the EMBARC study. J Psychiatr Res 2019;113:165–71.
31. Jha MK, Minhajuddin A, Gadad BS, et al. Can C-reactive protein inform antidepressant medication selection in depressed outpatients? Findings from the CO-MED trial. Psychoneuroendocrinology 2017;78:105–13.
32. Uher R, Tansey KE, Dew T, et al. An inflammatory biomarker as a differential predictor of outcome of depression treatment with escitalopram and nortriptyline. Am J Psychiatr 2014;171(12):1278–86.
33. Ejaz SM, Khawaja IS, Bhatia S, et al. Obstructive sleep apnea and depression: a review. Innovations in clinical neuroscience 2011;8(8):17.
34. Bschor T, Bauer M, Adli M. Chronic and treatment resistant depression: diagnosis and stepwise therapy. Deutsches Ärzteblatt International 2014;111(45):766.
35. Gottlieb DJ, Punjabi NM. Diagnosis and management of obstructive sleep apnea: a review. JAMA 2020;323(14):1389–400.
36. Sforza E, de Saint Hilaire Z, Pelissolo A, et al. Personality, anxiety and mood traits in patients with sleep-related breathing disorders: effect of reduced daytime alertness. Sleep Med 2002;3(2):139–45.
37. Netzer NC, Stoohs RA, Netzer CM, et al. Using the Berlin Questionnaire to identify patients at risk for the sleep apnea syndrome. Ann Intern Med 1999;131(7):485–91.
38. Chung FF, Abdullah HR, Liao P, et al. STOP-Bang Questionnaire: A Practical Approach to Screen for Obstructive Sleep Apnea. Chest 2016;149(3):631–8.
39. Iosifescu DV, Clementi-Craven N, Fraguas R, et al. Cardiovascular risk factors may moderate pharmacological treatment effects in major depressive disorder. Psychosom Med 2005;67(5):703–6.
40. Ohayon MM. Specific characteristics of the pain/depression association in the general population. J Clin Psychiatr 2004;65(suppl 12):5–9.

41. Hirschfeld R, Hasin D, Keller MB, et al. Depression and alcoholism: comorbidity in a longitudinal study. Comorbidity of Mood and Anxiety Disorders 1990;293–303.

42. Hagnell O, Gräsbeck A. Comorbidity of anxiety and depression in the Lundby 25-year prospective study: the pattern of subsequent episodes. Comorbidity of Mood and Anxiety Disorders 1990;139–52.

43. Murphy JM. Diagnostic comorbidity and symptom co-occurrence: The Stirling County Study. In: Maser JD, Cloninger CR, editors. Comorbidity of mood and anxiety disorders. American Psychiatric Association; 1990. p. 153–76.

44. McAllister-Williams RH, Arango C, Blier P, et al. The identification, assessment and management of difficult-to-treat depression: an international consensus statement. J Affect Disord 2020;267:264–82.

45. Davis LL, Rush JA, Wisniewski SR, et al. Substance use disorder comorbidity in major depressive disorder: an exploratory analysis of the Sequenced Treatment Alternatives to Relieve Depression cohort. Compr Psychiatr 2005;46(2):81–9.

46. Ostacher MJ. Comorbid alcohol and substance abuse dependence in depression: impact on the outcome of antidepressant treatment. Psychiatr Clin 2007; 30(1):69–76.

47. Worthington J, Fava M, Agustin C, et al. Consumption of alcohol, nicotine, and caffeine among depressed outpatients: relationship with response to treatment. Psychosomatics 1996;37(6):518–22.

48. Kessler RC, Berglund P, Demler O, et al. The epidemiology of major depressive disorder: results from the National Comorbidity Survey Replication (NCS-R). JAMA 2003;289(23):3095–105.

49. Kessler RC, Sampson NA, Berglund P, et al. Anxious and non-anxious major depressive disorder in the World Health Organization World Mental Health Surveys. Epidemiol Psychiatr Sci 2015;24(3):210–26.

50. Gaynes BN, Magruder KM, Burns BJ, et al. Does a coexisting anxiety disorder predict persistence of depressive illness in primary care patients with major depression? Gen Hosp Psychiatr 1999;21(3):158–67.

51. Van Valkenburg C, Akiskal HS, Puzantian V, et al. Anxious depressions: clinical, family history, and naturalistic outcome—comparisons with panic and major depressive disorders. J Affect Disord 1984;6(1):67–82.

52. Fagiolini A, Kupfer DJ. Is treatment-resistant depression a unique subtype of depression? Biol Psychiatr 2003;53(8):640–8.

53. Thase ME. The role of Axis II comorbidity in the management of patients with treatment-resistant depression. Psychiatr Clin 1996;19(2):287–309.

54. Shea MT, Widiger TA, Klein MH. Comorbidity of personality disorders and depression: implications for treatment. J Consult Clin Psychol 1992;60(6):857.

55. Fava M, Bouffides E, Pava JA, et al. Personality disorder comorbidity with major depression and response to fluoxetine treatment. Psychother Psychosom 1994; 62(3–4):160–7.

56. Gruber AJ, Hudson JI, Pope HG Jr. The management of treatment-resistant depression in disorders on the interface of psychiatry and medicine: fibromyalgia, chronic fatigue syndrome, migraine, irritable bowel syndrome, atypical facial pain, and premenstrual dysphoric disorder. Psychiatr Clin 1996;19(2):351–69.

57. Greden JF. The burden of disease for treatment-resistant depression. J Clin Psychiatr 2001;62:26–31.

58. Chandler GM, Iosifescu DV, Pollack MH, et al. RESEARCH: Validation of the Massachusetts General Hospital Antidepressant Treatment History Questionnaire (ATRQ). CNS Neurosci Ther 2010;16(5):322–5.

59. Sackeim HA. The definition and meaning of treatment-resistant depression. J Clin Psychiatr 2001;62:10–7.
60. Sackeim Harold A, Aaronson Scott T, Bunker Mark T, et al. The assessment of resistance to antidepressant treatment: Rationale for the Antidepressant Treatment History Form: Short Form (ATHF-SF). J Psychiatr Res 2019;113:125–36. ISSN 0022-3956.
61. Hazari H, Christmas D, Matthews K. The clinical utility of different quantitative methods for measuring treatment resistance in major depression. J Affect Disord 2013;150(2):231–6.
62. Frank E., Prien R.F., Jarrett R.B.,et al., Conceptualization and rationale for consensus definitions of terms in major depressive disorder: remission, recovery, relapse, and recurrence, Arch Gen Psychiatr, 48 (9), 1991, 851–855.
63. Rush AJ, Kraemer HC, Sackeim HA, et al. Report by the ACNP Task Force on response and remission in major depressive disorder. Neuropsychopharmacology 2006;31(9):1841–53.
64. Keller MB. Issues in treatment-resistant depression. J Clin Psychiatr 2005;66:5.
65. Rush AJ, Thase ME, Dubé S. Research issues in the study of difficult-to-treat depression. Biol Psychiatr 2003;53(8):743–53.
66. Judd LL, Akiskal HS, Maser JD, et al. Major depressive disorder: a prospective study of residual subthreshold depressive symptoms as predictor of rapid relapse. J Affect Disord 1998;50(2–3):97–108.
67. Rush AJ, Trivedi MH, Wisniewski SR, et al. Acute and longer-term outcomes in depressed outpatients requiring one or several treatment steps: a STAR* D report. Am J Psychiatr 2006;163(11):1905–17.
68. Fried EI, Nesse RM. The impact of individual depressive symptoms on impairment of psychosocial functioning. PLoS One 2014;9(2):e90311.
69. Ruberto VL, Jha MK, Murrough JW. Pharmacological treatments for patients with treatment-resistant depression. Pharmaceuticals 2020;13(6):116.
70. Mithawala PK. Managing Treatment-Resistant Depression. US Pharm 2020; 45(5):15–9.
71. Fava M. Augmentation and combination strategies in treatment-resistant depression. J Clin Psychiatr 2001;62:4–11.
72. Rush AJ, Trivedi MH, Wisniewski SR, et al. Acute and longer-term outcomes in depressed outpatients requiring one or several treatment steps: a STAR* D report. Am J Psychiatr 2006;1905–17.
73. Aan Het Rot M, Collins KA, Murrough JW, et al. Safety and efficacy of repeated-dose intravenous ketamine for treatment-resistant depression. Biol Psychiatr 2010;67(2):139–45.
74. Ibrahim L, Diazgranados N, Luckenbaugh DA, et al. Rapid decrease in depressive symptoms with an N-methyl-d-aspartate antagonist in ECT-resistant major depression. Prog Neuro Psychopharmacol Biol Psychiatr 2011;35(4):1155–9.
75. Murrough JW, Perez AM, Pillemer S, et al. Rapid and longer-term antidepressant effects of repeated ketamine infusions in treatment-resistant major depression. Biol Psychiatr 2013;74(4):250–6.
76. Xiong J, Lipsitz O, Chen-Li D, et al. The acute antisuicidal effects of single-dose intravenous ketamine and intranasal esketamine in individuals with major depression and bipolar disorders: A systematic review and meta-analysis. J Psychiatr Res 2021;134:57–68.
77. Janssen Announces US FDA approval of Spravato (esketamine) CIII nasal spray for adults with treatment-resistant depression (TRD) who have cycled through multiple treatments without relief, Available at: https://www.jnj.com/janssen-announces-

u-s-fda-approval-of-spravatotm-esketamine-ciii-nasal-spray-for-adults-with-treatment-resistant-depression-trd-who-have-cycled-through-multiple-treatments-without-relief. Accessed February 16, 2023.

78. Canuso CM, Singh JB, Fedgchin M, et al. Efficacy and safety of intranasal esketamine for the rapid reduction of symptoms of depression and suicidality in patients at imminent risk for suicide: results of a double-blind, randomized, placebo-controlled study. Am J Psychiatr 2018;175(7):620–30.

79. McIntyre RS, Rosenblat JD, Nemeroff CB, et al. Synthesizing the evidence for ketamine and esketamine in treatment-resistant depression: an international expert opinion on the available evidence and implementation. Am J Psychiatr 2021;5: 383–99.

80. Papakostas GI, Salloum NC, Hock RS, et al. Efficacy of esketamine augmentation in major depressive disorder: a meta-analysis. J Clin Psychiatr 2020;81: 19r12889.

81. Gelenberg AJ, Freeman MP, Markowitz JC, et al. Practice guideline for the treatment of patients with major depressive disorder. 3rd ed. Washington, DC: American Psychiatric Association; 2010.

82. Felipe RdM, Ferrão YA. Transcranial magnetic stimulation for treatment of major depression during pregnancy: a review. Trends in psychiatry and psychotherapy 2016;38(4):190–7.

83. Blumberger DM, Vila-Rodriguez F, Thorpe KE, et al. Effectiveness of theta burst versus high-frequency repetitive transcranial magnetic stimulation in patients with depression (THREE-D): a randomised non-inferiority trial. Lancet 2018; 391(10131):1683–92.

84. Blumberger DM, Vila-Rodriguez F, Dunlop K, et al. Intermittent theta-burst versus 10 Hz left dorsolateral prefrontal rTMS for treatment resistant depression: preliminary results from a two-site, randomized, single blind non-inferiority trial. Brain Stimul: Basic, Translational, and Clinical Research in Neuromodulation 2015; 8(2):329.

85. Huang Y-Z, Rothwell JC. The effect of short-duration bursts of high-frequency, low-intensity transcranial magnetic stimulation on the human motor cortex. Clinical neurophysiology 2004;115(5):1069–75.

86. Shelton RC, Osuntokun O, Heinloth AN, et al. Therapeutic options for treatment-resistant depression. CNS Drugs 2010;24(2):131–61.

87. Cleare A, Pariante CM, Young AH, et al. Evidence-based guidelines for treating depressive disorders with antidepressants: a revision of the 2008 British Association for Psychopharmacology guidelines. J Psychopharmacol 2015;29(5): 459–525.

88. Moeller S, Lücke C, Heinen C, et al. Vagus nerve stimulation as an adjunctive neurostimulation tool in treatment-resistant depression. JoVE 2019;7(143):e58264.

89. Aaronson ST, Conway CR. Vagus nerve stimulation: changing the paradigm for chronic severe depression? Psychiatric Clinics 2018;41(3):409–18.

90. Sackeim HA, Rush AJ, George MS, et al. Vagus nerve stimulation (VNS™) for treatment-resistant depression: efficacy, side effects, and predictors of outcome. Neuropsychopharmacology 2001;25(5):713–28.

91. Aaronson ST, Barber GS. VNS for treatment-resistant depression, Managing Treatment-Resistant Depression, 1. San Diego, CA: Elsevier; 2022. p. 319–29.

Pharmacotherapy for Treatment-Resistant Depression
Antidepressants and Atypical Antipsychotics

Collin Vas, MD[a], Ayush Jain[b], Mili Trivedi[c],
Manish Kumar Jha, MBBS[d],*, Sanjay J. Mathew, MD[e]

KEYWORDS

- Major depressive disorder • Antidepressants • Treatment-resistant depression
- Atypical antipsychotics • Aripiprazole • Brexpiprazole • Cariprazine • Quetiapine

KEY POINTS

- One in three adults with major depressive disorder (MDD) do not respond to commonly used antidepressants and may have treatment-resistant depression (TRD).
- Fewer than one in five patients will attain remission with commonly used antidepressants after nonresponse to two adequate trials in their current episode.
- In clinical practice, antidepressant monotherapy continues to predominate as the next-step option after inadequate improvement with first-line treatment.
- Atypical antipsychotics with approved indication for MDD include aripiprazole, brexpiprazole, cariprazine, quetiapine extended-release, and olanzapine-fluoxetine combination.
- The potential benefits of using atypical antipsychotics has to be weighed against their potential harm, especially in terms of weight gain, akathisia, and tardive dyskinesia.

INTRODUCTION

Major depressive disorder (MDD) is an often chronic and/or recurrent disorder that is associated with dysfunctions in multiple aspects of life including work and non-work-related productivity, psychosocial function, and quality of life.[1–5] It is widely prevalent and is estimated to affect one in five adults in the United States during their lifetime.[6] Although universal screening and use of measurement-based care can assist with

a UT Southwestern Medical Center, Dallas, TX, USA; b The Shri Ram School, Aravali, Gurgaon, Haryana, India; c Colleyville Heritage High School, Colleyville, TX, USA; d Center for Depression Research and Clinical Care, UT Southwestern Medical Center, 5323 Harry Hines Boulevard, Dallas, TX 75390-9119, USA; e Menninger Department of Psychiatry & Behavioral Sciences, Baylor College of Medicine, Michael E. DeBakey VA Medical Center, The Menninger Clinic, Houston, TX, USA
* Corresponding author.
E-mail address: manish.jha@utsouthwestern.edu

Psychiatr Clin N Am 46 (2023) 261–275
https://doi.org/10.1016/j.psc.2023.02.012
0193-953X/23/© 2023 Elsevier Inc. All rights reserved.
psych.theclinics.com

prompt identification of patients with MDD and initiation of evidence-based treatments,[7,8] as shown in the landmark Sequenced Treatment Alternatives to Relieve Depression (STAR*D) trial, one in three patients with MDD may not experience adequate improvement even after multiple sequential courses of antidepressants.[9] Findings from STAR*D further suggested patients with MDD who did not improve with two courses of antidepressant had low rates of remission, that is, attainment of none-to-minimal symptoms of depression, with a third or fourth course suggesting that they may have treatment-resistant depression (TRD).[9] Subsequent studies have found that the presence of TRD exacerbates the health care–related expenses associated with MDD and is associated with significantly higher rates of intentional self-harm and all-cause mortality.[10–12] However, clinical care of patients with TRD and management of individual patients is hindered by gaps in knowledge about the definition of TRD and its identification in clinical practice.

A recent systematic review for the Centers for Medicare & Medicaid Services and the Agency for Healthcare Research and Quality attempted to clarify how investigators and experts have defined TRD.[13] This review found that there was no consensus definition to define TRD. In the context of MDD, they found that TRD was defined as a minimum of two prior treatment failures with the confirmation of prior adequate dose and duration.[13] However, they found that only 17% of intervention studies enrolled samples that met the aforementioned specified criteria for TRD. Furthermore, the reports varied on the definition of nonresponse, adequacy of dose, and duration of prior treatment, and whether the treatments were used in the current episode or in a prior episode of depression.[13] In extant literature even when similar criteria were used for the dose and duration of antidepressants in the current episode, studies have differed in how they operationalized nonresponse. For example, in the phase 3 clinical trials of intranasal esketamine, nonresponse was defined as less than or equal to 25% improvement, whereas in the National Institute of Mental Health–funded dose-ranging study of intravenous ketamine, nonresponse was defined as less than 50% improvement in symptom.[14,15] Definitions of nonresponse have also relied on criterion symptoms of depression and often ignore the burden associated with symptoms, such as irritability and anxiety.[16–18] Because of the substantial heterogeneity in the conceptualization and definition of TRD, recent reports have undertaken a broader approach of considering an inadequate response to one course of antidepressant to evaluate the evidence of antipsychotic augmentation studies that included historical inadequate response to just one antidepressant in the current episode.[19] Additionally, the focus on short-term symptom improvements with the prevailing TRD definition has overlooked the chronic illness course of MDD and may warrant a shift in conceptualization toward "difficult-to-treat depression," which incorporates persistence of treatment response, the burden of side effects, and the impact on daily functioning and quality of life.[20,21]

Clinical care of patients with TRD starts with systematic measurement of symptom severity, side effects, and adherence using a measurement-based care approach.[22,23] This allows for tracking of changes in symptoms that is indexed to the dose and duration of antidepressant medication. When such prospective assessments are unavailable, structured assessments, such as the Massachusetts General Hospital–Antidepressant Treatment Response Questionnaire, is helpful in ascertaining the presence of TRD.[24] Systematic assessment of subthreshold hypomanic symptoms[25] and previously unrecognized bipolar depression should be considered in diagnostic work-up of patients with TRD. Consideration for comorbid conditions, such as systemic inflammation (as measured by levels of C-reactive protein) and obesity (measured with body mass index), is also important because these have been linked to inadequate response to commonly used selective serotonin reuptake inhibitors (SSRIs).[26,27] Systematic assessment of pain may also be warranted, using a simple measure, such as the Pain Frequency Intensity and Burden scale,[28] given the comorbidity of chronic pain with depression and its association with nonresponse to antidepressants.[29,30]

Regarding treatment options for TRD, several psychological treatments have been found to be effective including cognitive behavioral therapy and cognitive behavioral analysis system of psychotherapy.[31] Neuromodulation strategies, including electroconvulsive therapy, repetitive transcranial magnetic stimulation, and vagus nerve stimulation, are also effective for TRD.[32] However, this report is focused on pharmacologic treatments and does not discuss these psychotherapy and neuromodulation approaches (available elsewhere in this issue).

Data from real-world practices suggest that antidepressant medications continue to be predominantly used either as monotherapy or along with an augmentation agent after inadequate response to first-step treatment. In a recent analysis of a claims database, on average people underwent two prior steps of treatment before an adjunctive or augmentation treatment was tried.[33] A study using data from the Veterans Affairs (VA) system found that monotherapy with SSRI, serotonin norepinephrine reuptake inhibitor, bupropion, and mirtazapine was selected as the first-line treatment in 58.9%, 8.8%, 8.2%, and 7.8%, respectively. Although the proportion of individuals for whom monotherapy with these drugs declined with subsequent treatment steps, two in three patients who were on their third treatment step (which may serve as a proxy for the presence of TRD) were still on monotherapy with one of these antidepressants.[34] Anticonvulsants were the most common augmentation agent used, with their use significantly more common than the use of antipsychotics.[34] These findings suggest that patients undergo multiple trials of often ineffective treatments before TRD-specific interventions are used. In this report, we review the evidence regarding antidepressants and atypical antipsychotics with Food and Drug Administration (FDA)-approved indication for MDD and briefly discuss ketamine/esketamine and novel therapies that are in the pipeline.

EVIDENCE FOR ANTIDEPRESSANTS AFTER INITIAL NONRESPONSE TO ANOTHER ANTIDEPRESSANT
Citalopram

A recent open-label study randomized 104 patients with MDD who had not improved adequately with a 10-week course of imipramine (adjusted to plasma level) to either combination with citalopram versus augmentation with lithium.[35] This study found that the rate of remission (40.4% vs 21.1%) and the mean reduction in depression severity (58.8% vs 42.5%) were significantly greater with the combination of citalopram and imipramine as compared with augmentation of imipramine with lithium. Serious adverse events and dropouts caused by adverse events were similar between the two arms.[35] A prior small-scale study had demonstrated the augmentation with lithium among patients with MDD who did not respond to initial treatment with citalopram was associated with higher rates of treatment response as compared with augmentation with placebo.[36]

Fluoxetine

In a study of 101 patients with MDD who were either partial responders (n = 49) or nonresponders (n = 52) to 8 weeks of treatment with fluoxetine 20 mg/day, Fava and colleagues[37] randomized patients to 4 weeks of double-blind treatment with either high-dose fluoxetine (40–60 mg/d), fluoxetine plus lithium (300–600 mg/d), or fluoxetine plus desipramine (25–50 mg/d). They found no significant differences in response rates across the three treatment groups (high-dose fluoxetine, 42.4%; fluoxetine plus desipramine, 29.4%; fluoxetine plus lithium, 23.5%). There were also no significant differences in response rates across the three treatment groups among partial responders (high-dose fluoxetine, 50.0%; fluoxetine plus desipramine, 33.3%; fluoxetine plus lithium, 33.3%) and nonresponders (high-dose fluoxetine, 35.3%; fluoxetine plus desipramine, 26.3%; fluoxetine plus lithium, 12.5%).[37] These findings were similar to a previously smaller-scale study by Fava and colleagues[38] and argues for optimization of dose of initial antidepressant monotherapy before considering augmentation or combination approaches.

Bupropion

Bupropion has been widely studied as the next-step treatment option in individuals who did not respond adequately to initial SSRI treatment. In the STAR*D study, bupropion was a treatment option in switch (ie, individuals who elected to switch their treatment after initial citalopram treatment) and augmentation (ie, individuals who decided to continue their citalopram treatment and preferred for another medication to be added). In the switch arm, 727 patients with MDD were randomized for up to 14 weeks to either sustained-release (SR) bupropion (n = 239) at a maximal daily dose of 400 mg, sertraline (n = 238) at a maximal daily dose of 200 mg, or extended-release venlafaxine (n = 250) at a maximal daily dose of 375 mg.[39] Rates of remission and response on either clinician-rated or self-report measures were identical among the three treatment arms and did not demonstrate the superiority of switching to a nonserotonergic antidepressant (bupropion) after initial nonresponse to an SSRI.[39] In the augmentation arm of the second level of STAR*D, Trivedi and colleagues[40] randomized 565 patients with MDD without remission despite a mean of 11.9 weeks of citalopram therapy (mean final dose, 55 mg per day) to receive either bupropion SR (at a dose of up to 400 mg per day) or buspirone (at a dose of up to 60 mg per day) along with continuation of their initial antidepressant (citalopram). They found that rates of response (50% or greater reduction in symptom severity) and remission (presence of none-to-minimal symptoms) were similar between the two augmentation arms. However, augmentation with bupropion SR was associated with a greater reduction (from baseline to the second level of STAR*D) in self-reported depression severity than was buspirone (25.3% vs 17.1%), a lower self-reported depression severity score at the end of the second level of STAR*D, and a lower dropout rate caused by intolerance (12.5% vs 20.6%).[40] A recent study compared the augmentation with bupropion with a switch to bupropion in a study of adults with outpatients within the VA system and found that response and remission rates were similar for augmentation with bupropion versus switch to bupropion.[41]

In summary, these findings suggest that a trial of another antidepressant medication after optimizing (ie, attaining maximally tolerated dose) the initial antidepressant may be considered in the shared decision-making process of antidepressant treatments. However, remission rates in the second level of STAR*D were less than 30% and dropped lower than 20% in the third and fourth levels underscoring the need to consider other treatments, such as augmentation with atypical antipsychotics.

ATYPICAL ANTIPSYCHOTICS IN THE PHARMACOTHERAPY OF TREATMENT-RESISTANT DEPRESSION

Atypical antipsychotics were initially developed for schizophrenia but later found approval for multiple other indications including treatment of mania in bipolar disorder and irritability associated with autism. Four medications from this class are currently approved by the FDA as an augmentation treatment of MDD after inadequate response to an antidepressant: aripiprazole,[42] brexipiprazole,[43] cariprazine,[44] and quetiapine XR.[45] In contrast, the combination of olanzapine and fluoxetine (OFC) has been approved by the FDA specifically for the indication of TRD in patients with MDD.[46] OFC is also approved by FDA for the indication of bipolar depression.

Aripiprazole

Among atypical antipsychotics, aripiprazole was the first to receive regulatory approval from the FDA as an adjunctive treatment of MDD in 2007[42] and has the highest number of randomized controlled trials (RCTs) evaluating its efficacy. Initial RCTs enrolled individuals with historical nonresponse to greater than or equal to one but less than four antidepressants in a prospective treatment with antidepressants, and then randomized nonresponders (ie, those with <50% improvement) to double-blind augmentation for 6 weeks with either aripiprazole or placebo.[47–49] These studies demonstrated significantly greater improvement in depression severity with aripiprazole[47–49] with remission rates of 25.4%[47] and 26.0%[48] with aripiprazole versus 15.2%[47] and 15.7%[48] with placebo. The number needed to treat (NNT) for aripiprazole in these studies was 10 (ie, 10 additional individuals need to be treated with aripiprazole [vs placebo] to attain 1 additional remission). Subsequent similarly designed RCTs found similar NNTs for aripiprazole versus placebo (NNT range, 9–11).[50,51] In an influential study that was funded primarily by the National Institute of Mental Health, elderly individuals (aged 60 years or older) who did not attain remission with 12-week-long treatment with venlafaxine XR were randomized to receive either augmentation with aripiprazole or placebo for 12 weeks. In their study, Lenze and colleagues[52] found that augmentation with aripiprazole was associated with markedly higher rates of remission (44%) as compared with placebo (29%), thereby resulting in an NNT of seven. The use of aripiprazole was associated with more akathisia (27% of patients) and parkinsonism. However, aripiprazole did not differ from placebo in treatment-emergent suicidal ideation; prolongation of corrected QT interval; or increases in adiposity, glucose, insulin, or lipids. However, not all studies of aripiprazole augmentation have been positive. A small sample-sized study that used sequential parallel comparison design and treated individuals over two stages of 1-month each found an NNT of 44 for remission with aripiprazole versus placebo suggesting modest clinical benefit.[53]

The landmark STAR*D was conducted before the approval of atypical antipsychotics as augmentation agent for MDD, and therefore is limited in comparison of how augmentation of atypical antipsychotics may compare with augmentation or switch of antidepressants. Therefore, a consortium of investigators in the VA led a large multicenter trial entitled, VA Augmentation and Switching Treatments for Improving Depression Outcomes (VAST-D) of 1522 patients with nonpsychotic MDD who had historical nonresponse to first-line antidepressants in their current depressive episode. This study had three treatment arms: augmentation with aripiprazole, augmentation with bupropion SR, or switch to bupropion SR.[41] The investigators found that rates of remission with 12-week-long augmentation with aripiprazole (1–5 mg/kg; 28.9%) were higher than switch to bupropion SR (300–400 mg/d; 22.3%) but did not differ from augmentation with bupropion SR (300–400 mg/d; 26.9%). They found that augmentation arms of aripiprazole and bupropion SR were similar on most outcomes except for higher rates of response (74.3%) with aripiprazole augmentation as compared with bupropion augmentation (65.6%) with an NN of 12 favoring aripiprazole augmentation.[41] In summary, evidence from the industry-sponsored trials and the VA-based study of aripiprazole suggests that it is effective as an augmentation agent, although generalizability to patients with greater levels of medication resistance may be limited given that about two-thirds of individuals in prior RCTs of aripiprazole had only one prior historical nonresponse.[47,48,50,51]

Brexpiprazole

Brexpiprazole acts as a partial agonist of the dopamine D_2-receptor and serotonin 1A receptor (5-HT1A), and antagonist of the 5-HT2A receptor and seems to be pharmacologically similar to aripiprazole. It received regulatory approval by the FDA as an adjunctive treatment of MDD in 2015.[43,54] Initial RCTs enrolled patients with MDD with one to three prior antidepressant nonresponse and randomized those who did not respond to 8 weeks of open-label antidepressant to receive either brexpiprazole or placebo for 6 weeks.[55,56] These studies found significantly greater reductions in depressive symptoms with brexpiprazole 2 mg/d[55] and 3 mg/d[56] but not with 1 mg/d[56] augmentation after inadequate response to prospective antidepressant treatment. However, remission rates with brexpiprazole at all studied doses did not differ from placebo[55,56] and had very large NNT that ranged from 17 to 31. Follow-up acute-phase studies of brexpiprazole had similar results where reduction in overall depression symptom severity as a continuous measure was greater with adjunctive brexpiprazole (2 mg or 2–3 mg) versus placebo but the categorical outcome of remission did not differ between brexipiprazole versus placebo with NNT that ranged from 28 to 42.[57,58] Findings from a longer-term study of brexipiprazole were negative because there was no significant difference between brexipiprazole versus placebo in rates of remission (21.4% vs 24.9%) over a 24-week period. However, use of brexipiprazole was associated with higher rates of adverse event-related withdrawal (6.3%) as compared with placebo (3.4%).[59] Overall, these studies suggest that although there was statistically significant reduction in depressive symptoms with brexpiprazole, the clinical significance may be limited as indicated by high NNTs. Furthermore, the generalizability of these findings to individuals with TRD (ie, those who have two or more nonresponses in the current depressive episode) may be limited because more than 80% of individuals enrolled in these brexpiprazole studies had historical nonresponse to just one antidepressant before their enrollment in the trials.[55–59]

Cariprazine

Similar to aripiprazole and brexpiprazole, cariprazine is a partial D_2 receptor agonist. Partial agonists serve as antagonists when full agonists are present, whereas in the absence of full agonist, these medications have a functional agonist activity (albeit at lower levels).[60] Cariprazine is also a partial agonist of D_3 receptors and may have 10 times more preferential binding to D_3 over D_2, especially at lower doses.[61] Cariprazine has two major active metabolites, desmethyl-cariprazine and didesmethyl-cariprazine, which have long half-lives; thereby, resulting in the attainment of the steady state of 2 to 4 weeks.[62,63] It received regulatory approval from the FDA for augmentation of MDD in 2022.[44] An initial phase 2 study of cariprazine augmentation at low doses (0.1–0.3 mg/d or 1–2 mg/d) found no significant difference as compared with placebo.[64] Therefore, a subsequent study used higher doses and enrolled patients with MDD with inadequate historical response to one or two antidepressants, and randomized them to either placebo, cariprazine 1 to 2 mg/d, or cariprazine 2 to 4.5 mg/d.[65] The titration protocols differed between the two cariprazine dose with target dose of 1 mg/d achieved by Week 1 in the 1 to 2 mg/d group and dose of 2 mg/d achieved by Week 1 in the 2 to 4.5 mg group.[65] In this study, overall depression severity decreased significantly as compared with placebo with both doses (1–2 mg and 2–4.5 mg) by Week 2 but was maintained until Week 8 only in the 2- to 4.5-mg arm.[65] Similar to the findings of brexpiprazole studies where the categorical outcome of remission did not differ from placebo, rates of remission with both dose strengths of cariprazine were similar to placebo.[65] Augmentation with cariprazine did not significantly improve overall depressive symptoms as compared with placebo in a subsequent study of patients with MDD who received an 8-week-long prospective treatment with open-label antidepressant and those who did not respond adequately were then randomized to an 8-week-long augmentation with cariprazine (1.5–4.5 mg/d) or placebo.[66] According to the sponsor, a recent phase 3 trial of cariprazine demonstrated significantly greater improvement in overall depressive symptoms from baseline to Week 6 with cariprazine augmentation as compared with placebo.[44] According to sponsor, dosage titration at intervals of less than 14 days was associated with a higher incidence of adverse events with cariprazine.[44] Overall, these studies suggest that cariprazine may be effective in reducing depression severity but optimal dose may be unclear and clinical significance of these improvements may be uncertain.

Quetiapine XR

The precise pharmacologic effects of quetiapine remains unclear. However, it is known to target several neurotransmitter systems and demonstrates a high affinity for histamine 1, α_1-adrenergic, and 5-HT2A receptors and a low affinity for the dopamine D_2 receptor.[67,68] An active metabolite of quetiapine, N-desalkylquetiapine, is a potent inhibitor of norepinephrine reuptake and acts as a partial agonist of the 5-HT1A receptor.[69] Quetiapine XR received regulatory approval from the FDA as an adjunctive treatment of MDD in 2009.[45] The development program for quetiapine XR included monotherapy and augmentation studies but the approval by FDA was limited to its augmentation indication. As augmentation agents, two phase III trials evaluated its efficacy in patients with MDD who did not respond to one or more prior antidepressants.[70,71] Once-daily augmentation with quetiapine XR at 300 mg/d dose was associated with a significantly greater reduction of depression as compared with placebo in both studies.[71] However, the 150 mg/d dose was more effective in reducing depression severity as compared with the placebo in one[71] but not the other study.[70] When data from both the RCTs were pooled, remission rates were significantly higher with 150 mg/d (41.8%) and 300 mg/d (46.3%) of quetiapine XR as compared with placebo (32%) with an NNT of 11 and 7 for 150 mg/d and 300 mg/d doses, respectively.[72] In these studies, rates of withdrawal caused by adverse effects were significantly higher with both doses of quetiapine XR, 8.9% and 15.4% with 150 mg/d and 300 mg/d doses, respectively, as compared with 1.9% with placebo.[72] Overall, these findings suggest that quetiapine XR at the dose of 300 mg/d may result in clinically significant improvement in depressive symptoms. However, adverse-event-related withdrawal may occur in one in six patients suggesting poor tolerability profile.

Olanzapine Fluoxetine Combination

This combination received its regulatory approval from the FDA specifically for TRD in 2009.[46] Initial evidence for the efficacy of OFC was suggested by a pilot study of 28 patients with MDD where the use of OFC was associated with a greater reduction in symptom severity as compared with monotherapy with either olanzapine or fluoxetine.[73] Thereafter, larger RCTs were conducted to compare OFC with monotherapy with olanzapine and monotherapy with several antidepressants including fluoxetine, venlafaxine, and nortriptyline. Two of these RCTs were designed similarly and enrolled patients with TRD and found that in one study use of OFC was associated with significantly larger reductions in depression severity as compared with monotherapy with olanzapine or monotherapy with fluoxetine monotherapy, whereas the other study did not find any significant difference.[74] A separate study included monotherapy with venlafaxine as a fourth arm and found that OFC was superior only to monotherapy with olanzapine and not to monotherapy with either fluoxetine or venlafaxine.[75] Data from studies were combined to evaluate how acute-phase outcomes differ between OFC and monotherapy with either olanzapine or fluoxetine. This review found that remission rates with OFC (25.5%) were significantly higher as compared with the remission rate with olanzapine monotherapy (14.0%) or with fluoxetine monotherapy (17.3%).[76] Additionally, the time taken for attainment of remission was significantly shorted with OFC as compared with monotherapy with olanzapine or monotherapy with fluoxetine.[76] In longer-term studies where patients who were stabilized on OFC and were then switched to fluoxetine monotherapy, rates of relapse of depressive symptoms were significantly higher (31.8%) as compared with maintenance-phase continuation of OFC (15.8%). Furthermore, time to relapse was also shorter after switch to monotherapy with fluoxetine as compared with continuation of OFC.[77]

SIDE EFFECTS WITH ATYPICAL ANTIPSYCHOTICS IN PATIENTS WITH MAJOR DEPRESSIVE DISORDER

Use of atypical antipsychotics is associated with weight gain. Weight gain potential of quetiapine XR and OFC is considered to be higher than the weight gain liability of aripiprazole and brexipiprazole.[45,46] On average, the use of OFC was associated with a weight gain of 4.0 kg as compared with a weight loss of 0.3 kg with the placebo in acute-phase studies.[45,46] Clinically significant weight gain, operationalized greater than or equal to 7% weight gain, was observed in 22% of patients in acute-phase studies. With longer-term treatment, this clinically significant weight gain was present in 66% of patients with TRD who continued on OFC.[46] Clinically significant weight gain occurred in 3%, 7%, and 2% of patients with MDD who were treated with quetiapine XR 150 mg/d, quetiapine XR 300 mg/d or placebo, respectively, in acute-phase studies.[45] Studies that have used quetiapine XR for longer-term treatment have reported continued weight gain during the continuation phase.[78] Use of aripiprazole in clinical trials of individuals with MDD have found significantly greater weight gain with aripiprazole (+1.7 kg) versus placebo (+0.4 kg).[42,43] In acute-phase studies, clinically significant weight gain with aripiprazole was observed in 5.2% as compared with its presence in 0.6% for those treated with a placebo.[42] Similarly, the use of brexipiprazole has been associated with greater weight gain at all doses including 1 mg/d (1.3 kg), 2 mg/d (1.6 kg), and 3 mg/d (1.6 kg) as compared with placebo (0.3).[43] Clinically significant weight gain was noted in 30% of those treated with brexipiprazole in long-term open label studies of individuals with MDD.[43] According to the sponsor, use of cariprazine was associated with an average weight gain of less than 2 pounds and less than or equal to 3% of patients had a clinically significant weight increase.[44] Although abnormalities in metabolic function are not detailed, the patterns of changes are usually consistent with weight gain. Therefore, use of these medications should be accompanied by anthropometric measurements (including waist and hip circumference that allow for estimation of waist-to-hip ratio to ascertain visceral vs subcutaneous adiposity), physical examination, and laboratory testing for hyperglycemia and hyperlipidemia to detect changes in these parameters promptly.

According to prescribing labels, akathisia is common with the augmentation of aripiprazole with estimate rate of 25% as compared with 4% with placebo.[42] These rates of akathisia are similar to the high rates reported in the VAST-D study where 14.9% of those in the aripiprazole augmentation arm had akathisia as compared with the 5.3%

and 4.3% in bupropion SR augmentation and switch arms, respectively.[41] Akathisia rates are higher with higher doses of brexpiprazole; rates observed with 1 mg/d, 2 mg/d, and 3 mg/d doses were 4%, 7%, and 14%, respectively, as compared with the rate of 2% with placebo.[43] Akathisia was also reported in more than 5% of patients treated with cariprazine and this rate was at least two-fold higher than placebo, according to the sponsor.[44] Although atypical antipsychotics tend to have a lower annual prevalence of tardive dyskinesia, the annualized incidence of tardive dyskinesia with these medications ranges from 1.7% to 2.9%[79] and may warrant longer-term observation. It is noteworthy that atypical antipsychotics have typically been studied in acute-phase studies but their use may end up being long-term in real-world settings. This may be driving the phenomena where one in two patients with new-onset tardive dyskinesia were diagnosed with a mood disorder and most were prescribed atypical antipsychotics according to a recent analysis of insurance claims database.[80] Clinicians need to be vigilant about the incidence of tardive dyskinesia associated with the use of atypical antipsychotics for patients with MDD.

SUMMARY

Despite the limited efficacy of antidepressant medications, they are commonly used as pharmacotherapy agents for patients with TRD. After an inadequate response to a first-line antidepressant, there does not seem to be any significant difference between classes of antidepressants when switching is preferred. The recent VAST-D study suggests that augmenting with bupropion SR may be similar to switching to bupropion SR. This study demonstrated that augmentation with aripiprazole may be superior to switching to bupropion SR. With the FDA approval of several atypical antipsychotics for MDD, their use may be considered after inadequate response to one or two antidepressant treatments of adequate dose and duration. However, their benefits have to be weighed against the potential for harm, specifically weight gain, akathisia, and tardive dyskinesia. Future studies are needed for a head-to-head comparison of these atypical antipsychotics among each other and with other TRD-specific interventions, such as intranasal esketamine or repetitive transcranial magnetic stimulation.

CLINICS CARE POINTS

- Using measurement-based care approach of measuring symptom severity, side-effects, and adherence can help optimize outcomes of first-line treatments.
- Augmentation strategies with antipsychotics may be considered earlier in course of treatment as their efficacy in highly treatment-resistant depression is limited.
- Use of atypical antipsychotics beyond the acute-phase has to be weighed against their potential harm, especially in terms of weight gain, metabolic dysfunction, and tardive dyskinesia.

ACKNOWLEDGMENTS

Dr M.K. Jha is supported by a career development award from National Institute of Mental Health (MH126202), the O'Donnell Clinical Neuroscience Scholar Award from UT Southwestern Medical Center, and the resources from the Center for Depression Research and Clinical Care (CDRC) at UT Southwestern Medical Center. Dr S.J. Mathew is supported through the use of resources and facilities at the Michael E.

Debakey VA Medical Center, Houston, Texas and receives support from The Menninger Clinic.

DISCLOSURE

Dr C. Vas, A. Jain, and M. Trivedi have no conflicts to disclose. Dr M.K. Jha has received contract research grants from Acadia Pharmaceuticals, Neurocrine Bioscience, Navitor/Supernus and Janssen Research & Development; educational grant to serve as Section Editor of the Psychiatry & Behavioral Health Learning Network; consultant fees from Eleusis Therapeutics US, Inc, Janssen Global Services, Janssen Scientific Affairs, Worldwide Clinical Trials/Eliem and Inversargo, Boehringer Ingelheim, and Guidepoint Global; and honoraria from North American Center for Continuing Medical Education, Medscape/WebMD, Clinical Care Options, and Global Medical Education. Dr S.J. Mathew has served as a consultant to Allergan, Alkermes, Almatica Pharma, Axsome Therapeutics, Biohaven, BioXcel Therapeutics, Clexio Biosciences, COMPASS Pathways, Delix Therapeutics, Eleusis, EMA Wellness, Engrail Therapeutics, Greenwich Biosciences, Intra-Cellular Therapies, Janssen, Levo Therapeutics, Perception Neurosciences, Praxis Precision Medicines, Neumora, Neurocrine, Relmada Therapeutics, Sage Therapeutics, Seelos Therapeutics, Signant Health, and Sunovion; and received research support from Biohaven Pharmaceuticals, Boehringer Ingelheim, Janssen, Merck, Neurocrine, Sage Therapeutics, and Vistagen Therapeutics.

REFERENCES

1. Jha MK, Greer TL, Grannemann BD, et al. Early normalization of quality of life predicts later remission in depression: findings from the CO-MED trial. J Affect Disord 2016;206:17–22.

2. Jha MK, Teer RB, Minhajuddin A, et al. Daily activity level improvement with antidepressant medications predicts long-term clinical outcomes in outpatients with major depressive disorder. Neuropsychiatr Dis Treat 2017;13:803–13.

3. Jha MK, Minhajuddin A, Greer TL, et al. Early improvement in psychosocial function predicts longer-term symptomatic remission in depressed patients. PLoS One 2016;11:e0167901.

4. Jha MK, Minhajuddin A, Greer TL, et al. Early improvement in work productivity predicts future clinical course in depressed outpatients: findings from the CO-MED Trial. Am J Psychiatry 2016;173:1196–204.

5. Greer TL, Trombello JM, Rethorst CD, et al. Improvements in psychosocial functioning and health-related quality of life following exercise augmentation in patients with treatment response but nonremitted major depressive disorder: results from the tread study. Depress Anxiety 2016;33:870–81.

6. Hasin DS, Sarvet AL, Meyers JL, et al. Epidemiology of adult DSM-5 major depressive disorder and its specifiers in the United States. JAMA Psychiatr 2018;75:336–46.

7. Jha MK, Qamar A, Vaduganathan M, et al. Screening and management of depression in patients with cardiovascular disease: JACC State-of-the-Art Review. J Am Coll Cardiol 2019;73:1827–45.

8. Jha MK, Grannemann BD, Trombello JM, et al. A structured approach to detecting and treating depression in primary care: VitalSign6 Project. Ann Fam Med 2019;17:326–35.

9. Rush AJ, Trivedi MH, Wisniewski SR, et al. Acute and longer-term outcomes in depressed outpatients requiring one or several treatment steps: a STAR*D report. Am J Psychiatry 2006;163:1905–17.

10. Lundberg J, Cars T, Lööv S, et al. Association of treatment-resistant depression with patient outcomes and health care resource utilization in a population-wide study. JAMA Psychiatr 2022;80(2):167–75.

11. Pilon D, Joshi K, Sheehan JJ, et al. Burden of treatment-resistant depression in Medicare: a retrospective claims database analysis. PLoS One 2019;14: e0223255.

12. Zhdanava M, Pilon D, Ghelerter I, et al. The prevalence and national burden of treatment-resistant depression and major depressive disorder in the United States. J Clin Psychiatry 2021;82.

13. Gaynes BN, Lux L, Gartlehner G, et al. Defining treatment-resistant depression. Depress Anxiety 2020;37:134–45.

14. Daly EJ, Trivedi MH, Janik A, et al. Efficacy of esketamine nasal spray plus oral antidepressant treatment for relapse prevention in patients with treatment-resistant depression: a randomized clinical trial. JAMA Psychiatr 2019;76: 893–903.

15. Fava M, Freeman MP, Flynn M, et al. Double-blind, placebo-controlled, dose-ranging trial of intravenous ketamine as adjunctive therapy in treatment-resistant depression (TRD). Mol Psychiatry 2020;25:1592–603.

16. Jha MK, Minhajuddin A, Chin Fatt C, et al. Association between irritability and suicidal ideation in three clinical trials of adults with major depressive disorder. Neuropsychopharmacology 2020;45:2147–54.

17. Jha MK, Minhajuddin A, South C, et al. Irritability and its clinical utility in major depressive disorder: prediction of individual-level acute-phase outcomes using early changes in irritability and depression severity. Am J Psychiatry 2019;176: 358–66.

18. Fava M, Alpert JE, Carmin CN, et al. Clinical correlates and symptom patterns of anxious depression among patients with major depressive disorder in STAR*D. Psychol Med 2004;34:1299–308.

19. Jha MK, Mathew SJ. Pharmacotherapies for treatment-resistant depression: how antipsychotics fit in the rapidly evolving therapeutic landscape. Am J Psychiatry 2023;180. In press.

20. Rush AJ, Aaronson ST, Demyttenaere K. Difficult-to-treat depression: a clinical and research roadmap for when remission is elusive. Aust N Z J Psychiatry 2019;53:109–18.

21. Rush AJ, Sackeim HA, Conway CR, et al. Clinical research challenges posed by difficult-to-treat depression. Psychol Med 2022;52:419–32.

22. Jha MK, Trivedi MH. Experimental therapies for treatment-resistant depression: "how do you decide when to go to an unproven or experimental therapy with patients that are treatment-resistant depression? Focus 2018;16:279–84.

23. Trivedi MH, Rush AJ, Wisniewski SR, et al. Evaluation of outcomes with citalopram for depression using measurement-based care in STAR*D: implications for clinical practice. Am J Psychiatry 2006;163:28–40.

24. Desseilles M, Witte J, Chang TE, et al. Assessing the adequacy of past antidepressant trials: a clinician's guide to the antidepressant treatment response questionnaire. J Clin Psychiatry 2011;72:1152–4.

25. Jha MK, Malchow AL, Grannemann BD, et al. Do baseline sub-threshold hypomanic symptoms affect acute-phase antidepressant outcome in outpatients

with major depressive disorder? Preliminary findings from the randomized CO-MED trial. Neuropsychopharmacology 2018;43:2197–203.

26. Jha MK, Minhajuddin A, Gadad BS, et al. Can C-reactive protein inform antidepressant medication selection in depressed outpatients? Findings from the CO-MED trial. Psychoneuroendocrinology 2017;78:105–13.

27. Jha MK, Wakhlu S, Dronamraju N, et al. Validating pre-treatment body mass index as moderator of antidepressant treatment outcomes: findings from CO-MED trial. J Affect Disord 2018;234:34–7.

28. Jha MK, Schatzberg A, Minhajuddin A, et al. Cross-sectional associations among symptoms of pain, irritability, and depression and how these symptoms relate to social functioning and quality of life: findings from the EMBARC and STRIDE studies and the VitalSign6 Project. J Clin Psychiatry 2021;82.

29. Kubitz N, Mehra M, Potluri RC, et al. Characterization of treatment resistant depression episodes in a cohort of patients from a US commercial claims database. PLoS One 2013;8:e76882.

30. Roughan WH, Campos AI, García-Marín LM, et al. Comorbid chronic pain and depression: shared risk factors and differential antidepressant effectiveness. Front Psychiatry 2021;12:643609.

31. Scott F, Hampsey E, Gnanapragasam S, et al. Systematic review and meta-analysis of augmentation and combination treatments for early-stage treatment-resistant depression. J Psychopharmacol 2022. 2698811221104058.

32. Conroy SK, Holtzheimer PE. Neuromodulation strategies for the treatment of depression. Am J Psychiatry 2021;178:1082–8.

33. Jain R, Higa S, Keyloun K, et al. Treatment patterns during major depressive episodes among patients with major depressive disorder: a retrospective database analysis. Drugs Real World Outcomes 2022;9:477–86.

34. Zhao X, Karkare S, Nash AI, et al. Characteristics and current standard of care among veterans with major depressive disorder in the United States: a real-world data analysis. J Affect Disord 2022;307:184–90.

35. Navarro V, Boulahfa I, Obach A, et al. Lithium augmentation versus citalopram combination in imipramine-resistant major depression: a 10-week randomized open-label study. J Clin Psychopharmacol 2019;39:254–7.

36. Baumann P, Nil R, Souche A, et al. A double-blind, placebo-controlled study of citalopram with and without lithium in the treatment of therapy-resistant depressive patients: a clinical, pharmacokinetic, and pharmacogenetic investigation. J Clin Psychopharmacol 1996;16:307–14.

37. Fava M, Alpert J, Nierenberg A, et al. Double-blind study of high-dose fluoxetine versus lithium or desipramine augmentation of fluoxetine in partial responders and nonresponders to fluoxetine. J Clin Psychopharmacol 2002;22:379–87.

38. Fava M, Rosenbaum JF, McGrath PJ, et al. Lithium and tricyclic augmentation of fluoxetine treatment for resistant major depression: a double-blind, controlled study. Am J Psychiatry 1994;151:1372–4.

39. Rush AJ, Trivedi MH, Wisniewski SR, et al. Bupropion-SR, sertraline, or venlafaxine-XR after failure of SSRIs for depression. N Engl J Med 2006;354:1231–42.

40. Trivedi MH, Fava M, Wisniewski SR, et al. Medication augmentation after the failure of SSRIs for depression. N Engl J Med 2006;354:1243–52.

41. Mohamed S, Johnson GR, Chen P, et al. Effect of antidepressant switching vs augmentation on remission among patients with major depressive disorder unresponsive to antidepressant treatment: the VAST-D randomized clinical trial. JAMA 2017;318:132–45.

42. FDA. Aripirazole. Prescribing Label 2022. Available at: https://dailymed.nlm.nih.gov/dailymed/getFile.cfm?setid=c040bd1d-45b7-49f2-93ea-aed7220b30ac&type=pdf. Accessed on 19 December 2022.

43. FDA. Brexpiprazole. Prescribing Label 2022. Available at: https://dailymed.nlm.nih.gov/dailymed/getFile.cfm?setid=2d301358-6291-4ec1-bd87-37b4ad9bd850&type=pdf. 2021. Accessed on 19 December 2022.

44. AbbVie. U.S. FDA. Approves VRAYLAR® (cariprazine) as an adjunctive treatment for major depressive disorder. 2022. Available at: https://news.abbvie.com/article_display.cfm?article_id=12543. 2022. Accessed on 19 December 2022.

45. FDA. Quetiapine Extended-Release Prescribing Label. 2022. Available at: https://dailymed.nlm.nih.gov/dailymed/getFile.cfm?setid=473a3ac4-67f4-4782-baa9-7f9bdd8761f4&type=pdf. 2022. Accessed on 19 December 2022.

46. FDA. Olanzapine Fluoxetine Combination Prescribing Label. 2022. Available at: https://dailymed.nlm.nih.gov/dailymed/getFile.cfm?setid=6b28c424-0b7e-4b75-b090-f116b113554e&type=pdf. 2021. Accessed on 19 December 2022.

47. Marcus RN, McQuade RD, Carson WH, et al. The efficacy and safety of aripiprazole as adjunctive therapy in major depressive disorder: a second multicenter, randomized, double-blind, placebo-controlled study. J Clin Psychopharmacol 2008;28:156–65.

48. Berman RM, Marcus RN, Swanink R, et al. The efficacy and safety of aripiprazole as adjunctive therapy in major depressive disorder: a multicenter, randomized, double-blind, placebo-controlled study. J Clin Psychiatry 2007;68:843–53.

49. Berman RM, Fava M, Thase ME, et al. Aripiprazole augmentation in major depressive disorder: a double-blind, placebo-controlled study in patients with inadequate response to antidepressants. CNS Spectr 2009;14:197–206.

50. Kamijima K, Higuchi T, Ishigooka J, et al. Aripiprazole augmentation to antidepressant therapy in Japanese patients with major depressive disorder: a randomized, double-blind, placebo-controlled study (ADMIRE study). J Affect Disord 2013;151:899–905.

51. Kamijima K, Kimura M, Kuwahara K, et al. Randomized, double-blind comparison of aripiprazole/sertraline combination and placebo/sertraline combination in patients with major depressive disorder. Psychiatry Clin Neurosci 2018;72:591–601.

52. Lenze EJ, Mulsant BH, Blumberger DM, et al. Efficacy, safety, and tolerability of augmentation pharmacotherapy with aripiprazole for treatment-resistant depression in late life: a randomised, double-blind, placebo-controlled trial. Lancet 2015;386:2404–12.

53. Fava M, Mischoulon D, Iosifescu D, et al. A double-blind, placebo-controlled study of aripiprazole adjunctive to antidepressant therapy among depressed outpatients with inadequate response to prior antidepressant therapy (ADAPT-A Study). Psychother Psychosom 2012;81:87–97.

54. Maeda K, Sugino H, Akazawa H, et al. Brexpiprazole I: in vitro and in vivo characterization of a novel serotonin-dopamine activity modulator. J Pharmacol Exp Ther 2014;350:589–604.

55. Thase ME, Youakim JM, Skuban A, et al. Efficacy and safety of adjunctive brexpiprazole 2 mg in major depressive disorder: a phase 3, randomized, placebo-controlled study in patients with inadequate response to antidepressants. J Clin Psychiatry 2015;76:1224–31.

56. Thase ME, Youakim JM, Skuban A, et al. Adjunctive brexpiprazole 1 and 3 mg for patients with major depressive disorder following inadequate response to antidepressants: a phase 3, randomized, double-blind study. J Clin Psychiatry 2015;76:1232–40.

57. Hobart M, Skuban A, Zhang P, et al. Efficacy and safety of flexibly dosed brexpiprazole for the adjunctive treatment of major depressive disorder: a randomized, active-referenced, placebo-controlled study. Curr Med Res Opin 2018;34: 633–42.

58. Hobart M, Skuban A, Zhang P, et al. A randomized, placebo-controlled study of the efficacy and safety of fixed-dose brexpiprazole 2 mg/d as adjunctive treatment of adults with major depressive disorder. J Clin Psychiatry 2018;79.

59. Bauer M, Hefting N, Lindsten A, et al. A randomised, placebo-controlled 24-week study evaluating adjunctive brexpiprazole in patients with major depressive disorder. Acta Neuropsychiatr 2019;31:27–35.

60. Lieberman JA. Dopamine partial agonists: a new class of antipsychotic. CNS Drugs 2004;18:251–67.

61. Girgis RR, Slifstein M, D'Souza D, et al. Preferential binding to dopamine D3 over D2 receptors by cariprazine in patients with schizophrenia using PET with the D3/D2 receptor ligand [(11)C]-(+)-PHNO. Psychopharmacology (Berl) 2016;233: 3503–12.

62. Nakamura T, Kubota T, Iwakaji A, et al. Clinical pharmacology study of cariprazine (MP-214) in patients with schizophrenia (12-week treatment). Drug Des Devel Ther 2016;10:327–38.

63. Periclou A, Phillips L, Ghahramani P, et al. Population pharmacokinetics of cariprazine and its major metabolites. Eur J Drug Metab Pharmacokinet 2021;46: 53–69.

64. Fava M, Durgam S, Earley W, et al. Efficacy of adjunctive low-dose cariprazine in major depressive disorder: a randomized, double-blind, placebo-controlled trial. Int Clin Psychopharmacol 2018;33:312–21.

65. Durgam S, Earley W, Guo H, et al. Efficacy and safety of adjunctive cariprazine in inadequate responders to antidepressants: a randomized, double-blind, placebo-controlled study in adult patients with major depressive disorder. J Clin Psychiatry 2016;77:371–8.

66. Earley WR, Guo H, Németh G, et al. Cariprazine augmentation to antidepressant therapy in major depressive disorder: results of a randomized, double-blind, placebo-controlled trial. Psychopharmacol Bull 2018;48:62–80.

67. Roth BL, Sheffler DJ, Kroeze WK. Magic shotguns versus magic bullets: selectively non-selective drugs for mood disorders and schizophrenia. Nat Rev Drug Discov 2004;3:353–9.

68. Nemeroff CB, Kinkead B, Goldstein J. Quetiapine: preclinical studies, pharmacokinetics, drug interactions, and dosing. J Clin Psychiatry 2002;63(Suppl 13):5–11.

69. Jensen NH, Rodriguiz RM, Caron MG, et al. N-desalkylquetiapine, a potent norepinephrine reuptake inhibitor and partial 5-HT1A agonist, as a putative mediator of quetiapine's antidepressant activity. Neuropsychopharmacology 2008;33: 2303–12.

70. El-Khalili N, Joyce M, Atkinson S, et al. Extended-release quetiapine fumarate (quetiapine XR) as adjunctive therapy in major depressive disorder (MDD) in patients with an inadequate response to ongoing antidepressant treatment: a multicentre, randomized, double-blind, placebo-controlled study. Int J Neuropsychopharmacol 2010;13:917–32.

71. Bauer M, Pretorius HW, Constant EL, et al. Extended-release quetiapine as adjunct to an antidepressant in patients with major depressive disorder: results of a randomized, placebo-controlled, double-blind study. J Clin Psychiatry 2009;70:540–9.

72. Bauer M, El-Khalili N, Datto C, et al. A pooled analysis of two randomised, placebo-controlled studies of extended release quetiapine fumarate adjunctive to antidepressant therapy in patients with major depressive disorder. J Affect Disord 2010;127:19–30.

73. Shelton RC, Tollefson GD, Tohen M, et al. A novel augmentation strategy for treating resistant major depression. Am J Psychiatry 2001;158:131–4.

74. Thase ME, Corya SA, Osuntokun O, et al. A randomized, double-blind comparison of olanzapine/fluoxetine combination, olanzapine, and fluoxetine in treatment-resistant major depressive disorder. J Clin Psychiatry 2007;68:224–36.

75. Corya SA, Williamson D, Sanger TM, et al. A randomized, double-blind comparison of olanzapine/fluoxetine combination, olanzapine, fluoxetine, and venlafaxine in treatment-resistant depression. Depress Anxiety 2006;23:364–72.

76. Trivedi MH, Thase ME, Osuntokun O, et al. An integrated analysis of olanzapine/fluoxetine combination in clinical trials of treatment-resistant depression. J Clin Psychiatry 2009;70:387–96.

77. Brunner E, Tohen M, Osuntokun O, et al. Efficacy and safety of olanzapine/fluoxetine combination vs fluoxetine monotherapy following successful combination therapy of treatment-resistant major depressive disorder. Neuropsychopharmacology 2014;39:2549–59.

78. Liebowitz M, Lam RW, Lepola U, et al. Efficacy and tolerability of extended release quetiapine fumarate monotherapy as maintenance treatment of major depressive disorder: a randomized, placebo-controlled trial. Depress Anxiety 2010;27:964–76.

79. Carbon M, Kane JM, Leucht S, et al. Tardive dyskinesia risk with first- and second-generation antipsychotics in comparative randomized controlled trials: a meta-analysis. World Psychiatr 2018;17:330–40.

80. Loughlin AM, Lin N, Abler V, et al. Tardive dyskinesia among patients using antipsychotic medications in customary clinical care in the United States. PLoS One 2019;14:e0216044.

Pharmacotherapy
Ketamine and Esketamine

Anna Feeney, MD[a,b],*, George I. Papakostas, MD[a,b]

KEYWORDS

- Major depressive disorder • Treatment-resistant depression • Antidepressants
- Ketamine

KEY POINTS

- Ketamine and esketamine have rapid-onset antidepressant effects.
- They represent a novel adjunctive treatment option in treatment-resistant depression.
- Only IN esketamine currently has regulatory approval in the United States and European Union.
- The long-term safety and efficacy of ketamine/esketamine as antidepressants require further study.

INTRODUCTION/BACKGROUND

Antidepressant drug development in the twentieth and early twenty-first centuries focused on the modulation of monoaminergic neurotransmission.[1] Although many patients have greatly benefited from these treatments, their onset of action is typically delayed by weeks.[2,3] In addition, about 30% to 40% of depressed patients will remain depressed even with adequate antidepressant treatment trials.[4] These limitations of our current pharmacotherapies have prompted a new era of antidepressant research, a search for drugs with novel mechanisms of action and greater speed of onset. Ketamine, which has long been used in anesthesia, has emerged as a rapidly acting antidepressant with a target distinct from the monoaminergic system: an N-methyl-D-aspartate (NMDA) receptor antagonist. The antidepressant effects of intravenous (IV) ketamine and intranasal (IN) esketamine (the s-enantiomer of racemic ketamine) in major depressive disorder (MDD), including treatment-resistant depression (TRD), are now well-documented,[5–14] but the comparative efficacy of different formulations of ketamine remains unclear.[15]

IV ketamine, though not currently approved as an antidepressant by the Food and Drug Administration (FDA) in the United States (US), is increasingly being prescribed

[a] Department of Psychiatry, Clinical Trials Network and Institute, Massachusetts General Hospital, One Bowdoin Square, 9th Floor, Boston, MA 02114, USA; [b] Harvard Medical School, Boston, MA, USA
* Corresponding author.
E-mail address: feeneyac@tcd.ie

Psychiatr Clin N Am 46 (2023) 277–290
https://doi.org/10.1016/j.psc.2023.02.003
0193-953X/23/© 2023 Elsevier Inc. All rights reserved.

off-label by clinicians, often as an adjunctive therapy to patients with TRD and other psychiatric conditions.[16–19] IN esketamine is FDA-approved (when used with a standard oral antidepressant) for the treatment of adults with TRD and for depressive symptoms in adults with MDD and acute suicidal thoughts or actions.[20–24] It is also approved by the European Medicines Agency (EMA), when combined with an antidepressant, for TRD and for moderate to severe depressive episodes requiring acute emergency treatment.[25]

IV ketamine's potential as an antidepressant for MDD was initially established in two landmark studies. The first of these showed the benefit of a single infusion of IV ketamine (0.5 mg/kg) over IV saline placebo in a double-blinded, randomized trial[26]; this was followed by replication of these findings in a later randomized, placebo-controlled, double-blind crossover study of subjects with TRD.[27] Given the potential for unblinding in studies comparing IV ketamine with a saline placebo, the potential benefit of an "active" placebo which would better mimic the cognitive effects of ketamine than saline to optimize control conditions was clear. The rapid antidepressant effect of IV ketamine was validated in a randomized controlled trial of a larger group of TRD subjects, which compared a single infusion of IV ketamine to an "active" placebo, the anesthetic agent IV midazolam.[28] Another potential use of ketamine, as a rapid-acting anti-suicidal agent, was demonstrated in a randomized controlled trial of subjects with mood and anxiety disorders, in which ketamine-treated subjects experienced a greater reduction in suicidal ideation than those given a midazolam control up to 48 hours after the infusion.[29] The question of the optimum dose of ketamine as an antidepressant followed and was examined in a large randomized controlled trial which compared a range of subanesthetic doses of a single infusion of IV ketamine to a midazolam placebo. The findings supported the efficacy of the 0.5 mg/kg and 1.0 mg/kg doses of IV ketamine.[30] A further study demonstrated the maintained antidepressant efficacy of twice- and thrice-weekly administration of 0.5 mg/kg IV ketamine over 15 days.[31]

Given the logistical challenges associated with IV administration and that most patients with MDD are managed through outpatient care, the search for an alternative route of administration began. The bioavailability of IN ketamine was shown to be superior to oral and sublingual routes[32] and clinical trials of IN formulations for the treatment of depression followed. A randomized double-blind crossover trial of patients with MDD compared IN ketamine with placebo and showed significantly greater improvement in depressive symptoms 24 hours after ketamine compared with placebo, with minimal adverse effects.[33] Janssen subsequently launched their IN esketamine program for TRD and MDD with suicidal ideation.[34–36] A meta-analysis of five trials comparing adjunctive IN esketamine to placebo for the treatment of depressive symptoms found that esketamine was significantly more effective than placebo for depression severity change, response, and remission.[13]

The mechanism of action of ketamine is not yet fully understood; it is proposed to involve NMDA receptor blockade of γ-aminobutyric acid (GABA) interneurons on pre-synaptic glutamatergic neurons. This NMDA receptor blockade leads to a release of tonic inhibition of these interneurons, enabling a glutamate surge, activation of α-amino-3-hydroxy-5-methyl-4-isoxazolepropionic acid (AMPA) receptors, upregulation of brain-derived neurotrophic factor (BDNF), and activation of downstream signaling pathways, including mammalian target of rapamycin (mTOR) enhancement.[37–39] This sequence of events is suggested to facilitate synaptogenesis and synaptic potentiation, reversing synaptic deficits caused by stress in the depressed brain.[40,41] Although these pathways are still considered just a possible mechanism for ketamine's antidepressant effects, basic science work shows the utility of a metabolite of ketamine, (2R,6 R)-hydroxynorketamine (HNK), with direct AMPA activation.[42]

Given that ketamine's plasma terminal half-life is 2.5 hours,[43] perhaps HNK offers some explanation as to why ketamine's antidepressant effects are typically sustained for 1 to 2 weeks postinfusion.

PATIENT EVALUATION OVERVIEW
Assessment and Diagnosis

When assessing whether a patient is appropriate for IV ketamine treatment, a full psychiatric history and mental state examination should be completed. At present, most of the evidence base supports ketamine's use in MDD and TRD, as outlined above. A diagnosis of a current major depressive episode (MDE) should therefore be established in assessing suitability for treatment. Ketamine's efficacy in other psychiatric disorders is less clear. For depressive episodes in bipolar affective disorder, a single IV dose of ketamine leads to a greater response rate than placebo up to 24 hours.[44] Individual studies have reported low rates of ketamine-induced manic symptoms, though this issue is difficult to delineate due to the inclusion of subjects on mood stabilizers and other confounding variables.[45] Only preliminary evidence exists for the use of ketamine in obsessive compulsive disorder[46] and post-traumatic stress disorder.[47] A recent expert consensus recommended against the use of ketamine in those with an MDE with psychotic symptoms,[48] although some case reports suggest such patients may benefit.[49,50]

IN esketamine is now approved in the US and European Union (EU) with specific indications, based on data from three phase 3 trials in TRD.[34-36] In the US, it is approved for use in conjunction with an oral antidepressant for the treatment of adults with TRD and for depressive symptoms in adults with MDD and acute suicidal thoughts or actions.[24] In the EU, the EMA has specified the following narrower indications: esketamine should be prescribed in combination with a selective serotonin reuptake inhibitor (SSRI) or serotonin-noradrenaline reuptake inhibitor (SNRI) for adults with treatment-resistant MDD, who have not responded to at least two different treatments with antidepressants in the current moderate to severe depressive episode. It is also indicated, when coadministered with oral antidepressant therapy, for adults with a moderate to severe depressive episode as "acute short-term treatment, for the rapid reduction of depressive symptoms, which according to clinical judgment constitute a psychiatric emergency."[25]

Treatment Response History

A full history of antidepressant treatment response should be obtained to establish whether the current depressive episode is treatment resistant. Although variably defined, to be considered treatment-resistant patients should generally have had two or more failed trials of standard antidepressants at an adequate dose for an adequate duration.[51] Consideration should also be given to modifiable psychosocial factors, comorbid diagnoses, and current substance use in assessing treatment resistance.

Special Considerations

Patients with a current substance use disorder or history of ketamine abuse have generally been excluded from studies of ketamine in MDD. In such patients, the risk of abuse should be carefully weighed against the potential benefits of ketamine treatment. However, the evidence to date has not supported an increase in new-onset substance use disorders with single and repeated ketamine treatments.[48] In addition, certain factors may predict a more sustained antidepressant response such as a family history of alcohol use disorders.[52] Unlike what is observed with traditional antidepressants, whereby those with anxious depression have a lower response compared with those non-anxious depression,[53] response to ketamine may be similar[54] or possibly enhanced[55] in those with anxious depression.

DELIVERY OF TREATMENT
Clinician Experience

At present, there are no published guidelines or recommendations outlining the appropriate training required for clinicians to administer the sub-anesthetic doses of IV ketamine currently used to treat mood disorders.[17] A survey of US clinicians providing ketamine treatment for psychiatric disorders found that the majority (66.7%) were psychiatrists, with others trained in anesthesiology (22.8%), emergency medicine (3.5%), and family medicine (3.5%).[56]

Setting

Similarly, there are no established recommendations to guide the appropriate setting for and monitoring of IV ketamine treatment. The same survey described above reported that 73.7% of respondents administered ketamine in an office-based setting and 21.1% in a hospital-based setting or surgical/procedural suite.[19] An expert consensus recommended settings which can facilitate physical examination, body mass index (BMI) measurement, vital sign assessment, and cardiorespiratory monitoring during and posttreatment.[48] It also recommended that site staff can appropriately monitor for physical and psychiatric adverse events. The labeling for IN esketamine recommends measurement of blood pressure before and at least two hours after administration.[24]

Bioavailability and Formulation

Although most clinical trials have assessed the administration of IV and IN forms of ketamine/esketamine, other routes of administration have also been studied. As expected, ketamine's bioavailability differs based on the route of administration. A gradient of decreasing bioavailability is observed: IV, intramuscular, subcutaneous, IN, and oral forms.[48,57] The elimination of half-lives for racemic ketamine and esketamine is approximately 2 to 4 hours and 5 hours, respectively.[43] A recent meta-analysis compared IV, IN, and oral formulations of ketamine at various time points and concluded that it was not possible to arrive at any comparative efficacy claims given the significant heterogeneity across studies[15] (e.g., most IV ketamine studies have a examined a single infusion, whereas IN esketamine studies have included repeated doses). This analysis observed that the effect size was greatest for IV ketamine at 2 to 6 days, IN esketamine at 24 hours, and oral ketamine at 21 to 28 days. A separate recent meta-analysis compared IV ketamine with IN esketamine for the treatment of unipolar and bipolar depression. The authors concluded that IV ketamine outperformed IN esketamine: IV ketamine demonstrated significantly greater response and remission rates as well as lower rates of discontinuation due to adverse events.[14] However, a head-to-head comparison of the two formulations has never been conducted.

Dosage, Body Mass Index and Sex Differences

A randomized controlled trial which examined a single infusion of various doses of IV ketamine (0.1 mg/kg, 0.2 mg/kg, 0.5 mg/kg and 1.0 mg/kg) to IV midazolam placebo for the treatment of TRD (coadministered with a standard antidepressant) concluded that there was evidence for the antidepressant efficacy of the 0.5 mg/kg and 1.0 mg/kg doses of IV ketamine and no clear evidence for clinically meaningful efficacy of lower doses of IV ketamine.[30] Time to relapse among these subjects followed a dose–response relationship, whereby higher dosage was associated with increased time to relapse.[58] A post hoc analysis of this data set showed that obese patients (compared normal and overweight patients) had a more robust antidepressant response at 24 and 72 hours post-infusion.[59] A further post hoc examination of this data set showed no differential efficacy between men and women nor between premenopausal and postmenopausal women.[60]

For IN esketamine, a starting dose of 56 mg, administered twice weekly is recommended during an induction phase of 4 weeks; dosing can remain at 56 mg or increase to 84 mg based on response. Administration frequency is suggested to be reduced to once weekly during weeks 5 to 8, then biweekly or less frequently thereafter based on symptoms.[24]

Effect on Suicidal Ideation

Studies of the impact of a single infusion of IV ketamine on suicidal ideation in MDD have observed a rapid-onset anti-suicidal effect,[61–65] but weak durability.[62,63,66] When other psychiatric disorders are considered, IV ketamine's anti-suicidal effects also seem to be rapid in onset, but not sustained beyond 72 hours.[61] Multiple infusions of IV ketamine may be necessary to achieve a sustained anti-suicidal effect. To this end, a recent study examined the impact of repeated IV ketamine infusions on suicidal ideation following an initial single infusion.[67] Participants who received IV ketamine did not differ from those who received IV midazolam on Montgomery–Asberg Depression Rating Scale[68] (MADRS) suicide scores at 24 hours post-infusion; the maximal effect was seen at 7 days post-infusion, with cumulative decreases in suicidal ideation during six infusions over 2 weeks. The current literature is inconsistent on whether the anti-suicidal effect of IV ketamine is mediated through the antidepressant effect[65,69] or is at least partially an independent effect.[70–72] Based on currently available evidence, IV ketamine may have a role as an adjunct to standard treatments in patients with TRD and suicidal ideation. Of note, IN esketamine has consistently demonstrated significant efficacy (and is FDA-approved) in reducing depressive symptoms overall (though not suicidal thoughts or actions specifically) in patients with MDD with acute suicidal thoughts or behaviors.[20–24]

Maintaining Effects of Ketamine

As many studies of IV ketamine have examined a single infusion, it is unclear how best to maintain the observed rapid antidepressant effects beyond 24 to 72 hours, whether repeated infusions should be given and how frequently treatments should be administered. The effect size for a single infusion of IV ketamine drops to 0.38 (Hedges g) by day 5 and is no longer statistically significant after day 9.[73] A randomized, placebo-controlled trial which examined twice- and thrice-weekly IV 0.5 mg/kg ketamine infusions in subjects with TRD for up to 4 weeks found that both infusion frequencies similarly maintained antidepressant efficacy over 15 days.[31] In the twice-weekly dosing group, the mean change in MADRS score at day 15 from baseline was −18.4 versus −5.7 for ketamine and placebo. This corresponds to an approximate effect size of 1.14 (Cohen d) during 4 weeks, which is comparable to the effect size of a single dose of IV ketamine at 24 hours.[73] In the group that received three infusions per week, the mean change in MADRS score at day 15 was −17.7 versus −3.1 for ketamine and placebo, which corresponds to an effect size of 2.24 (Cohen d)—a much larger effect than that seen 24 hours after a single ketamine infusion. Although there was no significant difference on MADRS score change between the two frequencies tested, these results suggest that weekly ketamine infusions can maintain (if twice weekly) or even amplify (if three times weekly) rapid gains seen with single ketamine infusions in MDD. Of note, however, a subsequent smaller study of patients with TRD and chronic suicidal ideation did not replicate these findings. There was no significant difference in Hamilton Depression Rating Scale[74] scores between those who received twice weekly 0.5 mg/kg IV ketamine versus placebo for up to 3 weeks.[75]

Two studies have examined riluzole, another modulator of glutamatergic neurotransmission and a postsynaptic NMDA receptor blocker[76] as a potential agent to extend the effects of IV ketamine. Neither trial found a difference in efficacy between riluzole and placebo in extending the effects of a single infusion of ketamine.[77,78] Lithium has also been considered as potential option to maintain the early antidepressant effects of IV ketamine. However, a study which compared the addition of lithium or placebo in subjects with at least a partial response to an infusion of IV ketamine did not find a difference in depression severity, as measured by the MADRS, between the two groups.[79]

The evidence base for repeated administrations of IN esketamine is clearer, given that trials of esketamine have examined repeated rather than single inhalations.[34–36] An examination of subjects with TRD who had achieved stable response or remission with IN esketamine treatment showed that continuation of esketamine nasal spray combined with an oral antidepressant was associated with significantly longer time to relapse compared with antidepressant plus placebo.[80]

TREATMENT RESISTANCE/COMPLICATIONS
Prescribing Considerations

Patients with TRD are often prescribed several medications to treat their depressive and anxiety symptoms. It is therefore important to consider potential interactions between commonly co-prescribed medications for TRD. Most trials of ketamine and esketamine have examined these agents as adjuncts to standard antidepressants, in particular SSRIs and SNRIs, which act on the monoaminergic system rather than the glutamatergic system and are therefore unlikely to impact the efficacy of ketamine/esketamine.

Another class of medication commonly co-initiated with antidepressants in MDD is benzodiazepines.[81] GABAergic interneurons are a shared target of both ketamine and benzodiazepines; by blocking NMDA receptors on these interneurons, ketamine decreases inhibition enabling a glutamate surge, whereas on the other hand, benzodiazepines increase the inhibitory tone of these interneurons. These seemingly oppositional effects would suggest that benzodiazepines could interfere with or attenuate the antidepressant effects of ketamine.[82] Some studies have found that benzodiazepines do not impact ketamine/esketamine's antidepressant effects[83,84]; whereas conversely, other studies have concluded that benzodiazepines may attenuate or slow ketamine's antidepressant effects, particularly at higher benzodiazepine doses.[85–88] One of these studies found that a cutoff of 8 mg/day of diazepam distinguished ketamine responders from nonresponders, with higher benzodiazepine doses attenuating response to ketamine.[86] Regarding esketamine, in a secondary analysis of the ASPIRE I and II esketamine clinical trial data,[83] the antidepressant effects of esketamine were not attenuated or augmented by oral benzodiazepine use, with benzodiazepine use considered as a binary predictor, that is, without consideration of benzodiazepine dosage.

Adverse Effects

In addition to the practicalities of IV administration, Ketamine's side effects sometimes can present a barrier to its widespread use in daily clinical practice. Specifically, the dissociative effects of ketamine, which can include out-of-body experiences and perceptual disturbances, can be clinically prohibiting for some patients. However, it is also possible that a key mechanism by which ketamine's antidepressant effects are propagated may be through these dissociative properties,[89] that is, dissociation may be *necessary* for ketamine's antidepressant effects. Side effects associated with the use of ketamine for depression include psychiatric (eg, dissociative, psychotomimetic), cardiovascular/hemodynamic, neurologic, genitourinary, abuse potential, and other side effects.[48,90] Currently, there is a clear lack of data regarding adverse effects of repeated, long-term use as most trials have not extended beyond 2 months.

The labeling for IN esketamine notes that the most commonly observed adverse reactions in TRD patients treated with IN esketamine plus an oral antidepressant were dissociation, dizziness, nausea, sedation, vertigo, hypoesthesia, anxiety, lethargy, increase blood pressure, vomiting, and "feeling drunk."[24] It also makes some specific warnings, including in relation to sedation, dissociation, potential for misuse, suicidal thoughts in young adults, increased blood pressure, short-term cognitive impairment, and fetal toxicity. Some observed effects of recreational ketamine such as ulcerative/interstitial cystitis and long-term cognitive impairment have not been adequately evaluated with ketamine/esketamine prescribed for depression. At present, IN esketamine is only available through a restricted program, the Risk Evaluation and Mitigation Strategy, which requires health care settings in the United States to be certified to administer IN esketamine.

SUMMARY

IV, IN, and other forms of ketamine/esketamine have important potential clinical applications. Previously, clinicians lacked rapid-acting interventions, either pharmacological or psychological, for patients with TRD. Given ketamine and esketamine's potential to address this unmet need, many specialized treatment clinics have opened (particularly in the US) in recent years focusing on delivering these two treatments. Such clinics have offered a new treatment avenue to patients who have failed conventional treatments; however, given the lack of long-term safety data to support IV ketamine's use in depression beyond a few weeks, clinicians should continue to exercise caution when administering IV ketamine long term. Patients being considered for ketamine and esketamine must be adequately consented in respect of the unknowns of these treatments. In addition, there are currently no standard operating procedures for specialized clinics to guide the selection of patients, dosing and monitoring, and so forth, meaning there is likely great variability in how these clinics are organized.

Most importantly, ketamine and esketamine carry great importance as models for the discovery of other rapidly acting antidepressants, with similar mechanisms of action. Identifying ketamine and esketamine's antidepressant mechanism may also provide a pathway to understanding the pathophysiology of TRD. Future research should focus on further elucidating ketamine and esketamine's antidepressant mechanisms, efficacy and safety, and the exploration of other agents with similar antidepressant actions.

CLINICS CARE POINTS

- Ketamine and esketamine have more rapid antidepressant effects than standard antidepressants.

- IN esketamine has regulatory approval in the United States and European Union for major depressive disorder.
- IV ketamine is currently widely used 'off-label' as a rapid-acting antidepressant for major depression.

DISCLOSURE

A. Feeney: no disclosures. Dr G.I. Papakostas has served as a consultant for Abbott Laboratories, Acadia Pharmaceuticals, Inc*, Alkermes, Inc, Alphasigma USA*, Inc, AstraZeneca PLC, Avanir Pharmaceuticals, Axsome Therapeutics*, Boehringer Ingelheim, Boston Pharmaceuticals, Inc*, Brainsway Ltd, Bristol-Myers Squibb Company, Cala Health*, Cephalon Inc, Dey Pharma, L.P., Eleusis health solutions Ltd*, Eli Lilly Co, Genentech, Inc*, Genomind, Inc*, GlaxoSmithKline, Evotec AG, H. Lundbeck A/S, Inflabloc Pharmaceuticals, Janssen Global Services LLC*, Jazz Pharmaceuticals, Johnson & Johnson Companies*, Methylation Sciences Inc, Monopteros Therapeutics*, Mylan Inc*, Neurocentria, Novartis Pharma AG, One Carbon Therapeutics, Inc*, Osmotica Pharmaceutical Corp*, Otsuka Pharmaceuticals, PAMLAB LLC, Pfizer Inc, Pierre Fabre Laboratories, Praxis Precision Medicines*, Ridge Diagnostics (formerly known as Precision Human Biolaboratories), Sage Therapeutics*, Shire Pharmaceuticals, Sunovion Pharmaceuticals, Taisho Pharmaceutical Co, Ltd*, Takeda Pharmaceutical Company LTD, Theracos, Inc, and Wyeth, Inc. Dr G.I. Papakostas has received honoraria (for lectures or consultancy) from Abbott Laboratories, Acadia Pharmaceuticals Inc, Alkermes Inc, Alphasigma USA Inc, Asopharma America Central Y Caribe, Astra Zeneca PLC, Avanir Pharmaceuticals, Boehringer Ingelheim, Bristol-Myers Squibb Company, Brainsway Ltd, Cephalon Inc, Dey Pharma, L.P., Eli Lilly Co, Evotec AG, Forest Pharmaceuticals, GlaxoSmithKline, Inflabloc Pharmaceuticals, Grunbiotics Pty Ltd, Hypera S.A., Jazz Pharmaceuticals, H. Lundbeck A/S, Medichem Pharmaceuticals, Inc, Meiji Seika Pharma Co Ltd, Novartis Pharma AG, Otsuka Pharmaceuticals, PAMLAB LLC, Pfizer, Pharma Trade SAS, Pierre Fabre Laboratories, Ridge Diagnostics, Shire Pharmaceuticals, Sunovion Pharmaceuticals, Takeda Pharmaceutical Company LTD, Theracos, Inc, Titan Pharmaceuticals, and Wyeth Inc. Dr G.I. Papakostas has received research support (paid to hospital) from Alphasigma USA, Inc, AstraZeneca PLC, Bristol-Myers Squibb Company, Cala Health, Forest Pharmaceuticals, the National Institute of Mental Health, Mylan Inc, Neuralstem, Inc*, PAMLAB LLC, PCORI, Pfizer Inc, Johnson & Johnson Companies, Ridge Diagnostics (formerly known as Precision Human Biolaboratories), Sunovion Pharmaceuticals, Tal Medical, and Theracos, Inc. Dr G.I. Papakostas has served (not currently) on the speaker's bureau for Bristol Myers Squibb Co and Pfizer, Inc. *Asterisk denotes consulting activity undertaken on behalf of Massachusetts General Hospital.

REFERENCES

1. Lopez-Munoz F, Alamo C. Monoaminergic neurotransmission: the history of the discovery of antidepressants from 1950s until today. Curr Pharm Des 2009; 15(14):1563–86.
2. Papakostas GI, Perlis RH, Scalia MJ, et al. A meta-analysis of early sustained response rates between antidepressants and placebo for the treatment of major depressive disorder. J Clin Psychopharmacol 2006;26(1):56–60.

3. Stahl SM, Nierenberg AA, Gorman JM. Evidence of early onset of antidepressant effect in randomized controlled trials. J Clin Psychiatr 2001. Available at: https://pubmed.ncbi.nlm.nih.gov/11229783/. Accessed August 10, 2022.

4. Rush AJ, Trivedi MH, Wisniewski SR, et al. Acute and longer-term outcomes in depressed outpatients requiring one or several treatment steps: A STAR*D report. Am J Psychiatry 2006;163(11):1905–17.

5. Xu Y, Hackett M, Carter G, et al. Effects of low-dose and very low-dose ketamine among patients with major depression: a systematic review and meta-analysis. Int J Neuropsychopharmacology 2016;19(4):1–15.

6. Coyle CM, Laws KR. The use of ketamine as an antidepressant: a systematic review and meta-analysis. Hum Psychopharmacol Clin Exp 2015;30(3):152–63.

7. Lee EE, Della Selva MP, Liu A, et al. Ketamine as a novel treatment for major depressive disorder and bipolar depression: a systematic review and quantitative meta-analysis. Gen Hosp Psychiatry 2015;37(2):178–84.

8. McGirr A, Berlim MT, Bond DJ, et al. A systematic review and meta-analysis of randomized, double-blind, placebo-controlled trials of ketamine in the rapid treatment of major depressive episodes. Psychol Med 2015;45(4):693–704.

9. Fond G, Loundou A, Rabu C, et al. Ketamine administration in depressive disorders: a systematic review and meta-analysis. Psychopharmacology (Berl) 2014;231(18):3663–76.

10. Bobo WV, Vande Voort JL, Croarkin PE, et al. Ketamine for treatment-resistant unipolar and bipolar major depression: critical review and implications for clinical practice. Depress Anxiety 2016;33:698–710.

11. Schwartz J, Murrough JW, Iosifescu DV. Ketamine for treatment-resistant depression: recent developments and clinical applications. Evid Based Ment Health 2016;19(2):35–8.

12. Serafini G, Howland R, Rovedi F, et al. The role of ketamine in treatment-resistant depression: a systematic review. Curr Neuropharmacol 2014;12(5):444–61.

13. Papakostas GI, Salloum NC, Hock RS, et al. Efficacy of esketamine augmentation in major depressive disorder: a meta-analysis. J Clin Psychiatry 2020;81(4). https://doi.org/10.4088/JCP.19r12889.

14. Bahji A, Vazquez GH, Zarate CA. Comparative efficacy of racemic ketamine and esketamine for depression: a systematic review and meta-analysis. J Affect Disord 2021;278:542–55.

15. McIntyre RS, Carvalho IP, Lui LMW, et al. The effect of intravenous, intranasal, and oral ketamine in mood disorders: A meta-analysis. J Affect Disord 2020;276:576–84.

16. Skånland SS, Cieślar-Pobuda A. Off-label uses of drugs for depression. Eur J Pharmacol 2019;865:172732.

17. Sanacora G, Frye MA, McDonald W, et al. A consensus statement on the use of ketamine in the treatment of mood disorders. JAMA Psychiatr 2017;74(4):399–405.

18. Wilkinson ST, Sanacora G. Considerations on the off-label use of ketamine as a treatment for mood disorders. JAMA 2017;318(9):793.

19. Wilkinson ST, Toprak M, Turner M, et al. A survey of the clinical, off-label use of ketamine as a treatment for psychiatric disorders. Am J Psychiatry 2017;174(7):695.

20. Canuso CM, Singh JB, Fedgchin M, et al. Efficacy and safety of intranasal esketamine for the rapid reduction of symptoms of depression and suicidality in patients at imminent risk for suicide: results of a double-blind, randomized, placebo-controlled study. Am J Psychiatry 2018;175:620–30.

21. Fu D.J., Ionescu D.F., Li X., et al., Esketamine nasal spray for rapid reduction of major depressive disorder symptoms in patients who have active suicidal ideation with intent, J Clin Psychiatry, 81 (3), 2020, 19m13191.

22. Ionescu D.F., Fu D.J., Qiu X., et al., Esketamine Nasal Spray for Rapid Reduction of Depressive Symptoms in Patients with Major Depressive Disorder Who Have Active Suicide Ideation with Intent: Results of a Phase 3, Double-Blind, Randomized Study (ASPIRE II), Int J Neuropsychopharmacology, 24(1), 2021, 22-31.

23. Singh JB, Daly EJ, Mathews M, et al. Approval of esketamine for treatment-resistant depression. Lancet Psychiatr 2020;7(3):232–5.

24. SPRAVATO ® (esketamine) nasal spray, CIII HIGHLIGHTS OF PRESCRIBING INFORMATION. Available at: https://www.accessdata.fda.gov/drugsatfda_docs/label/2020/211243s004lbl.pdf. Accessed August 31, 2022.

25. EMA. Spravato. European Medicines Agency. Available at: https://www.ema.europa.eu/en/medicines/human/EPAR/spravato. Accessed August 24, 2022.

26. Berman RM, Cappiello A, Anand A, et al. Antidepressant effects of ketamine in depressed patients. Biol Psychiatry 2000;47(4):351–4.

27. Zarate CA, Singh JB, Carlson PJ, et al. A randomized trial of an N-methyl-D-aspartate antagonist in treatment-resistant major depression. Arch Gen Psychiatry 2006;63(8):856–64.

28. Murrough JW, Iosifescu DV, Chang LC, et al. Antidepressant efficacy of ketamine in treatment-resistant major depression: a two-site randomized controlled trial. Am J Psychiatry 2013;170(10):1134–42.

29. Murrough JW, Soleimani L, Dewilde KE, et al. Ketamine for rapid reduction of suicidal ideation: a randomized controlled trial. Psychol Med 2015;45(16):3571–80.

30. Fava M, Freeman MP, Flynn M, et al. Double-blind, placebo-controlled, dose-ranging trial of intravenous ketamine as adjunctive therapy in treatment-resistant depression (TRD). Mol Psychiatry 2020;25(7):1592 603.

31. Singh JB, Fedgchin M, Daly EJ, et al. A double-blind, randomized, placebo-controlled, dose-frequency study of intravenous ketamine in patients with treatment-resistant depression. Am J Psychiatry 2016;173(8):816–26.

32. Yanagihara Y, Ohtani M, Kariya S, et al. Plasma concentration profiles of ketamine and norketamine after administration of various ketamine preparations to healthy Japanese volunteers. Biopharm Drug Dispos 2003;24(1):37–43.

33. Lapidus KAB, Levitch CF, Perez AM, et al. A randomized controlled trial of intranasal ketamine in major depressive disorder. Biol Psychiatry 2014;76(12):970–6.

34. Fedgchin M, Trivedi M, Daly EJ, et al. Efficacy and safety of fixed-dose esketamine nasal spray combined with a new oral antidepressant in treatment-resistant depression: results of a randomized, double-blind, active-controlled study (TRANSFORM-1). Int J Neuropsychopharmacology 2019;22(10):616–30.

35. Popova V, Daly EJ, Trivedi M, et al. Efficacy and safety of flexibly dosed esketamine nasal spray combined with a newly initiated oral antidepressant in treatment-resistant depression: a randomized double-blind active-controlled study. Am J Psychiatry 2019;176:428–38.

36. Ochs-Ross R, Daly EJ, Zhang Y, et al. Efficacy and safety of esketamine nasal spray plus an oral antidepressant in elderly patients with treatment-resistant depression-TRANSFORM-3. Am J Geriatr Psychiatry 2020;28(2):121–41.

37. Strasburger SE, Bhimani PM, Kaabe JH, et al. What is the mechanism of Ketamine's rapid-onset antidepressant effect? A concise overview of the surprisingly large number of possibilities. J Clin Pharm Ther 2017;42:147–54.

38. Irwin MN, VandenBerg A. Retracing our steps to understand ketamine in depression: a focused review of hypothesized mechanisms of action. Ment Health Clin 2021;11(3):200.

39. Abdallah CG, Adams TG, Kelmendi B, et al. Ketamine's mechanism of action: a path to rapid-acting antidepressants. Depress Anxiety 2016;33(8):689.

40. Duman RS, Aghajanian GK. Synaptic dysfunction in depression: potential therapeutic targets. Science 2012;338(6103):68.

41. Duman RS, Aghajanian GK, Sanacora G, et al. Synaptic plasticity and depression: new insights from stress and rapid-acting antidepressants. Nat Med 2016;22(3):238.

42. Zanos P, Moaddel R, Morris PJ, et al. NMDAR inhibition-independent antidepressant actions of ketamine metabolites. Nat 2016;533(7604):481-6.

43. Zhao X, Venkata SLV, Moaddel R, et al. Simultaneous population pharmacokinetic modelling of ketamine and three major metabolites in patients with treatment-resistant bipolar depression. Br J Clin Pharmacol 2012;74(2):304.

44. Dean RL, Marquardt T, Hurducas C, et al. Ketamine and other glutamate receptor modulators for depression in adults with bipolar disorder. Cochrane Database Syst Rev 2021;2021(10). https://doi.org/10.1002/14651858.CD011611.

45. Singh B, Vande Voort JL, Frye MA, et al. Can ketamine be a safe option for treatment-resistant bipolar depression? Expert Opin Drug Saf 2022;21(6):717-20.

46. Rodriguez CI, Kegeles LS, Levinson A, et al. Randomized controlled crossover trial of ketamine in obsessive-compulsive disorder: proof-of-concept. Neuropsychopharmacology 2013;38(12):2475-83.

47. Feder A, Parides MK, Murrough JW, et al. Efficacy of intravenous ketamine for treatment of chronic posttraumatic stress disorder: a randomized clinical trial. JAMA Psychiatr 2014;71(6):681-8.

48. McIntyre RS, Rosenblat JD, Nemeroff CB, et al. Synthesizing the evidence for ketamine and esketamine in treatment-resistant depression: an international expert opinion on the available evidence and implementation. Am J Psychiatry 2021; 178(5):383-99.

49. Ribeiro CM da F, Sanacora G, Hoffman R, et al. The Use of Ketamine for the Treatment of Depression in the Context of Psychotic Symptoms: To the Editor. Biol Psychiatry 2016;79(9):e65-6. https://doi.org/10.1016/j.biopsych.2015.05.016.

50. Ajub E, Lacerda ALT. Efficacy of esketamine in the treatment of depression with psychotic features: a case series. Biol Psychiatry 2018;83(1):e15-6.

51. Chandler GM, Iosifescu DV, Pollack MH, et al. Validation of the massachusetts general hospital Antidepressant Treatment History Questionnaire (ATRQ). CNS Neurosci Ther 2010;16(5):322-5.

52. Niciu MJ, Luckenbaugh DA, Ionescu DF, et al. Ketamine's antidepressant efficacy is extended for at least four weeks in subjects with a family history of an alcohol use disorder. Int J Neuropsychopharmacology 2014;18(1):pyu039.

53. Fava M, Uebelacker LA, Alpert JE, et al. Major depressive subtypes and treatment response. Biol Psychiatry 1997;42(7):568-76.

54. Salloum NC, Fava M, Freeman MP, et al. Efficacy of intravenous ketamine treatment in anxious versus nonanxious unipolar treatment-resistant depression. Depress Anxiety 2019;36(3):235-43.

55. Ionescu DF, Luckenbaugh DA, Niciu MJ, et al. Effect of baseline anxious depression on initial and sustained antidepressant response to ketamine. J Clin Psychiatry 2014;75(9). e932-8.

56. Zhang MW, Harris KM, Ho RC. Is Off-label repeat prescription of ketamine as a rapid antidepressant safe? Controversies, ethical concerns, and legal implications. BMC Med Ethics 2016;17(1). https://doi.org/10.1186/S12910-016-0087-3.

57. Zanos P, Moaddel R, Morris PJ, et al. Ketamine and ketamine metabolite pharmacology: insights into therapeutic mechanisms. Pharmacol Rev 2018;70(3): 621–60.

58. Salloum NC, Fava M, Hock RS, et al. Time to relapse after a single administration of intravenous ketamine augmentation in unipolar treatment-resistant depression. J Affect Disord 2019. https://doi.org/10.1016/j.jad.2019.09.017.

59. Freeman MP, Hock RS, Papakostas GI, et al. Body mass index as a moderator of treatment response to ketamine for major depressive disorder. J Clin Psychopharmacol 2020;40(3):287–92.

60. Freeman MP, Papakostas GI, Hoeppner B, et al. Sex differences in response to ketamine as a rapidly acting intervention for treatment resistant depression. J Psychiatr Res 2019;110:166–71.

61. Witt K, Potts J, Hubers A, et al. Ketamine for suicidal ideation in adults with psychiatric disorders: a systematic review and meta-analysis of treatment trials 883341A NP ANZJP ArticlesWitt et al. ANZJP Artic Aust N Z J Psychiatry 2020; 54(1):29–45.

62. Burger J, Capobianco M, Lovern R, et al. A double-blinded, randomized, placebo-controlled sub-dissociative dose ketamine pilot study in the treatment of acute depression and suicidality in a military emergency department setting. Mil Med 2016;181(10):1195–9.

63. Domany Y, Shelton RC, Mccullumsmith CB. Ketamine for acute suicidal ideation. An emergency department intervention: a randomized, double-blind, placebo-controlled, proof-of-concept trial. Depress Anxiety 2020;37:224–33.

64. Grunebaum MF, Galfalvy HC, Choo TH, et al. Ketamine for rapid reduction of suicidal thoughts in major depression: a midazolam-controlled randomized clinical trial. Am J Psychiatry 2018;175(4):327–35.

65. Price RB, Iosifescu DV, Murrough JW, et al. Effects of ketamine on explicit and implicit suicidal cognition: a randomized controlled trial in treatment-resistant depression. Depress Anxiety 2014;31(4):335–43.

66. Feeney A, Hock RS, Freeman MarleneP, et al. The effect of single administration of intravenous ketamine augmentation on suicidal ideation in treatment-resistant unipolar depression: results from a randomized double-blind study. Eur Neuropsychopharmacology J Eur Coll Neuropsychopharmacol 2021;49:122–32.

67. Phillips JL, Norris S, Talbot J, et al. Single and repeated ketamine infusions for reduction of suicidal ideation in treatment-resistant depression. Neuropsychopharmacology 2020;45(4):606–12.

68. Montgomery SA, Asberg M. A new depression scale designed to be sensitive to change. Br J Psychiatry 1979;134(4):382–9.

69. Price RB, Nock MK, Charney DS, et al. Effects of intravenous ketamine on explicit and implicit measures of suicidality in treatment-resistant depression. Biol Psychiatry 2009;66(5):522–6.

70. Ballard ED, Ionescu DF, Vande Voort JL, et al. Improvement in suicidal ideation after ketamine infusion: relationship to reductions in depression and anxiety. J Psychiatr Res 2014;58:161–6.

71. Wilkinson ST, Ballard ED, Bloch MH, et al. The effect of a single dose of intravenous ketamine on suicidal ideation: a systematic review and individual participant data meta-analysis. Am J Psychiatr 2018;175:150–8. https://doi.org/10.1176/appi.ajp.2017.17040472. American Psychiatric Association.

72. Zheng W, Zhou YL, Liu WJ, et al. Investigation of medical effect of multiple ketamine infusions on patients with major depressive disorder. J Psychopharmacol 2019;33(4):494–501.

73. Kishimoto T, Chawla JM, Hagi K, et al. Single-dose infusion ketamine and non-ketamine N-methyl-D-aspartate receptor antagonists for unipolar and bipolar depression: a meta-analysis of efficacy, safety and time trajectories. Psychol Med 2016;46(7):1459–72.

74. Hamilton M. A rating scale for depression. J Neurol Neurosurg Psychiatr 1960; 23(1):56–62.

75. Ionescu DF, Bentley KH, Eikermann M, et al. Repeat-dose ketamine augmentation for treatment-resistant depression with chronic suicidal ideation: A randomized, double blind, placebo controlled trial. J Affect Disord 2019;243:516–24.

76. Doble A. The pharmacology and mechanism of action of riluzole. Neurology 1996;47(6 Suppl 4):S233–41.

77. Mathew SJ, Murrough JW, aan het Rot M, et al. Riluzole for relapse prevention following intravenous ketamine in treatment-resistant depression: a pilot randomized, placebo-controlled continuation trial. Int J Neuropsychopharmacol Off Sci J Coll Int Neuropsychopharmacol CINP 2010;13(1). https://doi.org/10.1017/S1461145709000169.

78. Ibrahim L, DiazGranados N, Franco-Chaves J, et al. Course of Improvement in Depressive Symptoms to a Single Intravenous Infusion of Ketamine vs Add-on Riluzole: Results from a 4-Week, Double-Blind, Placebo-Controlled Study. Neuropsychopharmacology 2012;37(6):1526–33.

79. Costi S, Soleimani L, Glasgow A, et al. Lithium continuation therapy following ketamine in patients with treatment resistant unipolar depression: a randomized controlled trial. Neuropsychopharmacology 2019;44(10):1812–9.

80. Daly EJ, Trivedi MH, Janik A, et al. Efficacy of Esketamine Nasal Spray Plus Oral Antidepressant Treatment for Relapse Prevention in Patients With Treatment-Resistant Depression. JAMA Psychiatr 2019;76(9):893–903.

81. Bushnell GA, Stürmer T, Gaynes BN, et al. Simultaneous Antidepressant and Benzodiazepine New Use and Subsequent Long-term Benzodiazepine Use in Adults With Depression, United States, 2001-2014. JAMA Psychiatr 2017;74(7):747–55.

82. Veraart JKE, Smith-Apeldoorn SY, Bakker IM, et al. Pharmacodynamic interactions between ketamine and psychiatric medications used in the treatment of depression: a systematic review. Int J Neuropsychopharmacol 2021;25. https://doi.org/10.1093/IJNP/PYAB039.

83. Diekamp B, Borentain S, Fu DJ, et al. Effect of Concomitant Benzodiazepine Use on Efficacy and Safety of Esketamine Nasal Spray in Patients with Major Depressive Disorder and Acute Suicidal Ideation or Behavior: Pooled Randomized, Controlled Trials. Neuropsychiatr Dis Treat 2021;17:2347–57.

84. Shiroma PR, Thuras P, Wels J, et al. A randomized, double-blind, active placebo-controlled study of efficacy, safety, and durability of repeated vs single subanesthetic ketamine for treatment-resistant depression. Transl Psychiatry 2020;10(1). https://doi.org/10.1038/S41398-020-00897-0.

85. Albott C.S., Shiroma P.R., Cullen K.R., et al., The antidepressant effect of repeat dose intravenous ketamine is delayed by concurrent benzodiazepine use, *J Clin Psychiatry*, 78 (3), 2017, e308-e309.

86. Andrashko V, Novak T, Brunovsky M, et al. The antidepressant effect of ketamine is dampened by concomitant benzodiazepine medication. Front Psychiatry 2020; 11:1.

87. Frye MA, Blier P, Tye SJ. Implications for large scale study design and clinical development. J Clin Psychopharmacol 2015;35(3):334–6.
88. Ford N, Ludbrook G, Galletly C. Benzodiazepines may reduce the effectiveness of ketamine in the treatment of depression. Aust N Z J Psychiatry 2015;49(12): 1227.
89. Luckenbaugh DA, Niciu MJ, Ionescu DF, et al. Do the dissociative side effects of ketamine mediate its antidepressant effects? J Affect Disord 2014;159:56–61.
90. Short B, Fong J, Galvez V, et al. Side-effects associated with ketamine use in depression: a systematic review. Lancet Psychiatr 2018;5(1):65–78.

Role of Psychedelics in Treatment-Resistant Depression

Shubham Kamal, MBBS[a], Manish Kumar Jha, MBBS[b],
Rajiv Radhakrishnan, MD[a,c],*

KEYWORDS

- Psychedelic • Psilocybin • LSD • MDMA • Ayahuasca • DMT
- Treatment-resistant depression • Pharmacology

KEY POINTS

- The relatively short-duration of action and potential long-lasting antidepressant effects of psychedelics make them attractive as a therapeutic option in patient with treatment-resistant depression (TRD).
- The evidence for the efficacy of psychedelics in TRD is limited at the present time, although initial studies of small sample size are promising.
- The long-lasting effects of psychedelics are proposed to be due to their altering synaptic plasticity, modulating default mode network and increasing cognitive flexibility.
- The role of psychotherapy and expectancy in the antidepressant effects of psychedelics remain to be delineated.
- There is a need for large, randomized controlled trials in diverse population groups with standardized protocols.

INTRODUCTION

Major depressive disorder (MDD) is a serious psychiatric disorder that is characterized by feelings of sadness and/or loss of interest in pleasurable activities. MDD can affect all age groups, ranging from childhood through old age, and is approximately two times more common in females.[1] It is the leading cause of disability, affecting more than 300 million people worldwide.[2] Apart from disability, MDD is one of the leading causes of suicide and is comorbid with many medical conditions, including diabetes, Parkinson's disease, hepatitis C, endocrine disorders, and obesity.[1,3]

[a] Department of Psychiatry, School of Medicine, Yale University, 300 George Street, Suite 901, New Haven, CT 06511, USA; [b] Department of Psychiatry, University of Texas Southwestern Medical Center, 5323 Harry Hines Boulevard, Dallas, TX 75390-9119, USA; [c] Department of Radiology and Biomedical Imaging, New Haven, CT 06511, USA
* Corresponding author. 300 George Street, Suite 901, New Haven, CT 06511.
E-mail address: rajiv.radhakrishnan@yale.edu

Psychiatr Clin N Am 46 (2023) 291–305
https://doi.org/10.1016/j.psc.2023.02.004
0193-953X/23/© 2023 Elsevier Inc. All rights reserved.

psych.theclinics.com

Although there are multiple treatment options, such as antidepressant medications, psychotherapies, and brain stimulation protocols, finding the right treatment for MDD often involves trial and error.[4,5] A significant proportion of MDD patients, however, fail to respond adequately despite adequate trials with at least two antidepressants, and are therefore deemed to have treatment-resistant depression (TRD).[6,7] The current treatment options for TRD include ketamine,[8] esketamine, switching antidepressant medications, augmentation (with adjunctive atypical antipsychotics, thyroid hormones, dopamine compounds (modafinil and lisdexamfetamine) and lithium),[9] combination of antidepressants, brain stimulation, and electroconvulsive therapy,[10] and have been discussed in other reports in this issue of the *Clinics*.

Interest in examining the role of "psychedelics" as a potential treatment for TRD has mushroomed in recent years. In this article, we consider the current state of the evidence for the use of psychedelics in TRD, explore the challenges associated with their use, and suggest future directions for the development of these compounds as viable treatments.

What Are Psychedelics?

The term psychedelic (Greek: "mind manifesting"), refers to a group of compounds that produce "various (often profound) psychological effects characterized by altered states of perception, thoughts, feelings, and consciousness."[11] Although there is no consensus on what compounds belong to the class "psychedelics", they have been traditionally classified as "classic sertoninergic psychedelics" that are thought to exert their effects via serotonin 5HT2A agonism (or partial agonism) and "atypical psychedelics" that have non-serotoninergic mechanisms of action.[12]

The classic psychedelics comprise three broad classes, based on their chemical structure (1) tryptamines (including psilocybin (a prodrug of psilocin (4-OH-dimethyltryptamine)); *N,N*-dimethyltryptamine [DMT], the active constituent contained in ayahuasca; 5-methoxy-DMT, DMT fumarate)), (2) ergolines (including lysergic acid diethylamide [LSD] and ᴅ-lysergic acid amide [LSA]), and (3) phenethylamines (including mescaline, 2,5-dimethoxy-4-iodoamphetamine (DOI), 2,5-dimethoxy-4-methylamphetamine (DOM), 4-bromo-2,5-dimetoxyphenethylamine (2C-B), and 2-(4-iodo-2,5-dimethoxyphenyl)-N-[(2-methoxyphenyl)methyl]ethanamine (25I-NBOMe)).[12] (**Table 1**).

The atypical psychedelics comprise (a) 3,4-methylenedioxymethamphetamine (MDMA), (also a phenethylamine), that acts via the release of presynaptic serotonin and to a lesser extent via norepinephrine and dopamine through interactions with the corresponding monoamine transporter, including trace amine-associated receptor 1 (TAAR1) and vesicular monoamine transporter 2 (VMAT2) (b) ketamine, an NMDA receptor antagonist, (c) muscimol (derived from the mushroom, Amanita muscaria), a potent GABA-A receptor agonist (d) salvinorin A, a kappa-opioid receptor agonist, and (e) ibogaine/noribogaine, a potent serotonin reuptake inhibitor and moderate kappa-opioid receptor agonist.[12]

Psychedelics in the Treatment of Major Depressive Disorder/Treatment-Resistant Depression

Psychedelics that have been studied in individuals with MDD/TRD include (a) psilocybin, (b) DMT/ayahuasca, and (c) ketamine. Studies of LSD have examined its safety and efficacy in anxiety associated with the life-threatening disease with depression as a secondary outcome measure.[13] In addition, animal studies suggest that salvinorin-A, ibogaine, LSD, 5-MeO-DMT, and DMT fumarate may have antidepressant properties.[14] Notably, clinical trials with salvinorin-A, ibogaine, LSD,

Table 1
Classification of psychedelics

Classic Psychedelics

Tryptamines	Proposed Mechanism of Action
Psilocybin	5-HT$_{2A}$ agonism
DMT (N,N-dimethyltryptamine)	5-HT$_{2A}$ agonism, TAAR and sigma-1 agonism
5-methoxy-DMT	Non-selective 5-HT agonism
DMT Fumarate	Non-selective 5-HT agonism

Ergolines	Proposed Mechanism of Action
LSD (lysergic acid diethylamide)	5-HT$_{2A}$ partial agonism; 5-HT$_{1A}$ agonism
LSA (D-lysergic acid amide)	5-HT$_{2A}$ partial agonism

Phenethylamines	Proposed Mechanism of Action
Mescaline	5-HT$_{2A}$ agonism
DOI (2,5-dimethoxy-4-iodoamphetamine)	5-HT$_{2A,B,C}$ receptor agonism
DOM (2,5-dimethoxy-4-methylamphetamine)	Selective 5-HT$_{2A,B}$ agonism
2C-B (4-bromo-2,5-dimetoxyphenethylamine)	5-HT$_{2C}$ partial agonism
25I-NBOMe (2-(4-iodo-2,5-dimethoxyphenyl)-N-[(2-methoxyphenyl)methyl]ethanamine)	5-HT$_{2C}$ partial agonism; 5-HT$_{2A}$ antagonism; 5-HT$_{2A}$ agonism

Atypical Psychedelics

Compound/Chemical Name	Proposed Mechanism of Action
MDMA[a] (3,4-methylenedioxymethamphetamine)	Inhibits reuptake: NET > SERT > DAT; VMAT2 inhibition and TAAR-1 agonism
Ketamine	NMDA receptor antagonist
Muscimol	GABA-A receptor agonist
Salvinorin A	Kappa-opioid receptor agonist; Inhibits reuptake: SERT
Ibogaine/noribogaine	Kappa-opioid receptor agonist

[a] MDMA is also a phenethylamine.

5-MeO-DMT, and DMT-fumarate in the treatment of MDD/TRD are currently underway.[15]

We will focus on human clinical studies with psilocybin, DMT/ayahuasca, and LSD in the remaining portion of the review. Although the role of ketamine in TRD is covered elsewhere in this special issue, it is interesting to note that the commonly used dose of ketamine (0.5 mg/kg) may not produce symptoms of partial dissociation (or psychedelic-like effects). This in turn results in uptitration of dose in clinical practice, despite paucity of evidence that a psychedelic-like response is necessary for a clinical response.[16,17]

Mechanisms of Antidepressant Effects of Psychedelics

As noted earlier, classic psychedelics (including psilocybin, DMT/ayahuasca and LSD) are thought to exert their psychedelic effects via serotonin 5-HT2A agonism (or partial agonism).[18–22] Consistent with this hypothesis, pretreatment with 5-HT2A receptor antagonists (such as ketanserine, MDL-100,907) has been shown to nullify the effects of psychedelics across many preclinical[23,24] and clinical studies,[21,25,26] with some notable exceptions.[27,28] Serotonin 5-HT2A receptors are rich in frontal and paralimbic regions of the brain; regions that are part of the default mode network (DMN), which is involved in emotional regulation, introspection, and rumination. Resting-state functional magnetic resonance imaging (fMRI) studies suggest that the antidepressant effect of psychedelics may be related to the modulation of the DMN.[29,30] There is however significant heterogeneity in resting-state fMRI studies that have made it difficult to draw consistent conclusions across studies.[31]

However, emerging evidence suggests the potential role of alternate mechanisms. Classic psychedelics such as psilocybin and DMT bind to several other receptors, including 5-HT1A, 5-HT2B, 5-HT6, 5-HT2C receptor, alpha-adrenergic receptors, sigma-1 receptor, trace amine-associated receptor (TAAR-1), and may alter levels of dopamine and glutamate.[32,33] Atypical psychedelics seem to exert their effect via non-serotoninergic mechanisms. In addition, some animal studies show that antidepressant response is retained despite pre-treatment with ketanserin (a 5-HT2A antagonist),[28] suggesting the possibility a more complex mechanism that involves synaptic plasticity. In preclinical studies, psilocybin has been shown to result in rapid increase in dendritic spines within 24 hours, in the frontal cortex (in a mouse model of learned helplessness).[34] Notably, this increase in dendritic spines was persistent when examined at 1 month.[34] Such a psychoplastogenic mechanism (ie, mediating an increase in synaptic plasticity) is also attractive in being able to explain the seemingly long-lasting effects (ie, as long as 6 months) seen after treatment with a single dose of psilocybin.[35] Consistent with this hypothesis, studies of psilocybin have also shown an increase in the synthesis of brain-derived neurotrophic factor (BDNF).[36]

Psychological mechanisms such as openness to experience, ego-dissolution, and cognitive flexibility have been associated with improvements in symptoms of MDD with psychedelics.[30] Psychedelics induce several different subjective experiences encompassing changes in mood, thought, cognition, and perception, which are sometimes experienced as a dream-like state, or memory flashes.[37,38] Subjects also report ego-dissolution, audio-visual synesthesia, derealization, depersonalization, and profound mystical experiences characterized by feelings of boundarylessness and enhanced introspection.[2–4] These psychedelic or mystical experiences may have an important role in mediating the antidepressant response.[39] It is, however, not entirely clear that a psychedelic response is necessary or sufficient for an anti-depressant response.[40] For example, studies have shown that ketamine administered intraoperatively improved postoperative mood, even though patients were unconscious at the time of administration.[41–43]

Synthesis of compounds with a similar mechanism of antidepressant action as psychedelics but without hallucinogenic properties are in development and tested in mice models. One such compound is "Tabernanthalog," a non-toxic, non-hallucinogenic analog of Ibogaine. In mice models, it promoted dendritic growth and increased dendritic spine density. These changes in neural plasticity have been previously reported with ketamine and suggest a similar antidepressant mechanism of action.[44]

Evidence for the Efficacy of Psychedelics in Treatment-Resistant Depression

Although there are a large number of studies with psychedelics in MDD, currently, to date there are only 5 published studies in TRD (**Table 2**).

Efficacy of psilocybin in treatment-resistant depression

There is 1 randomized controlled trial (RCT) of psilocybin in TRD.[45] In a large phase 2, double-blind, randomized clinical trial conducted by COMPASS Pathways, adults ($n = 233$) with TRD, across 10 countries, were randomized to receive one of three doses of psilocybin: 25 mg psilocybin ($n = 79$), 10 mg psilocybin ($n = 75$) and 1 mg psilocybin (active control) ($n = 79$). All participants received psychedelic-assisted psychotherapy in addition to drug/placebo. Depression severity was assessed using Montgomery–Åsberg Depression Rating Scale (MADRS) at baseline and at 3 weeks. The mean MADRS score at baseline was 31.9 ± 5.4 in the 25 mg psilocybin arm, 33.0 ± 6.3 in the 10 mg psilocybin arm, and 32.7 ± 6.2 in the 1 mg psilocybin (active placebo) arm. Least-squares mean change in score from baseline to week 3 were -12.0 ± 1.3 in 25 mg psilocybin arm; -7.9 ± 1.4 in 10 mg psilocybin arm and -5.4 ± 1.4 in 1 mg psilocybin (active placebo) arm. The highest dose of psilocybin (25 mg), but not the intermediate dose (10 mg), resulted in significantly lower levels of depressive symptoms (95% confidence interval [CI], -10.2 to -2.9; $P < .001$) after 3 weeks compared with the active control (1 mg psilocybin). The incidence of response with the 25 mg psilocybin (37%) was however numerically lower than that seen in TRD trials of other antidepressants, such as citalopram (54.12%) or desipramine (55.22%).[46,47] In addition, study participants were noted to initiate antidepressant treatment at a rate of 12% between baseline and 3-week post-dose ($n = 27$) and 26% between week 3 and week 12 ($n = 60$), probably reflective of limited efficacy.[45]

Of relevance to the limited efficacy seen in the above trial, psilocybin and escitalopram were compared in a phase 2, double-blind, randomized, controlled trial in patients with a moderate-to-severe MDD. The psilocybin group received 25 mg of psilocybin 3 weeks apart plus 6 weeks of daily placebo. The escitalopram group received 1 mg of psilocybin 3 weeks apart plus 6 weeks of daily escitalopram. Quick Inventory of Depressive Symptomatology–Self-Report (QIDS-SR-16) was used to assess the symptoms at baseline and 6 weeks. The trial did not find any significant difference in the antidepressant effects between psilocybin and escitalopram.[48]

Carhart-Harris and colleagues[49] conducted an open-label study in n= 12 patients (6 women, 6 men) with TRD. Participants received 2 oral doses of psilocybin (10 mg and 25 mg, 1 week apart). The study design included an assisted-psychotherapy paradigm comprising 3 separate psychotherapy sessions—a preparatory session (before dosing), non-directive supportive therapy (during the dosing session), and psychological debriefing or integrative session (1 week after the dosing session). During the preparatory session, patients were encouraged to discuss their opinion about the origin of their depression, followed by information about psilocybin's psychological effects and

Table 2
Summary of studies of psychedelics in treatment-resistant depression

Study	Study Design	N	Diagnosis	Mean Age (SD)	Intervention	Measurement Time Points	Assessment	Mean Depression Score at Baseline	Mean Reduction in Depression (SD)	Effect Size	Dropout
Carhart-Harris et al,[49] 2016	Open-label	12	TRD	42.7 (10.2)	Psilocybin 10 mg, then 25 mg 7 d later	Week 1,2,3,5, 3 mo	QIDS, BDI	QIDS: 19.2 (2.0) BDI: 33.7 (7.1)	QIDS: 1 wk (−11.8); 3 mo (−9.2) BDI: 1 wk (−25.0), 3 mo (−18.5)	Hedges' g 1 wk = 3.1 (QIDS), 2.5 (BDI), 3 mo = 2.0 (QIDS), 2.0 (BDI)	0
Carhart-Harris et al,[50] 2018	Open-label	19	TRD	44.1 (11.0)	Psilocybin 10 mg, then 25 mg 7 d later	Week 1,2,3,5, 3 mo and 6 mo	QIDS, BDI	QIDS: 19 (2.7) BDI: 35 (7.4)	BDI: 6 mo −14.9 (12.0)	Cohen's d 6 mo = 1.6 (QIDS), 1.4 (BDI)	0
Palhano-Fontes et al,[51] 2019	Randomized, placebo controlled	29	TRD	39.7 (11.3)	Ayahuasca 0.36 mg/kg	Baseline, Days 1, 2 and 7	HAMD, MADRS	HAMD: 24.1 (5.3) MADRS: 36.1 (6.1)	HAMD: Day 7: −14.4 MADRS: Day 7: −24.6	Cohen's d HAMD: 2.2 at Day 7 MADRS:2.9 at day 7 (1.49 between-group)	1
D'Souza et al,[52] 2022	Open-label	10	TRD	43.5 (13.9)	DMT 0.1 mg/kg, 0.3 mg/kg 48 h apart	Baseline, 1 d after 0.1 mg/kg, 1 d after 0.3 mg/kg	HAMD-17	HAMD-17: 23.86 (4.45)	HAMD-17: Day 1 after 0.1 mg/kg: −1 Day 1 after 0.3 mg/kg: −4.5	Hedges' g = 0.75 after 0.3 mg/kg dose	0
Goodwin et al,[45] 2022	Phase 2 double-blind, randomized	233	TRD	39.8 (12.2)	Psilocybin 25 mg, 10 mg, 1 mg (control)	Baseline, 3 wk	MADRS	MADRS: 31.9 (5.4) in 25 mg arm 33.0 (6.3) in 10 mg arm 32.7 (6.2) in 1 mg arm	MADRS: −12.0 (1.3) in 25 mg arm −7.9 (1.4) in 10 mg arm −5.4 (1.4) in 1 mg arm	24 by week 12	

Abbreviations: BDI, beck depression inventory; HAMD-17, Hamilton Depression Rating scale-17 item; MADRS, Montgomery–Asberg Depression Rating Scale; QIDS, the dosing session. During the dosing- session, participants listened to music while wearing eyeshades. Depressive symptoms were assessed using the Quick Inventory of Depressive Symptoms (QIDS) at 1 week and 3 months of treatment. Depressive symptoms were significantly reduced at 1 week (mean QIDS difference $-11 \cdot 8$, 95% CI $-9 \cdot 15$ to $-14 \cdot 35$, $P = 0 \cdot 002$, Hedges' g = $3 \cdot 1$) and 3 months ($-9 \cdot 2$, 95% CI $-5 \cdot 69$ to $-12 \cdot 71$, $P = 0 \cdot 003$, Hedges' g = 2) as compared with baseline. Improvement in anhedonia and anxiety was also noted.[49]

The group conducted a follow-up study which included additional participants (n = 20). Participants were assessed 6 months following treatment using self-rated QIDS (QIDS-SR16) and Beck Depression Inventory (BDI). Sustained reduction in depressive symptoms was noted at the 6-month follow-up period (QIDS: Cohen's d = 1.6, P = .004; BDI: mean reduction = -14.9, Cohen's d = 1.4, P < .001).[50]

Efficacy of Ayahuasca/N,N-Dimethyltryptamine in treatment-resistant depression
Palhano-Fontes and colleagues[51] conducted a RCT investigating Ayahuasca in patients with TRD (n= 29). A 14 patients received 0.36 mg/kg DMT; and15 patients received placebo. On the dosing day, subjects were reminded of the expected experience, and were asked to remain quiet with their eyes closed during the dosing session. They were also allowed to listen to a predefined music playlist and received support from at least two investigators throughout the session. Depression severity was assessed using the Hamilton Depression Rating Scale and the Montgomery-Åsberg Depression Rating Scale (MADRS) at baseline, day 1 (D1), day 2 (D2), and day 7 (D7) after dosing. As compared with placebo, Ayahuasca was reported to have significant antidepressant effects at all-time points. The ayahuasca group had significantly lower MADRS scores on D1, D2 (P = .04), and D7 (P < .0001). The between-group effect size was reported to increase from D1 to D7 (D1: Cohen's d = 0.84; D7: Cohen's d = 1.49). Response and remission rates were also higher in the ayahuasca group. At D7, the response rate for ayahuasca was significantly higher [OR 4.95 (95% CI 1.11 to 21.02); P = .04]. Remission rates showed a trend toward significance [OR 7.78 (95% CI 0.81 to 77.48); P = .054].

D'Souza and colleagues[52] conducted an open-label, fixed order, dose escalation (0.1 mg/kg then 0.3 mg/kg) exploratory study to investigate the safety, efficacy, and tolerability of intravenous DMT in patients with MDD (n = 7) and healthy controls (n = 3). The study was conducted in a hospital setting with minimal psychotherapy support. The two dosing sessions (0.1 and 0.3 mg/kg) were at least 48 hours apart. HAMD-17 was used to assess the symptoms of depression at baseline and 1 day after each dosing session. Although there was no significant reduction in depression severity following the 0.1 mg/kg session as compared with the baseline, there was a significant reduction in depression severity scores post-0.3 mg/kg session as compared with baseline (20.20 [SD 7.82]) (difference -4.5 [95% CI: -7.80 to -1.20] $t = -3.50$, P = .017; Hedge's g = 0.75). There was also a significant difference in HAMD-17 scores between the 0.1 mg/kg and 0.3 mg/kg dose (difference -3.5 [95% CI: -6.87 to -0.013] $t = -2.67$, P = .044; Hedge's g = 0.55).

Efficacy of lysergic acid diethylamide in treatment-resistant depression
No published RCTs have evaluated the efficacy of LSD in TRD to date. One small pilot study (n = 12) compared 2 moderate LSD doses (200 µg) to active placebo LSD (20 µg) in patients experiencing anxiety associated with life-threatening diseases.[38] In total, 7 of the 12 participants had a comorbid diagnosis of a depressive disorder and an anxiety disorder. Compared with placebo, LSD-assisted psychotherapy was associated with a reduction in mean scores from baseline (10.0 ± 4.5) to 2 months

postintervention (7.5 ± 3.3) on the HADS-D. These results were largely sustained at the 12-month follow-up (7.6 ± 4.7). Measures of depressive symptoms were considered secondary in this study; therefore, to reduce multiplicity, the authors did not conduct significance testing or control for depressive symptoms at baseline.[38] The conclusions that can be drawn from these results regarding LSD-assisted psychotherapy for depressive symptoms associated with life-threatening diseases are limited.

Efficacy of 3,4-methylenedioxymethamphetamine in treatment-resistant depression

No published RCTs have evaluated the efficacy of MDMA in TRD to date. MDMA has been designated as a "Breakthrough Therapy" in treating post-traumatic stress disorder (PTSD) by the US Food and Drug Administration (FDA). Although anxiety disorders have had the majority of focus in clinical research, MDMA has also been investigated in treating mood disorders such as depression. Wolfson and colleagues[53] conducted a randomized, double-blind, controlled trial investigating the effects of MDMA for the treatment of anxiety disorders with the impact on depression as a secondary outcome. $N = 18$ participants (F = 14 and M = 4) were enrolled in the study, out of which $N = 13$ received MDMA, and $N = 5$ received a placebo. $N = 14$ participants were diagnosed with depression. Depression was assessed using Beck Depression Inventory II (BDI-II) and Montgomery-Asberg Depression Rating Scale (MADRS) at baseline, post two sessions, treatment exit, and 6 and 12-month follow-up. Although there were no statistically significant differences in depressive symptoms post two experimental sessions as compared with baseline ($P > .05$), there was a significant decrease in depressive symptoms at the following time points-treatment exit, 6-month follow-up, and 12-month follow-up ($P < .0001$).

Neurobiological Correlates of Response to Psychedelics

There has been increasing interest in understanding the neurobiological effects of psychedelics and their relationship to treatment response. In human studies using fMRI, psychedelics have been shown to primarily affect amygdala activation and altered functional connectivity in default-mode network (DMN) (primarily with psilocybin, DMT) and the thalamocortical salience network (primarily with LSD).[54,55] In three studies with psilocybin, these changes correlated with treatment response.[29,56,57] However, there is variability across studies with respect to the brain regions that correlate with treatment response. Preliminary evidence suggests that the DMN and limbic networks may be a target for future research on the neural mechanisms of psychedelics.[54,55] These changes have also been variously interpreted as a change in brain modularity and an increase in cognitive flexibility. There is however, recognition that there's wide heterogeneity in fMRI paradigms and analysis methods such as thalamus seed-based connectivity and DMN functional connectivity, which may be contributing to inconsistent results across studies.[31] Further work in the area with standardized paradigms and independent replication is warranted to identify specific neurobiological effects that are causally linked to treatment response.

Role of Psychedelic-Assisted Therapy

One of the criticisms of current clinical trials with psychedelics is that the inclusion of psychedelic-assisted therapy may inflate the expectancy response.[58,59] Nevertheless, psychedelic-assisted therapy may have an important role in clinical treatment settings. Psychedelic-assisted therapy typically comprises of 3 components (1) preparatory sessions, (2) supportive psychotherapy during the psychedelic experience, and (3) integration sessions following the experience[49,60] (**Box 1**). The preparatory session typically involves a discussion about the individual's experience with depression,

Box 1	
Components of psychedelic psychotherapy	
Session	**Components**
Preparatory session (1 or more sessions before the psychedelic experience)	Involves discussion about the individual's experience with depression, exploration of psychological origins of depression and a discussion of the psychedelic experience.
	May also include simulation of aspects of the dosing session (eg, familiarizing subjects with the room, wearing eyeshades and listening to music that will be used during the dosing session)
Supportive psychotherapy session (during the psychedelic experience)	Involves a therapist being physically present and incorporates aspects of empathetic listening, reassurance, and the use of grounding techniques
Integration session (1 or more sessions following the psychedelic experience)	Involves debriefing of the subject's experience and an effort at making meaning of the experience; advice about psychological reframing and cultivating change for the future

exploration of psychological origins of depression, and a discussion of the psychedelic experience. The preparatory session may also include a simulation of aspects of the dosing session (eg, familiarizing subjects with the room, wearing eyeshades, and listening to music that will be used during the dosing session). The supportive psychotherapy session during dosing typically involves a therapist being physically present and incorporates aspects of empathetic listening, reassurance, and the use of grounding techniques. The integration session that occurs following the dosing session involves debriefing of the subject's experience and an effort at making meaning of the experience and advice about psychological reframing and cultivating change for the future.

Potential Risks Associated with Use of Psychedelics

One of the challenges with the use of psychedelics is the risk of serotonin-syndrome (albeit small) when given in combination with other serotoninergic antidepressants.[61] Currently, studies typically require a washout period (approximately 2 to 4 weeks[48,50] or 5 half-lives[62]) during which antidepressants are tapered and stopped to minimize the risk of serotonin syndrome. There is thus a risk of discontinuation symptoms (constellation of new-onset symptoms after discontinuation of serotonergic antidepressants) and/or worsening of depressive symptoms (which can occur from the loss of therapeutic effects of antidepressant).[63-65] Therefore, greater monitoring and psychological support is needed during this period.

In clinical trials, elevated blood pressure was the most common physiologic adverse effect with Psilocybin and MDMA but did not require medical intervention. The one RCT of psilocybin in TRD noted a high rate of adverse events (77%) including headache, nausea, dizziness and suicidal ideation/behavior.[45] The rate of worsening of suicidal ideation/behavior between baseline and week 3 was 14% in the 25 mg psilocybin arm ($n = 11$), 17% in the 10 mg psilocybin arm ($n = 13$), and 9% in the 1 mg psilocybin (active control arm) ($n = 7$).[45] Anxiety, confusion and nausea were other prevalent acute adverse effects associated with psilocybin, ayahuasca, LSD.[49,51,66] Anxiety was mostly reported before sessions whereas confusion occurred at the peak of the session. Headache was a late adverse effect, reported in the high-dose psilocybin (25 mg) group and MDMA studies.[49,67] Another long-term effect of psychedelics, although rare is "Hallucinogen Persisting Perception Disorder" (HPPD). This may comprise of visual, sensory-perceptual disturbances that may result in functional impairment.[68–70] There also appears to be a small risk of psychosis that has been reported in the literature.

Limitations of the Current Evidence

One of the limitations of the current evidence is the small sample size of most of the studies that have been conducted to date. Although the small open-label studies have shown large effects, the effects in larger RCTs have been modest. The heterogeneity in clinical-trial design, the difficulty with adequate blinding for a compound associated with profound subjective effects, and the effects of psychedelic-assisted psychotherapy make it challenging to discern whether the large effect sizes in the studies is because of a true effect of the psychedelic, the effects of psychotherapy or an inflated expectancy response. It is also important to note that participants in the current studies have been able to successfully tolerate an antidepressant washout period of 2 to 4 weeks. This may not be generalizable to all patients with MDD, some of whom have dramatic worsening of mood and suicidal ideation when off antidepressants. The majority of participants in current studies are Caucasian individuals treated in controlled research settings. A crucial question remains whether people from diverse racial, ethnic, socioeconomic backgrounds and history of trauma will respond and benefit from psychedelic therapy. There's thus a need for larger, adequately powered RCTs of longer duration and independent replication of findings in diverse populations.

There are several ongoing studies using psychedelics, including salvinorin-A, ibogaine, LSD, 5-MeO-DMT, and DMT-fumarate in the treatment of MDD/TRD.[15] COMPASS pathways, a mental health care company is developing COMP360 Psilocybin, and is involved in clinical trials for TRD in Europe and North America. Clinicaltrials. gov has listed 7 studies investigating the effects of COMP360 psilocybin in TRD, 1 in PTSD, 2 in anorexia nervosa, and 1 in body dysmorphic disorder.

There is also increasing recognition that psychedelic research is currently "trapped in a hype bubble driven largely by media and industry interests" as exemplified by the Gartner Hyper Cycle that is thought to represent phases of public perception following new technological advancements.[71] The trajectory of the hype cycle begins with a new innovation ("technological trigger") followed by a steep increase in enthusiasm and unrealistic expectations ("peak of inflated expectations"), that reverses steeply following negative results ("trough of disillusionment") and morphs into a more, gentle period where realistic expectations are better crystallized ("slope of enlightenment") and stabilizes into a period when mainstream adoption begins to take place ("period of productivity"). The challenge for the field is to overcome the hyper bubble and hyped claims of miraculous cure and delineate strategies that capitalize on the therapeutic potential of these compounds and minimize risks.

SUMMARY AND FUTURE DIRECTIONS

Psychedelics offer promise as a treatment for TRD but the current evidence is limited.

Amidst the fervid enthusiasm for the utility of these compounds, a few critical questions remain to be answered before psychedelic treatments can transform the treatment of TRD. First, it is unclear whether a psychedelic response is necessary or sufficient for an antidepressant response. This would be important for identification of the ideal dose that maximizes benefits and minimizes side-effects. Second, it is unclear whether psychedelics can produce as robust an antidepressant response in the absence of assisted psychotherapy. The addition of psychedelic psychotherapy if it isn't necessary for the therapeutic effects, incurs additional logistical challenges, especially in the use of short-acting psychedelics, such as DMT. Third, it is not known whether repeated dosing is required to maximize benefits and whether repeated dosing would result in the development of tolerance. This information is important to help design a more effective treatment protocol. Answers to these questions would accelerate the clinical development of psychedelics from research settings to the clinic.

CLINICS CARE POINTS

- Psychedelics offer promise as a treatment for treatment-resistant depression (TRD) but the current evidence is limited.

- While small studies with psilocybin, and DMT/ayahuasca show improvements in depression, the individual contribution of psychotherapy and patient expectancy remain to be delineated.

- The proposed neurobiological mechanisms underlying the effect of psychedelics include altered synaptic plasticity, functional connectivity and cognitive flexibility.

- There is also increasing recognition that psychedelic research is currently subject to the effects of the Hype Cycle that is "driven largely by media and industry interests".

DISCLOSURE

Dr S. Kamal has nothing to disclose. Dr R. Radhakrishnan has received research funding/support from Wallace Research Foundation, United States, Neurocrine Biosciences and Jazz Pharmaceuticals. Dr M. Jha has received contract research grants from ACADIA Pharmaceuticals, United States, Neurocrine Bioscience, Navitor/Supernus, and Janssen Research & Development, United States, an educational grant to serve as Section Editor of the Psychiatry & Behavioral Health Learning Network, consultant fees from Eleusis Therapeutics US, Inc, Janssen Global Services, Janssen Scientific Affairs, Worldwide Clinical Trials/Eliem and Inversargo, and Guidepoint Global, and honoraria from North American Center for Continuing Medical Education, Medscape/WebMD, Clinical Care Options, and Global Medical Education.

REFERENCES

1. Akil H, Gordon J, Hen R, et al. Treatment resistant depression: A multi-scale, systems biology approach. Neurosci Biobehav Rev 2018;84:272–88.
2. World Health O. Depression and other common mental disorders: global health estimates. Geneva: World Health Organization; 2017.
3. Dwyer JB, Aftab A, Radhakrishnan R, et al. Hormonal Treatments for Major Depressive Disorder: State of the Art. Am J Psychiatry 2020;177(8):686–705.
4. Jha MK, Trivedi MH. Pharmacogenomics and Biomarkers of Depression. Handb Exp Pharmacol 2019;250:101–13.
5. The evidence-based guide to antidepressant medications. Arlington, VA: American Psychiatric Publishing, Inc; 2012.
6. McIntyre RS, Filteau MJ, Martin L, et al. Treatment-resistant depression: definitions, review of the evidence, and algorithmic approach. J Affect Disord 2014; 156:1–7.

7. Sforzini L, Worrell C, Kose M, et al. A Delphi-method-based consensus guideline for definition of treatment-resistant depression for clinical trials. Mol Psychiatry 2022;27(3):1286–99.
8. Alnefeesi Y, Chen-Li D, Krane E, et al. Real-world effectiveness of ketamine in treatment-resistant depression: A systematic review & meta-analysis. J Psychiatr Res 2022;151:693–709.
9. Nunez NA, Joseph B, Pahwa M, et al. Augmentation strategies for treatment resistant major depression: A systematic review and network meta-analysis. J Affect Disord 2022;302:385–400.
10. Li H, Cui L, Li J, et al. Comparative efficacy and acceptability of neuromodulation procedures in the treatment of treatment-resistant depression: a network meta-analysis of randomized controlled trials. J Affect Disord 2021;287:115–24.
11. Hosanagar A, Cusimano J, Radhakrishnan R. Therapeutic Potential of Psychedelics in the Treatment of Psychiatric Disorders, Part 1: Psychopharmacology and Neurobiological Effects. J Clin Psychiatry 2021;82(2):20ac13786.
12. Kelmendi B, Kaye AP, Pittenger C, et al. Psychedelics. Curr Biol 2022;32(2):R63–7.
13. Gasser P, Holstein D, Michel Y, et al. Safety and efficacy of lysergic acid diethylamide-assisted psychotherapy for anxiety associated with life-threatening diseases. J Nerv Ment Dis 2014 Jul;202(7):513–20.
14. Harden MT, Smith SE, Niehoff JA, et al. Antidepressive effects of the kappa-opioid receptor agonist salvinorin A in a rat model of anhedonia. Behav Pharmacol 2012 Oct;23(7):710–5.
15. Siegel AN, Meshkat S, Benitah K, et al. Registered clinical studies investigating psychedelic drugs for psychiatric disorders. J Psychiatr Res 2021 Jul;139:71–81.
16. O'Brien B, Wilkinson ST, Mathew SJ. An Update on Community Ketamine Practices. Am J Psychiatry 2022 May;179(5):393–4.
17. Oliver PA, Snyder AD, Feinn R, et al. Clinical Effectiveness of Intravenous Racemic Ketamine Infusions in a Large Community Sample of Patients With Treatment-Resistant Depression, Suicidal Ideation, and Generalized Anxiety Symptoms: A Retrospective Chart Review. J Clin Psychiatry 2022 Sep 12;83(6):21m14336.
18. Kometer M, Schmidt A, Bachmann R, et al. Psilocybin Biases Facial Recognition, Goal-Directed Behavior, and Mood State Toward Positive Relative to Negative Emotions Through Different Serotonergic Subreceptors. Biol Psychiatr 2012;72(11):898–906.
19. Preller KH, Pokorny T, Hock A, et al. Effects of serotonin 2A/1A receptor stimulation on social exclusion processing. Proc Natl Acad Sci USA 2016;113(18):5119–24.
20. Preller KH, Duerler P, Burt JB, et al. Psilocybin Induces Time-Dependent Changes in Global Functional Connectivity. Biol Psychiatr 2020;88(2):197–207.
21. Vollenweider FX, Vollenweider-Scherpenhuyzen MFI, Bäbler A, et al. Psilocybin induces schizophrenia-like psychosis in humans via a serotonin-2 agonist action. Neuroreport 1998;9(17):3897–902.
22. Madsen MK, Fisher PM, Burmester D, et al. Psychedelic effects of psilocybin correlate with serotonin 2A receptor occupancy and plasma psilocin levels. Neuropsychopharmacology 2019 2019/06/01;44(7):1328–34.
23. Catlow BJ, Song S, Paredes DA, et al. Effects of psilocybin on hippocampal neurogenesis and extinction of trace fear conditioning. Exp Brain Res 2013 Aug;228(4):481–91.

24. Tyls F, Palenicek T, Kaderabek L, et al. Sex differences and serotonergic mechanisms in the behavioural effects of psilocin. Behav Pharmacol 2016 Jun;27(4): 309–20.

25. Quednow BB, Kometer M, Geyer MA, et al. Psilocybin-induced deficits in automatic and controlled inhibition are attenuated by ketanserin in healthy human volunteers. Neuropsychopharmacology 2012 Feb;37(3):630–40.

26. Kraehenmann R, Pokorny D, Vollenweider L, et al. Dreamlike effects of LSD on waking imagery in humans depend on serotonin 2A receptor activation. Psychopharmacology (Berl) 2017 Jul;234(13):2031–46.

27. Carter OL, Hasler F, Pettigrew JD, et al. Psilocybin links binocular rivalry switch rate to attention and subjective arousal levels in humans. Psychopharmacology (Berl) 2007 Dec;195(3):415–24.

28. Hesselgrave N, Troppoli TA, Wulff AB, et al. Harnessing psilocybin: antidepressant-like behavioral and synaptic actions of psilocybin are independent of 5-HT2R activation in mice. Proc Natl Acad Sci U S A 2021 Apr 27; 118(17). e2022489118.

29. Carhart-Harris RL, Roseman L, Bolstridge M, et al. Psilocybin for treatment-resistant depression: fMRI-measured brain mechanisms. Sci Rep 2017 Oct 13; 7(1):13187.

30. Doss MK, Povazan M, Rosenberg MD, et al. Psilocybin therapy increases cognitive and neural flexibility in patients with major depressive disorder. Transl Psychiatry 2021 Nov 8;11(1):574.

31. McCulloch DE, Knudsen GM, Barrett FS, et al. Psychedelic resting-state neuroimaging: A review and perspective on balancing replication and novel analyses. Neurosci Biobehav Rev 2022 Jul;138:104689.

32. De Gregorio D, Enns JP, Nunez NA, et al. d-Lysergic acid diethylamide, psilocybin, and other classic hallucinogens: Mechanism of action and potential therapeutic applications in mood disorders. Prog Brain Res 2018;242:69–96.

33. Nichols DE. Psychedelics. Pharmacological Reviews 2016;68(2):264–355.

34. Shao LX, Liao C, Gregg I, et al. Psilocybin induces rapid and persistent growth of dendritic spines in frontal cortex in vIvo. Neuron 2021 Aug 18;109(16):2535–2544 e2534.

35. Calder AE, Hasler G. Towards an understanding of psychedelic-induced neuroplasticity. Neuropsychopharmacology 2022;48(1):104–12.

36. de Almeida RN, Galvao ACM, da Silva FS, et al. Modulation of Serum Brain-Derived Neurotrophic Factor by a Single Dose of Ayahuasca: Observation From a Randomized Controlled Trial. Front Psychol 2019;10:1234.

37. Grinspoon L, Bakalar JB. Psychedelic drugs reconsidered. New York: Basic Books; 1979.

38. Gasser P, Holstein D, Michel Y, et al. Safety and Efficacy of Lysergic Acid Diethylamide-Assisted Psychotherapy for Anxiety Associated With Life-threatening Diseases. J Nerv Ment Dis 2014;202(7):513–20.

39. Yaden DB, Griffiths RR. The Subjective Effects of Psychedelics Are Necessary for Their Enduring Therapeutic Effects. ACS Pharmacol Transl Sci 2021;4(2):568–72.

40. Olson DE. The Subjective Effects of Psychedelics May Not Be Necessary for Their Enduring Therapeutic Effects. ACS Pharmacol Transl Sci 2021 Apr 9;4(2): 563–7.

41. Liu P, Li P, Li Q, et al. Effect of Pretreatment of S-Ketamine On Postoperative Depression for Breast Cancer Patients. J Invest Surg 2021 Aug;34(8):883–8.

42. Kudoh A, Takahira Y, Katagai H, et al. Small-dose ketamine improves the postoperative state of depressed patients. Anesth Analg 2002;95(1):114–8, table of contents.

43. Jiang M, Wang MH, Wang XB, et al. Effect of intraoperative application of ketamine on postoperative depressed mood in patients undergoing elective orthopedic surgery. J Anesth 2016;30(2):232–7.

44. Cameron LP, Tombari RJ, Lu J, et al. A non-hallucinogenic psychedelic analogue with therapeutic potential. Nature 2021;589(7842):474–9.

45. Goodwin GM, Aaronson ST, Alvarez O, et al. Single-Dose Psilocybin for a Treatment-Resistant Episode of Major Depression. N Engl J Med 2022;387(18):1637–48.

46. Souery D, Serretti A, Calati R, et al. Citalopram versus desipramine in treatment resistant depression: effect of continuation or switching strategies: a randomized open study. World J Biol Psychiatry 2011;12(5):364–75.

47. Madras BK. Psilocybin in Treatment-Resistant Depression. N Engl J Med 2022;387(18):1708–9.

48. Carhart-Harris R, Giribaldi B, Watts R, et al. Trial of Psilocybin versus Escitalopram for Depression. N Engl J Med 2021;384(15):1402–11.

49. Carhart-Harris RL, Bolstridge M, Rucker J, et al. Psilocybin with psychological support for treatment-resistant depression: an open-label feasibility study. Lancet Psychiatr 2016;3(7):619–27.

50. Carhart-Harris RL, Bolstridge M, Day CMJ, et al. Psilocybin with psychological support for treatment-resistant depression: six-month follow-up. Psychopharmacology 2018;235(2):399–408.

51. Palhano-Fontes F, Barreto D, Onias H, et al. Rapid antidepressant effects of the psychedelic ayahuasca in treatment-resistant depression: a randomized placebo-controlled trial. Psychological medicine 2019;49(4):655–63.

52. D'Souza DC, Syed SA, Flynn LT, et al. Exploratory study of the dose-related safety, tolerability, and efficacy of dimethyltryptamine (DMT) in healthy volunteers and major depressive disorder. Neuropsychopharmacology 2022;47(10):1854–62.

53. Wolfson PE, Andries J, Feduccia AA, et al. MDMA-assisted psychotherapy for treatment of anxiety and other psychological distress related to life-threatening illnesses: a randomized pilot study. Sci Rep 2020;10(1):20442.

54. Kuburi S, Di Passa AM, Tassone VK, et al. Neuroimaging Correlates of Treatment Response with Psychedelics in Major Depressive Disorder: A Systematic Review. Chronic Stress (Thousand Oaks) 2022;6. 24705470221115342.

55. Avram M, Muller F, Rogg H, et al. Characterizing Thalamocortical (Dys)connectivity Following D-Amphetamine, LSD, and MDMA Administration. Biol Psychiatry Cogn Neurosci Neuroimaging 2022 Sep;7(9):885–94.

56. Mertens LJ, Wall MB, Roseman L, et al. Therapeutic mechanisms of psilocybin: Changes in amygdala and prefrontal functional connectivity during emotional processing after psilocybin for treatment-resistant depression. J Psychopharmacol 2020 Feb;34(2):167–80.

57. Roseman L, Demetriou L, Wall MB, et al. Increased amygdala responses to emotional faces after psilocybin for treatment-resistant depression. Neuropharmacology 2018 Nov;142:263–9.

58. Reiff CM, Richman EE, Nemeroff CB, et al. Psychedelics and Psychedelic-Assisted Psychotherapy. Am J Psychiatry 2020 May 1;177(5):391–410.

59. Hosanagar A, Cusimano J, Radhakrishnan R. Therapeutic Potential of Psyche-delics in Treatment of Psychiatric Disorders, Part 2: Review of the Evidence. J Clin Psychiatry 2021;82(3):20ac13787.
60. Schenberg EE. Psychedelic-Assisted Psychotherapy: A Paradigm Shift in Psychi-atric Research and Development. Front Pharmacol 2018;9:733.
61. Malcolm B, Thomas K. Serotonin toxicity of serotonergic psychedelics. Psycho-pharmacology (Berl) 2022 Jun;239(6):1881–91.
62. Davis AK, Barrett FS, May DG, et al. Effects of Psilocybin-Assisted Therapy on Major Depressive Disorder: A Randomized Clinical Trial. JAMA Psychiatr 2021 May 1;78(5):481–9.
63. Jha MK, Rush AJ, Trivedi MH. When Discontinuing SSRI Antidepressants Is a Challenge: Management Tips. Am J Psychiatry 2018 Dec 1;175(12):1176–84.
64. Waldvogel N, Akira A. Antidepressant Discontinuation Syndrome Resulting in a Suicide Attempt: A Case Report. J Clin Psychiatry 2022;83(6):22cr14562.
65. Jha MK. Discontinuing Antidepressants: How Can Clinicians Guide Patients and Drive Research? J Clin Psychiatry 2019 Nov 26;80(6).
66. Gasser P, Kirchner K, Passie T. LSD-assisted psychotherapy for anxiety associ-ated with a life-threatening disease: a qualitative study of acute and sustained subjective effects. J Psychopharmacol 2015 Jan;29(1):57–68.
67. Breeksema JJ, Kuin BW, Kamphuis J, et al. Adverse events in clinical treatments with serotonergic psychedelics and MDMA: A mixed-methods systematic review. J Psychopharmacol 2022;36(10):1100–17.
68. Lerner AG, Gelkopf M, Skladman I, et al. Flashback and Hallucinogen Persisting Perception Disorder: clinical aspects and pharmacological treatment approach. Isr J Psychiatry Relat Sci 2002;39(2):92–9.
69. A GL, Goodman C, Rudinski D, et al. LSD Flashbacks - The Appearance of New Visual Imagery Not Experienced During Initial Intoxication: Two Case Reports. Isr J Psychiatry Relat Sci 2014;51(4):307–9.
70. A GL, Rudinski D, Bor O, et al. Flashbacks and HPPD: A Clinical-oriented Concise Review. Isr J Psychiatry Relat Sci 2014;51(4):296–301.
71. Yaden DB, Potash JB, Griffiths RR. Preparing for the Bursting of the Psychedelic Hype Bubble. JAMA Psychiatr 2022 Oct 1;79(10):943–4.

Noninvasive Brain Stimulation Techniques for Treatment-Resistant Depression

Transcranial Magnetic Stimulation and Transcranial Direct Current Stimulation

Andrea Boscutti, MD[a,b,1],
Juliana Mendonca De Figueiredo, MD[a,1], Dana Razouq, MD[a],
Nicholas Murphy, PhD[c,d], Raymond Cho, MD[c,d],
Sudhakar Selvaraj, MBBS, DPhil (Oxon), FRCPsych[a,*]

KEYWORDS

- Noninvasive brain stimulation • Transcranial magnetic stimulation
- Transcranial direct current stimulation • Treatment-resistant depression
- Neuromodulation • TMS • tDCS • Neuroplasticity

KEY POINTS

- Transcranial magnetic stimulation is a noninvasive neurostimulation technique approved for treatment-resistant depression (TRD).
- The main advantage over pharmacologic treatments is the low incidence of side effects.
- Open challenges include localization of the stimulation target and selection of stimulation parameters.
- Newer stimulation approaches are shorter, tailored and biomarker-based.
- Transcranial direct current stimulation is a promising alternative for TRD, but it is not currently approved in the United States for clinical use.

[a] Louis. A. Faillace, MD, Department of Psychiatry and Behavioral Sciences, The University of Texas Health Science Center at Houston, Houston, TX, USA; [b] Department of Pathophysiology and Transplantation, University of Milan, Milan, Italy; [c] Baylor College of Medicine, Menninger Department of Psychiatry and Behavioral Sciences, Houston, TX, USA; [d] The Menninger Clinic, Houston, TX, USA
[1] These authors contributed equally to this study.
* Corresponding author. Louis. A. Faillace, MD, Department of Psychiatry and Behavioral Sciences, The University of Texas Health Science Center at Houston, 1941 East Road, Houston, TX.
E-mail address: Sudhakar.selvaraj@uth.tmc.edu

Psychiatr Clin N Am 46 (2023) 307–329
https://doi.org/10.1016/j.psc.2023.02.005
0193-953X/23/© 2023 Elsevier Inc. All rights reserved.

INTRODUCTION

Major depressive disorder is a highly prevalent and debilitating disease, and a leading cause of the global health-related burden.[1] The first treatment approach consists of either psychotherapy and/or pharmacologic interventions, but leads to remission in only one-third of patients. Moreover, these interventions require weeks or months to be effective.[2] In many cases, patients will go on to fail multiple treatments.[3] Depression is defined as treatment-resistant (treatment-resistant depression [TRD]) after a failure to respond to 2 or more antidepressants.[4]

Currently, no validated biomarkers are available to inform clinician decisions,[5] so they rely solely on trial-and-error approaches. The heterogeneity in remission rates among the most commonly prescribed treatments indicates that treatment resistance might be a failing to target the correct underlying neural mechanism. The theory of neural biotyping for depression[6] emphasizes that depression symptomology rarely depends on a singular circuit, and instead results from divergent patterns of synaptic dysfunction within and between cognitive domains. More specifically, the ability to interact with these circuits is available to clinicians due to advances in the field of neuromodulation.

US Food and Drug Administration (FDA)-approved techniques for TRD include transcranial magnetic stimulation (TMS), electroconvulsive therapy (ECT), and vagus nerve stimulation. Transcranial direct current stimulation (tDCS) has undergone a relatively large body of investigation but the technique is not currently FDA-approved for depression.

TMS was approved for clinical use in 2008 and has since become an increasingly popular approach for TRD. Its antidepressant action is thought to depend on the neuroplastic changes induced by the electromagnetic field. Its main clinical advantages include a good safety profile and a low rate of mild side effects. Open challenges include optimizing target localization, selecting parameters of stimulation, and adopting accelerated protocols to improve the rapidity of action. Future directions point toward personalized treatment based on individual biomarkers, such as functional magnetic resonance imaging (fMRI) connectivity measures.

This review will mainly focus on the clinical application of Repetitive Transcranial Magnetic Stimulation (rTMS), covering patient selection, stimulation parameters selection and considerations on safety, side effects, and cost-effectivity. The TMS mechanism of action and future directions are also briefly covered. tDCS is a promising treatment option for TRD; however, it is not currently FDA-approved for clinical use. An overview of this neuromodulation technique is provided in the section "Transcranial direct current stimulation".

NEUROBIOLOGY OF TRANSCRANIAL MAGNETIC STIMULATION
Physical Principles

TMS uses dynamic magnetic fields to influence the activity of small brain regions. Brain stimulation is based on Faraday's law of electromagnetism induction, by which a magnetic field interacts with a conductor to generate an electrical current in the circuit. Ultimately, an action potential is elicited in the neurons of the targeted brain region.[7]

Magnetic fields are generated by passing an electrical current through a coil of wire. Because the coil is placed tangential to the scalp, the resulting magnetic field is normal to the surface of the coil and to the scalp's surface. The magnetic field, in turn, induces an electric field perpendicular to it and parallel to the coil itself. The direction of the generated field is, therefore, highly dependent on the orientation and shape of the coil. Key parameters influenced by the coil shape are the electrical field depth of penetration and focality. All coils follow a depth-focality tradeoff: coils with larger depth are less focal than those with smaller depth, and vice versa.[8] Modern stimulation protocols are typically based on the use of a figure-eight coil design. In this design, 2 circular coils are placed side by side with opposite directions of current flow. The intersection of the 2 coils causes an enhanced magnetic field at the center of the device, improving focality by reducing the degradation of the magnetic field with distance from the coil. Each magnetic field strength can be as high as 2 T at the coil's surface, lasting about 100 microseconds. Notably, the extent of the cortical area stimulated is remarkably small, around 2 mm in diameter.[9]

Action Potential Generation and Neuroplasticity Induction

The magnetic field effect on neuronal activity can be mediated by 2 mechanisms. Although the voltage of the magnetic field can directly generate currents in neurons, the most crucial effect depends on the induced electrical field. Each magnetic pulse causes voltage-gated sodium channels of cortical pyramidal neurons to open, generating bursts of action potential in groups of neurons.[10] The resulting effect can be one of transient neuronal activation or inhibition. The ultimate response to a TMS stimulus is complex, being influenced by the nature of the stimulated neuronal population (excitatory vs inhibitory), the orientation of the electromagnetic field, and, especially, by the functional state of the stimulated brain region.[9,11–13]

In the clinical setting, trains of pulses are delivered at high frequency, with a cumulative effect on the underlying brain tissue. Repetitive, high-frequency stimulation leads to a delayed opening of voltage-gated calcium channels, increasing intracellular calcium levels.[10] Voltage-dependent calcium channels are a key component of TMS-induced synaptic plasticity, an important factor in TMS antidepressant effects.[14] Synaptic plasticity is a property that describes the brain's ability to modify the strength of synaptic transmission.[15] Long-term potentiation and long-term depression involve a persistent increase or decrease in synaptic strength. A series of seminal studies[16,17] showed that while high-frequency (>5 Hz) stimulation is associated with long-term potentiation, low-frequency stimulation (0.2–1 Hz) induces long-term depression of the stimulated area. The ultimate effect on brain plasticity also depends on the stimulation's temporal pattern. For example, intermittent theta-burst stimulation (a specific high-frequency stimulation paradigm) induces long-term potentiation, and continuous theta-burst stimulation is associated with long-term depression.[18]

Transcranial Magnetic Stimulation Target Regions

Left dorsolateral prefrontal cortex

The main stimulation target in clinical settings is the Left dorsolateral prefrontal cortex (LDLPFC). This area is involved in a wide range of demanding task conditions,[19] such as cognitive control and executive functions,[20] emotional processing,[21] top–down attentional control[22] and goal prioritizations,[23] among others. This cortical region is hypoactive in depression,[24] and both pharmacologic[25] and psychotherapy[26] interventions are associated with a functional normalization of LDLPFC. Therefore, high-frequency (ie, excitatory) stimulation of the LDLPFC is the most common TMS protocol used in clinical practice.

Right dorsolateral prefrontal cortex

Another approach is to target the right Dorsolateral prefrontal cortex (DLPFC) (RLPFC) with a low-frequency (i.e., inhibitory) stimulation. Historically, left DLPFC was chosen as the target of excitatory because lesion studies from patients with strokes showed how left-side lesions were associated with higher rates of depression.[27] In comparison, right-side lesions were associated with higher rates of manic symptoms.[28] When the Right dorsolateral prefrontal cortex (RDLPFC) is stimulated with high-frequency TMS, dysphoric symptoms emerge.[29]

A series of neuroimaging studies supported a lateralization component as a putative neurobiological feature of depression. fMRI studies showed an imbalance of left and RDLPFC during emotional judgment tasks, with left hypoactivity and right hyperactivity in depressed patients compared with healthy controls.[30] For this reason, both unilateral low-frequency RDLPFC stimulation and bilateral DLPFC stimulation (high frequency on the left, low frequency on the right) are considered valid stimulation protocols for depression.

Other stimulation targets

The orbitofrontal cortex is a region involved in cognitive reappraisal, emotion regulation, and rewards reversal learning.[31,32] Hyperactivation and hyperconnectivity of this cortical region have been described in depressed patients.[33,34] Recent reports suggest inhibitory, low-frequency stimulation of the right lateral orbitofrontal cortex may provide clinical benefit in patients refractory to stimulation in the above sites. These results, although promising, are based on an open-label trial with small samples,[35,36] and therefore require validation.

Stimulation of the dorsomedial Prefontal Cortex (PFC) (dmPFC) has been proposed as another potential stimulation target.[37] The neurobiological rationale is that dmPFC in patients with depression is a region of increased connectivity between the cognitive control network, default mode network, and affective network.[38] For this reason, randomized sham-controlled targeting of the dmPFC included both stimulatory and inhibitory stimulation arms. However, no significant differences between any of the active stimulation arms and sham treatment arm were found.[39,40] Other potential stimulation targets include the ventromedial PFC[41] and the ventrolateral PFC.[42]

CLINICAL EVIDENCE OF TRANSCRANIAL MAGNETIC STIMULATION EFFICACY IN TREATMENT-RESISTANT DEPRESSION
Randomized Clinical Trials

The first report about the potential therapeutic effect of TMS in depression dates back to 1995.[43] Since then, several clinical studies have been published; however, these were small, and many did not include a sham stimulation arm.[44]

The results of the randomized clinical trial that led to the FDA approval of TMS for TRD were published [45] in 2007. This was the first large, multisite, double-blind, randomized, sham-controlled trial of TMS in TRD. About 325 patients that failed at least one pharmacologic treatment (but not more than 4) were randomized to receive active or sham high-frequency TMS for 6 weeks (5 sessions a week). A figure-eight coil generated a magnetic field with an intensity of 120% relative to the patient's motor threshold (MT). The frequency of stimulation was 10 Hz, with a stimulus train duration of 4 seconds and an intertrain interval of 26 seconds. The session duration was 37.5 minutes, with a total of 3000 magnetic pulses delivered per session. LDLPFC was localized through anatomic landmarks. Both response and remission rates were significantly higher in the active group, with a good safety profile.

The results of this study were replicated in 2010.[46] The inclusion criteria and the stimulation parameters were essentially the same between the two trials. However, some methodological improvements were introduced, including MRI-guided localization of the stimulation target and a sham condition that better mimicked the somatosensory experience of TMS.

Another relatively large (127 patients), multicentric, sham-controlled TMS study was published in 2007. This study aimed to assess whether TMS could be used as an augmentation strategy to antidepressants. The proportion of treatment resistance was about 15%, but in this case, treatment resistance was defined as treatment failure with 2 or more antidepressants. Moreover, the stimulation dose was lower compared to previous trials[45] (2000 stimuli per session, 15 sessions in total). The investigators did not find any significant difference between the active and sham stimulations arms, suggesting that TMS did not significantly accelerate or augment the pharmacologic response.

Meta-Analyses

During the last 30 years, more than 80 clinical trials on TMS in depression have been published. These trials are often heterogeneous in terms of population characteristics (severity of symptoms, treatment-resistance status), study design, regions stimulated and their localization, stimulation parameters, and design of the sham stimulation. Most importantly, the sample size, and therefore the statistical power, significantly differs across studies. For these reasons, meta-analyses have been performed to provide synthetic measures of the treatment efficacy and explain the heterogeneity observed.

A network meta-analysis published in 2016 compared 88 randomized control trials (RCTs) investigating different TMS paradigms (high frequency, low frequency, bilateral, theta-burst, deep, synchronized, accelerated, priming low-frequency).[47] The authors found that high-frequency, low-frequency (with or without priming), bilateral, and theta-burst TMS paradigms were more effective than a sham, whereas deep, synchronized, and accelerated TMS did not reach statistical significance. In general, estimates of the efficacy were imprecise. Moreover, only a few trials were available for the more recent TMS interventions (deep, synchronized, and accelerated). When compared one to one, few differences were found in the efficacy and safety of the different TMS modalities.

Another, more recent, comprehensive meta-analysis was published in 2019 and compared different nonsurgical brain stimulation techniques.[48] TMS techniques, the results were consistent with the previous meta-analysis [47] in that high-frequency, low-frequency (with or without priming), bilateral, and theta-burst TMS paradigms were found to be more effective than placebo. In contrast, newer TMS techniques (deep, synchronized, and accelerated TMS) failed to reach statistical significance. Again, estimates for the latter techniques were influenced by the limited number of available studies. In a separate commentary, the authors of this meta-analysis pointed out that most trials (64%) included participants with at least 2 failed pharmacologic treatments. Moreover, only 3 trials (n = 49 patients) included only non–treatment-resistant patients. This leads to various considerations. First, valuable information regarding the efficacy of TMS in non–treatment-resistant patients is needed. TMS is a highly safe treatment associated with very low rates of side effects, and newer, shorter TMS paradigms are being introduced (ie, theta-burst stimulation[49]), making the intervention suitable for treatment-naive patients. Second, the high degree of treatment resistance found in TMS RCT may have biased the clinical reputation of TMS, since the efficacy of TMS is influenced by the degree of pharmacologic treatment resistance.[50]

CLINICAL APPLICATION
Patients' Selection

1. TMS treatment is approved by FDA for patients who failed to respond to at least one course of antidepressant treatment with an adequate dosage and duration.[51]

2. In patients with psychotic symptoms or acutely suicidal ideation, other, well-established treatments such as ECT should be considered.[52]
3. TMS is approved only for the treatment of the acute phase because not enough evidence is available to support its clinical efficacy as a maintenance treatment.[53]
4. TMS is not currently approved for treating depression in children or adolescents or women with perinatal depression.[52]

Contraindications to Transcranial Magnetic Stimulation

1. Any magnetic-sensitive objects implanted in the head and/or neck.[54]
2. Caution should be exercised in patients with implanted devices such as deep brain stimulation devices, cochlear implants, aneurysm clips, pacemakers, intracardiac lines, or medication pumps because excessive heating of the device could lead to tissue damage.[55]
3. Patients at high risk of epileptic seizures.[56]

Safety and Side Effects

TMS is a safe procedure. Although magnetic stimulation produces tissue heating, the effect is minimal ($<0.1^{\circ}C$)[57] and devoid of any significant biological impact. No evidence of brain tissue damage has been reported during any rTMS session,[52] even for accelerated protocols.[58] The most common side effects include transient headache, local pain, and paresthesia. Side effects associated with TMS are summarized in **Table 1**.

A major side effect is the induction of tonic-clonic seizures, resulting from direct or indirect excitation of the motor cortex. However, this is an extremely rare occurrence, with one event occurring every 30,000 treatment exposures.[59,60] The risk of TMS-induced seizures can be minimized with a comprehensive evaluation of the patient's health history. Risk factors for TMS-induced seizures include[54] the following:

1. Personal and family history of seizure or epilepsy.
2. History of head trauma or stroke with neurologic sequela.
3. Decreased seizure threshold due to
   a. Substance abuse (eg, stimulants).
   b. Tapering down medications with anticonvulsant properties (eg, benzodiazepines) or substance abuse withdrawal.
   c. Neurologic or medical disorders, such as sleep deprivation, increased intracranial pressure, or electrolyte imbalance.

Treatment Parameters

Coil selection

The first FDA-approved coil was the figure-eight-shaped coil, characterized by good focality at the intersection of the 2 "rounds" of the eight-shape.

Because the intensity of the electrical field generated with standard coils (round or 8-shaped) drops steeply with distance,[61] the stimulation of deep regions would require stimulation intensities that exceed the safety threshold. Hesed (H) coils generate electric fields with a significantly lower decay rate at the expense of reduced focality.[62] This allows for relatively selective stimulation of deeper (but broader) regions.[63] The use of the H1-coil has been shown to be effective and safe for treating depression,[64,65] and it is FDA-approved for TRD. Another type of H-coil (H7) is FDA-approved for obsessive-compulsive disorder, and represents a promising treatment of comorbid depression and Obsessive Compulsive Disorder (OCD).[66]

Table 1
Side effects associated with transcranial magnetic stimulation treatment

Side Effect	Frequency	Comments
Transient headache, local pain, paresthesia	Frequent (up to 40%)	• Most common side effect • Pain should subside shortly after the session has ended • Headache that persist beyond the duration of the session can be treated with oral analgesics

Transient hearing changes	Possible, but not reported when hearing protection are adopted	• Recommendation to reduce risk:
		  a. Hearing protection
		  b. Patients complaining of acute hearing impairment or tinnitus should be promptly referred for auditory assessment
		  c. Risk/benefit should be weighed for subjects with noise-induced hearing loss or taking ototoxic medications
		  d. TMS is contraindicated in patients with cochlear implants

Seizure induction	Possible in epileptic patients (1.4%) Extremely rare in general population ($\sim$0.003%)	• Comprehensive pretreatment evaluation for risk factors assessment
Syncope	Possible	• Vasodepressor (neurocardiogenic) • Can mimic seizures if positive phenomena are present (tonic stiffening, jerking, oral or motor automatisms) • Rapid recovery of consciousness within seconds
Treatment emergent mania (TEM)	Uncommon (<1%) Occurs only with LDLPFC stimulation	• Risk factors include patients with a history of TEM induced by other antidepressants, or undiagnosed bipolar disorder
Transient neuropsychological changes	Negligible	• No reports of long-term neuropsychological changes
Burns from scalp electrodes	Rare	• Skin burns can occur due to eddy (or loop) currents • Using low-conductivity plastic electrodes and titanium skull plates can reduce the risk of burns

(continued on next page)

Table 1 (continued)		
Side Effect	Frequency	Comments
Induced currents in implanted devices	Rare, occurs only if TMS is delivered in the proximity of the device	
Transient thyroid stimulating hormone, blood lactate levels changes	Rare	

Adapted from Rossi S, Antal A, Bestmann S, et al. Safety and recommendations for TMS use in healthy subjects and patient populations, with updates on training, ethical and regulatory issues: Expert Guidelines. Clin Neurophysiol. 2021;132(1):269-306. https://doi.org/10.1016/j.clinph.2020. 10.003.

Motor threshold determination

MT is defined as the magnetic pulse intensity that elicits a motor response of the first dorsal interosseous or the abductor pollicis brevis of the hand contralateral to the stimulation site. The motor response can be assessed visually or through electromyographic measurement. MT is reached when more than 5 out of 10 trials elicit a valid motor response.

Parameter selection

FDA-approved protocols involve high-frequency stimulation of the LDLPFC. Low-frequency (inhibitory) stimulation of the RDLPFC has been suggested to be equally effective. Alternative, opposite strategies (high-frequency stimulation of RDLPFC or low-frequency stimulation of left DLPFC) did not result in satisfactory results.[48] Bilateral stimulation (high frequency on the left, low frequency on the right) has been proposed to augment the efficacy of stimulation. However, several trials did not find significant differences between unilateral and bilateral approaches.[67–69]

High-frequency protocols for the 2 FDA-approved coils are described in **Table 2**.

A relatively recent stimulation protocol is the intermittent theta burst stimulation (iTBS) of the left DLPFC. The term "theta" refers to the Electroencephalography (EEG) theta range (4–7 Hz), whereas the word "bursts" refers to a series of TMS pulses delivered at a higher frequency compared to traditional high-frequency TMS. The neurophysiological rationale of these stimulation parameters derives from the burst discharge at the theta range registered from the rat hippocampus during exploratory behavior.[70] This was validated by findings about TBS being very efficacious in inducing LTP animal brain slices.[71] With this stimulation technique, triplet 50 Hz bursts are delivered at 5 Hz for 2 seconds, followed by an interval of 8 seconds in which no pulse is delivered. In this way, 600 pulses are delivered in just 3 minutes, whereas a traditional high-frequency TMS session lasts 37.5 minutes.[72] This technique would therefore allow broadened accessibility and reduce the costs of TMS treatment. In 2016[49] the results of a large, multisite RCT were published, showing noninferiority of iTBS compared with traditional high-frequency TMS for TRD.

Stimulation site targeting

Although some methods theoretically allow for more precise localization of the DLPFC, it needs to be clarified whether this translates to increased clinical efficacy. Therefore, the choice of the stimulation site is still an open challenge, with novel approaches discussed at the end of the manuscript (see "Future Directions" section).

Table 2
Stimulation parameters Food and Drug Administration-approved protocols for the figure-eight and the H1 coil

Protocol	High Frequency	High Frequency	Intermittent Theta Burst Stimulation
Coil shape	Figure-eight	Hesed-coil (H1)	Figure eight
Target region	Left dorsolateral prefrontal cortex		
Intensity (% of MT)	120	120	120
Pulses frequency	10 Hz	18 Hz	Triplet 50 Hz bursts, repeated at 5 Hz
Train duration (s)	4	2	2
Intertrain interval (s)	26	20	8
Pulses per session	3000	1980	600
Session duration	37.5 min	30 min	3 min 9 s

- The most common method is the 5-cm rule, in which the coil is placed 5 cm anterior to the primary motor cortex on a parasagittal plane.
- In a newer approach, DLPFC is assumed to correspond to the position of the F3 electrode in the 10 to 20 international system. F3 point located through a set of individual scalp measures.
- Frameless stereotactic positioning methods based on structural MRI allow for the most accurate localization of DLPFC. However, this approach requires a dedicated MRI session and a neuronavigation device, which can result impractical.

Duration of transcranial magnetic stimulation treatment
The recommended duration for the standard is 5 daily sessions for 4 to 6 weeks. Continuation of treatment of 1 or 2 additional weeks can be considered in some situations, such as[73,74] (a) patients with a known history of late or slow response to antidepressants, and (b) highly treatment-resistant patients.

Transcranial Magnetic Stimulation Availability and Costs

TMS treatment is widely available at clinics across the United States. Most of the major insurance companies cover the cost of TMS for TRD. However, the payment amount for the patient will vary and depend on the insurance policy regarding deductibles and copays.

Several reports indicate that TMS is cost-effective after a single failed antidepressant medication trial compared with other treatment modalities.[75,76]

TRANSCRANIAL DIRECT CURRENT STIMULATION

tDCS is a noninvasive brain stimulation technique that delivers low electrical current through the scalp. During tDCS, a weak electrical current is administered transcranially through electrodes (anode and cathode) placed on the scalp. Current flows through the electrodes, with the brain tissues acting as conductors to close the circuit. The direction of the current flow can be controlled to produce either anodal or cathodal stimulation. Traditionally, the former is associated with membrane depolarization and enhanced excitability of the underlying region, and the latter with membrane hyperpolarization and decreased excitability. However, for behavioral measures, this is probably a simplification, with inconsistent results between motor and cognitive domains.[77] Moreover, recent reports suggest a more complex spatial relationship, with electrical fields being as strong as the ones immediately under the electrodes.[78]Anodal stimulation of the left DLPFC is the most common therapeutic approach for depression.

Neuromodulatory Effects of Transcranial Direct Current Stimulation

A major difference between tDCS and TMS is that tDCS does not generate action potentials in the stimulated neurons. The traditional paradigm is that tDCS-induced tonic subthreshold depolarization and hyperpolarization modulate neuronal excitability.[79] In support of this, numerous studies have documented changes in neuronal in various brain regions, such as changes in motor and visual evoked potentials.[80,81] However, some have suggested that short-term cortical excitability is *directly* altered by tDCS only for current densities higher than those used in conventional human protocols.[82,83] *Indirect* mechanisms have been proposed to explain how weak currents can modulate neuronal activity. At a cellular level, these include tDCS-induced changes in neuronal spike timing and probability,[84] and modulation (but not induction) of endogenous synaptic plasticity.[85] At a network level, these reflect stochastic and rhythm resonance mechanisms that influence neural information coding.[84] This could help to restore the integrity of frontal networks in patients with depression,[86] and to normalize connectivity between prefrontal regions and other regions involved in affective regulation.[87,88]

Clinical Evidence of Efficacy in Depression

Early randomized, sham-controlled trials reported heterogeneous results but suggested greater antidepressant efficacy of active stimulation.[89]

In 2013, the results of a trial with a 2 × 2 factorial design (sertraline/placebo, active/sham tDCS) were published.[90] Results were suggestive of a cumulative effect of tDCS when combined with the pharmacologic intervention and of similar efficacy of the 2 active interventions. In a similar but more powered study published by the same author in 2017 tDCS failed to show noninferiority to escitalopram.[91] However, blinding efficacy was unbalanced between treatments, being higher for tDCS versus sham than for escitalopram versus placebo; this could have inflated the effectiveness of the pharmacologic intervention, invalidating the noninferiority comparison.

Recent meta-analyses support the efficacy of tDCS in patients with depression.[92–96] Evidence from one meta-analysis was of significant impact because it was based on individual patient data.[92] Other meta-analyses emphasized that tDCS may augment the effect of pharmacologic interventions, and that antidepressant effects persist during follow-ups.[96]

Finally, sham controlling in tDCS studies is particularly challenging, given the somatosensory experience associated with active stimulation. Strategies to ensure blinding include a continuous low-intensity active stimulation, or a gradual increase in current (ie, ramp-up), shortly followed by a decrease in intensity (ramp-down). Some suggest that these techniques do not achieve acceptable blinding.[97,98] However, the delivery of electrical current at higher intensities may compromise the intrinsic nature of the sham-condition, given the relatively large antidepressant effect registered in patients included in the sham arms among tDCS RCTs.[98]

The Effect of Transcranial Direct Current Stimulation on Cognition

Several reports suggested that tDCS may exert cognitive enhancement effects. Specifically, stimulation may facilitate verbal fluency,[99] improve working memory,[100] inhibitory control,[101] cognitive control,[102] and motor learning.[103] Evidence from meta-analyses suggests that tDCS may have a small but significant effect on working memory and attention/vigilance across several psychiatric and neurologic diagnoses, including depression.[104]

Safety and Side Effects

tDCS is considered a safe treatment. There is no need for anesthesia or sedation during the procedure. No serious adverse events have been reported in more than 18,000 sessions of stimulation in various populations (healthy subjects, neurologic, and psychiatric patients). Common side effects are mild and include headache, fatigue, and paresthesia (burning, prickling sensations) at the stimulation site. Notably, these side effects are also frequently reported by patients receiving sham stimulation.[105] The incidence of side effects does not appear to increase with higher levels of tDCS exposure.[106]

Optimization of Stimulation Parameters

In standard therapeutic protocols, currents of 1 to 2 mA are delivered through electrodes sized between 25 and 35 cm^2, resulting in charge densities of approximately 0.03 to 0.09 C/cm^2. Each session lasts about 20 to 30 minutes; a treatment course includes 10 to 20 sessions (5 sessions/wk).[53]

Because the effect of stimulation on cortical excitability seems to vary significantly across individuals,[107] tailored approaches are probably needed to maximize antidepressant efficacy. Parameters that may need to be fine-tuned based on individual characteristics include current waveform[108] and intensity,[109] session duration,[110] spacing of treatment sessions,[111] size and number of electrodes and electrode positioning (montage).[112]

A notable example of individualized treatment is the reconstruction of realistic head models based on individual MRI. This allows us to estimate anatomic factors (such as electrode-to-cortex distance) and simulate tDCS-induced electrical fields. Both have been found to explain part of the variability of the neuromodulatory effect of tDCS across subjects.[113] The coupling of a multichannel tDCS setting with simulation of electrical fields allows for selective stimulation of designated regions with higher current intensities, while reducing side effects and tingling/burning sensations.[114]

FUTURE DIRECTIONS

Several approaches have been proposed to optimize TMS treatment efficacy.

They involve new stimulation protocols in terms of priming, duration of treatment (accelerated TMS), stimulation site selection and target localization, and treatment personalization based on various biomarkers (structural MRI, functional MRI, electroencephalography).

Priming Stimulation

According to the Bienenstock-Cooper-Munro theory, the probability of plasticity induction partially depends on the previous synaptic activity.[115] Based on this, it has been suggested that a more significant reduction in the excitability of the RDLPFC can be achieved if a low-frequency stimulation session is preceded by a period of higher frequency stimulation of the same area.[116]

In a trial involving 60 patients, low-frequency stimulation of RDLPFC preceded by twenty 5 seconds trains of 6 Hz stimulation produced a greater reduction of depressive symptoms than sham-priming condition.[117] A subsequent trial by the same research group, comparing right unilateral primed stimulation with bilateral nonprimed stimulation, reported no differences in antidepressant efficacy between the 2 groups.[68]

EEG-Informed Treatment: Synchronized Transcranial Magnetic Stimulation

One putative mechanism of action underlying the TMS antidepressant effect is the influence of stimulation on cortical rhythms. Reports suggest that TMS may modulate endogenous oscillatory dynamics, such as the power in the alpha band and the alpha:-gamma phase synchrony.[118] This could, in turn, reset thalamocortical oscillators and induce plastic changes, ultimately resulting in an antidepressant effect.[119] With this rationale, a method has been proposed to deliver a low-field stimulation with a sinusoidal waveform personalized based on the individual's alpha frequency. This is achieved using rotating magnets positioned on the scalp's midsagittal line. Because stimulation is synchronized with the alpha-rhythm frequency, lower intensity magnetic fields are required, hence the low-field (subthreshold) stimulation.

The results of a sham-controlled RCT were published in 2015.[120] The trial included 202 patients heterogeneous in their treatment-resistance status. There was no statistical difference between the active and sham groups in the intention to treat analysis; however, a greater reduction in depressive scores was observed in the active treatment group when the individuals that received a suboptimal treatment dose were excluded from the analysis.

Shorter Course of Treatment: Accelerated Transcranial Magnetic Stimulation

A typical course of TMS treatment with the FDA-approved protocol requires 4 to 6 weeks of daily stimulation sessions. This limits accessibility to treatment and its use in acutely suicidal patients and/or in inpatient settings.

Various accelerated TMS protocols have been proposed. The rationale for accelerated protocols relies on 2 assumptions. First, that a densely scheduled session enhances the effect on cortical excitability.[121] Second, that a shorter course of treatment has comparable long-term efficacy to longer duration protocols.[121] The short duration of iTBS sessions makes this technique particularly suitable for this goal but accelerated variations of traditional high-frequency stimulation have been proposed as well.

A large, two-site, sham-controlled RCT tested the efficacy of a short course of high-frequency (10 Hz) stimulation (three 30-minute sessions for 3 days, for a total of 54,000 stimuli) in a sample of depressed, suicidal inpatients.[58] This dose (18,000 stimuli/d) represented a 6-fold increase in the daily dose administered in the FDA-approved protocol. Notably, no major side effects were registered, with the incidence of side effects being similar between the active and sham arms. Although the planned analysis did not show any significant difference between active and sham groups in terms of efficacy on suicidal symptom reduction, post hoc analyses of completers suggested a greater and more immediate effect in the active arm.

Toward an Individualized Stimulation Target

It has been suggested that a significant proportion of heterogeneity in the clinical efficacy of TMS may be attributable to nonoptimal localization of the putative "ideal" site for stimulation. Two challenges with increasing degrees of complexity develop. First, how to correctly localize the DLPFC. Second, how to identify the "ideal" site for stimulation inside this region. In fact, the left DLPFC encompasses a relatively large area: within this region, several subregions have been identified that vary significantly in their cytoarchitectonic characteristics and in their connectivity patterns.[122,123]

Targeting DLPFC with scalp measurements does not adjust for differences in individual neuroanatomy. This leads to stimulation of adjacent regions in a significant proportion of patients,[124] such that some authors suggested systematically moving the area of stimulation more anteriorly and laterally.[125] A newer localization method has been developed based on the 10 to 20 EEG systems. Based on coregistration of EEG electrode position with anatomic MRI, it has been suggested that the area antero-lateral to F3 correctly localizes the DLPFC.[126] Although performing better in terms of DLPFC localization,[127,128] evidence supporting an incremental value in terms of clinical efficacy is still lacking.

MRI-based localization accounts for individual variations in neuroanatomy and is gaining popularity in clinical practice. However, a clear superiority of this approach to other non-MRI-based localization methods is still to be proven because initial hints of MRI-based incremental value on antidepressant efficacy compared with the 5-cm rule[129] were not replicated in a subsequent trial.[130] However, both studies were probably underpowered.

A recent proof of concept study implemented electrical field modeling to improve localization, correcting for individual differences in neuroanatomy (and thus conductivity) and coil orientation.[131] Indeed, it has been shown that coil orientation influences the direction of stimulation as much as coil location.[132]

An emerging approach is the identification of the target region based on its functional connectivity metrics. This is based on the following assumptions: (1) depression is associated with alterations in various large-scale brain networks,[133] (2) TMS can alter the dynamics of brain networks,[134] and (3) different DLPFC subregions display different functional connectivity patterns.[122]

The most consistent relationship between TMS efficacy and functional connectivity measures involves the functional connectivity between DLPFC and the subgenual anterior cingulate cortex (sgACC). This area is involved in affective and emotional regulation and arousal.[135] It is also one of the targets of deep brain stimulation in depression.[136] Several studies reported how stimulation efficacy increases when the anticorrelation between the stimulated region and the sgACC is stronger,[137] or when the distance between the stimulated site and the DLPFC site most anticorrelated with the sgACC is minimized.[138] These results were also validated in a prospective study.[139] A series of studies have tried to implement this concept into a personalized treatment based on individualized connectivity, with promising results.[140–142]

Stanford Accelerated Intelligent Neuromodulation Therapy: an Innovative, Integrated Approach

In 2020, a TMS protocol was proposed that integrated many of the aspects mentioned above, the Stanford Accelerated Intelligent Neuromodulation Therapy. The stimulation protocol was an accelerated its paradigm with 10 sessions of 50 min/d, 1800 pulses/session, 18,000 pulses/d for 5 consecutive days, and 90,000 pules in total. The stimulation target was identified using an ad hoc algorithm that localized the DLPFC subunit most anticorrelated with sgACC. Stimulation intensity was corrected for the coil-cortex index. An open-label study on 20 patients with TRD showed very-high remission rates (90%) and, notably, a good safety profile with a low rate of side effects, given the high temporal density of stimulation.[143] In a subsequent sham-controlled trial performed on 32 participants with the same protocol (renamed Stanford Neuromodulation Therapy [SNT]),[144] a 52.5% reduction in Montgomery-Asberg Depression Rating Scale score 4 weeks after treatment was achieved in the active stimulation group, against 11.1% reduction in the sham group. In September 2022, FDA cleared SNT for clinical use. The SNT protocol may therefore represent the first successful model of noninvasive, accelerated, biomarker-based, personalized neuromodulation.

CLINICS CARE POINTS

- TMS is FDA approved in depression for patients that failed to respond to at least one antidepressant.

- TMS is a safe procedure, even when a high number of pulses are delivered in a short time window (ie, accelerated protocols). There is a very-low risk for induction of tonic-clonic seizures, but this can be reduced further with a thorough patient pretreatment evaluation and screening for risk factors.

- Localization of the stimulation can be done with scalp measurements (5 cm anterior to motor cortex, F3 position in the 10–20 system), or with frameless stereotactic positioning (MRI-guided).

- Standard stimulation protocols include high-frequency stimulation of the LDLPFC. iTBS sessions are significantly shorter (30 vs 3 minutes) and allow for accelerated protocols.

- A new accelerated protocol (SNT), based on fMRI connectivity measures, has recently received FDA approval for use in TRD.

- tDCS, although not currently FDA-approved for clinical use, is a promising neuromodulation technique for TRD, especially for the treatment of cognitive symptoms.

DISCLOSURE STATEMENT

Funding: S. Selvaraj has received grants/research support from NIMH, United States (1R21MH119441-01A1), NIMH (1R21MH129888-01A1), NICHD 1R21HD106779-01A1, and Anne and Don Fizer Foundation, United States. N. Murphy has received grants/research support from NIMH (1R21MH119441-01A1); REAM Misophonia Research Fund (The REAM Foundation - YR01); Caroline Wiess Law Fund for Research in Molecular Medicine. Role of Funder: The content of this study is solely the responsibility of the authors and does not necessarily represent the official views of the NIH, NIMH, and NICHD. The UT Health institution played no role in the design and conduct of the study; collection, management, analysis, and interpretation of the data; preparation, review, or approval of the article; and decision to submit the article for publication.

DECLARATION OF INTEREST

S. Selvaraj has received honoraria from the British Medical Journal Publishing Group and Psychiatry Education Forum LLC. He has received research support as a Principal investigator or study/subinvestigator for clinical research for Flow Neuroscience, COMPASS Pathways, LivaNova, Janssen, and Relmada. N. Murphy has received research support as a subinvestigator for clinical research for Neurocrine Biosciences Inc.

REFERENCES

1. Global, regional, and national burden of 12 mental disorders in 204 countries and territories, 1990–2019: a systematic analysis for the Global Burden of Disease Study 2019. Lancet Psychiatr 2022;9(2):137–50.
2. Machado-Vieira R, Baumann J, Wheeler-Castillo C, et al. The Timing of Antidepressant Effects: A Comparison of Diverse Pharmacological and Somatic Treatments. Pharmaceuticals 2010;3(1):19–41.

3. Rush AJ, Trivedi MH, Wisniewski SR, et al. Acute and Longer-Term Outcomes in Depressed Outpatients Requiring One or Several Treatment Steps: A STAR*D Report. Am J Psychiatry 2006;163(11):1905–17.

4. Sforzini L, Worrell C, Kose M, et al. A Delphi-method-based consensus guideline for definition of treatment-resistant depression for clinical trials. Mol Psychiatry 2022;27(3):1286–99.

5. Carvalho AF, Solmi M, Sanches M, et al. Evidence-based umbrella review of 162 peripheral biomarkers for major mental disorders. Transl Psychiatry 2020; 10(1):152.

6. Williams LM. Defining biotypes for depression and anxiety based on large-scale circuit dysfunction: a theoretical review of the evidence and future directions for clinical translation. Depress Anxiety 2017;34(1):9–24.

7. Hallett M. Transcranial magnetic stimulation and the human brain. Nature 2000; 406(6792):147–50.

8. Deng ZD, Lisanby SH, Peterchev AV. Electric field depth–focality tradeoff in transcranial magnetic stimulation: Simulation comparison of 50 coil designs. Brain Stimul 2013;6(1):1–13.

9. Romero MC, Davare M, Armendariz M, et al. Neural effects of transcranial magnetic stimulation at the single-cell level. Nat Commun 2019;10(1):2642.

10. Banerjee J, Sorrell ME, Celnik PA, et al. Immediate Effects of Repetitive Magnetic Stimulation on Single Cortical Pyramidal Neurons. In: Choi J, editor. PLoS One 2017;12(1):e0170528.

11. Ye H, Chen V, Hendee J. Cellular mechanisms underlying state-dependent neural inhibition with magnetic stimulation. Sci Rep 2022;12(1):12131.

12. Siebner HR, Funke K, Aberra AS, et al. Transcranial magnetic stimulation of the brain: What is stimulated? – A consensus and critical position paper. Clin Neurophysiol 2022;140:59–97.

13. Yang H, Wang H, Guo L, et al. Dynamic responses of neurons in different states under magnetic field stimulation. J Comput Neurosci 2022;50(1):109–20.

14. Sridharan PS, Lu Y, Rice RC, et al. Loss of Cav1.2 channels impairs hippocampal theta burst stimulation-induced long-term potentiation. Channels 2020;14(1): 287–93.

15. Citri A, Malenka RC. Synaptic Plasticity: Multiple Forms, Functions, and Mechanisms. Neuropsychopharmacology 2008;33(1):18–41.

16. Pascual-Leone A, Tormos JM, Keenan J, et al. Study and Modulation of Human Cortical Excitability With Transcranial Magnetic Stimulation. J Clin Neurophysiol 1998;15(4):333–43.

17. Kimbrell TA, Little JT, Dunn RT, et al. Frequency dependence of antidepressant response to left prefrontal repetitive transcranial magnetic stimulation (rTMS) as a function of baseline cerebral glucose metabolism. Biol Psychiatry 1999; 46(12):1603–13.

18. Huang YZ, Edwards MJ, Rounis E, et al. Theta Burst Stimulation of the Human Motor Cortex. Neuron 2005;45(2):201–6.

19. Duncan J. The Structure of Cognition: Attentional Episodes in Mind and Brain. Neuron 2013;80(1):35–50.

20. Friedman NP, Robbins TW. The role of prefrontal cortex in cognitive control and executive function. Neuropsychopharmacology 2022;47(1):72–89.

21. Nejati V, Majdi R, Salehinejad MA, et al. The role of dorsolateral and ventromedial prefrontal cortex in the processing of emotional dimensions. Sci Rep 2021; 11(1):1971.

22. Brosnan MB, Wiegand I. The Dorsolateral Prefrontal Cortex, a Dynamic Cortical Area to Enhance Top-Down Attentional Control. J Neurosci 2017;37(13):3445–6.

23. Turnbull A, Wang HT, Murphy C, et al. Left dorsolateral prefrontal cortex supports context-dependent prioritisation of off-task thought. Nat Commun 2019; 10(1):3816.

24. Pizzagalli DA, Roberts AC. Prefrontal cortex and depression. Neuropsychopharmacology 2022;47(1):225–46.

25. Fales CL, Barch DM, Rundle MM, et al. Antidepressant treatment normalizes hypoactivity in dorsolateral prefrontal cortex during emotional interference processing in major depression. J Affect Disord 2009;112(1–3):206–11.

26. Yang Z, Oathes DJ, Linn KA, et al. Cognitive Behavioral Therapy Is Associated With Enhanced Cognitive Control Network Activity in Major Depression and Posttraumatic Stress Disorder. Biol Psychiatry Cogn Neurosci Neuroimaging 2018;3(4):311–9.

27. Grajny K, Pyata H, Spiegel K, et al. Depression Symptoms in Chronic Left Hemisphere Stroke Are Related to Dorsolateral Prefrontal Cortex Damage. J Neuropsychiatry Clin Neurosci 2016;28(4):292–8.

28. Barahona-Corrêa JB, Cotovio G, Costa RM, et al. Right-sided brain lesions predominate among patients with lesional mania: evidence from a systematic review and pooled lesion analysis. Transl Psychiatry 2020;10(1):139.

29. Pascual-Leone A, Catala MD, Pascual APL. Lateralized effect of rapid-rate transcranial magnetic stimulation of the prefrontal cortex on mood. Neurology 1996;46(2):499–502.

30. Grimm S, Beck J, Schuepbach D, et al. Imbalance between Left and Right Dorsolateral Prefrontal Cortex in Major Depression Is Linked to Negative Emotional Judgment: An fMRI Study in Severe Major Depressive Disorder. Biol Psychiatry 2008;63(4):369–76.

31. Rolls ET, Deco G. Non-reward neural mechanisms in the orbitofrontal cortex. Cortex 2016;83:27–38.

32. Wager TD, Davidson ML, Hughes BL, et al. Prefrontal-Subcortical Pathways Mediating Successful Emotion Regulation. Neuron 2008;59(6):1037–50.

33. Cheng W, Rolls ET, Qiu J, et al. Medial reward and lateral non-reward orbitofrontal cortex circuits change in opposite directions in depression. Brain 2016; 139(12):3296–309.

34. McTeague LM, Huemer J, Carreon DM, et al. Identification of Common Neural Circuit Disruptions in Cognitive Control Across Psychiatric Disorders. Am J Psychiatry 2017;174(7):676–85.

35. van der Vinne N, van Oostrom I, Arns M. Right orbitofrontal TMS as a fallback after unsuccessful DLPFC rTMS? Brain Stimul 2021;14(6):1687–8.

36. Feffer K, Fettes P, Giacobbe P, et al. 1 Hz rTMS of the right orbitofrontal cortex for major depression: Safety, tolerability and clinical outcomes. Eur Neuropsychopharmacol 2018;28(1):109–17.

37. Bakker N, Shahab S, Giacobbe P, et al. rTMS of the Dorsomedial Prefrontal Cortex for Major Depression: Safety, Tolerability, Effectiveness, and Outcome Predictors for 10 Hz Versus Intermittent Theta-burst Stimulation. Brain Stimul 2015;8(2):208–15.

38. Sheline YI, Price JL, Yan Z, et al. Resting-state functional MRI in depression unmasks increased connectivity between networks via the dorsal nexus. Proc Natl Acad Sci U S A 2010;107(24):11020–5.

39. Kreuzer PM, Schecklmann M, Lehner A, et al. The ACDC Pilot Trial: Targeting the Anterior Cingulate by Double Cone Coil rTMS for the Treatment of Depression. Brain Stimul 2015;8(2):240–6.
40. Dunlop K, Sheen J, Schulze L, et al. Dorsomedial prefrontal cortex repetitive transcranial magnetic stimulation for treatment-refractory major depressive disorder: A three-arm, blinded, randomized controlled trial. Brain Stimul 2020; 13(2):337–40.
41. Junghofer M, Winker C, Rehbein MA, et al. Noninvasive Stimulation of the Ventromedial Prefrontal Cortex Enhances Pleasant Scene Processing. Cereb Cortex 2017;27(6):3449–56.
42. Downar J, Daskalakis ZJ. New Targets for rTMS in Depression: A Review of Convergent Evidence. Brain Stimul 2013;6(3):231–40.
43. George MS, Wassermann EM, Williams WA, et al. Daily repetitive transcranial magnetic stimulation (rTMS) improves mood in depression. Neuroreport 1995; 6(14):1853–6.
44. Burt T, Lisanby SH, Sackeim HA. Neuropsychiatric applications of transcranial magnetic stimulation: a meta analysis. Int J Neuropsychopharmacol 2002;5(1).
45. O'Reardon JP, Solvason HB, Janicak PG, et al. Efficacy and Safety of Transcranial Magnetic Stimulation in the Acute Treatment of Major Depression: A Multisite Randomized Controlled Trial. Biol Psychiatry 2007;62(11):1208–16.
46. George MS, Lisanby SH, Avery D, et al. Daily Left Prefrontal Transcranial Magnetic Stimulation Therapy for Major Depressive Disorder: A Sham-Controlled Randomized Trial. Arch Gen Psychiatry 2010;67(5):507.
47. Brunoni AR, Chaimani A, Moffa AH, et al. Repetitive Transcranial Magnetic Stimulation for the Acute Treatment of Major Depressive Episodes: A Systematic Review With Network Meta-analysis. JAMA Psychiatr 2017;74(2):143.
48. Mutz J, Vipulananthan V, Carter B, et al. Comparative efficacy and acceptability of non-surgical brain stimulation for the acute treatment of major depressive episodes in adults: systematic review and network meta-analysis. BMJ 2019;27: l1079. Published online March.
49. Blumberger DM, Vila-Rodriguez F, Thorpe KE, et al. Effectiveness of theta burst versus high-frequency repetitive transcranial magnetic stimulation in patients with depression (THREE-D): a randomised non-inferiority trial. Lancet 2018; 391(10131):1683–92.
50. Mutz J, Edgcumbe DR, Brunoni AR, et al. Efficacy and acceptability of non-invasive brain stimulation for the treatment of adult unipolar and bipolar depression: A systematic review and meta-analysis of randomised sham-controlled trials. Neurosci Biobehav Rev 2018;92:291–303.
51. Cohen SL, Bikson M, Badran BW, et al. A visual and narrative timeline of US FDA milestones for Transcranial Magnetic Stimulation (TMS) devices. Brain Stimul 2022;15(1):73–5.
52. McClintock SM, Reti IM, Carpenter LL, et al. Consensus Recommendations for the Clinical Application of Repetitive Transcranial Magnetic Stimulation (rTMS) in the Treatment of Depression: (Consensus Statement). J Clin Psychiatry 2018; 79(1):35–48.
53. Lefaucheur JP, Aleman A, Baeken C, et al. Evidence-based guidelines on the therapeutic use of repetitive transcranial magnetic stimulation (rTMS): An update (2014–2018). Clin Neurophysiol 2020;131(2):474–528.
54. Rossi S, Antal A, Bestmann S, et al. Safety and recommendations for TMS use in healthy subjects and patient populations, with updates on training, ethical and regulatory issues: Expert Guidelines. Clin Neurophysiol 2021;132(1):269–306.

55. Rossi S, Hallett M, Rossini PM, et al. Safety, ethical considerations, and application guidelines for the use of transcranial magnetic stimulation in clinical practice and research. Clin Neurophysiol 2009;120(12):2008–39.

56. Stultz DJ, Osburn S, Burns T, et al. Transcranial Magnetic Stimulation (TMS) Safety with Respect to Seizures: A Literature Review. Neuropsychiatr Dis Treat 2020;16:2989–3000.

57. Sabouni A, Honrath M, Khamechi M. Thermal Effects in the Brain During Transcranial Magnetic Stimulation. IEEE Magn Lett 2017;8:1–3.

58. George MS, Raman R, Benedek DM, et al. A Two-site Pilot Randomized 3 Day Trial of High Dose Left Prefrontal Repetitive Transcranial Magnetic Stimulation (rTMS) for Suicidal Inpatients. Brain Stimul 2014;7(3):421–31.

59. Carpenter LL, Janicak PG, Aaronson ST, et al. Transcranial magnetic stimulation (tms) for major depression: a multisite, naturalistic, observational study of acute treatment outcomes in clinical practice. Depress Anxiety 2012;29(7):587–96.

60. Taylor JJ, Newberger NG, Stern AP, et al. Seizure risk with repetitive TMS: Survey results from over a half-million treatment sessions. Brain Stimul 2021;14(4):965–73.

61. Maccabee PJ, Eberle L, Amassian VE, et al. Spatial distribution of the electric field induced in volume by round and figure '8' magnetic coils: relevance to activation of sensory nerve fibers. Electroencephalogr Clin Neurophysiol 1990;76(2):131–41.

62. Roth Y, Amir A, Levkovitz Y, et al. Three-Dimensional Distribution of the Electric Field Induced in the Brain by Transcranial Magnetic Stimulation Using Figure-8 and Deep H-Coils. J Clin Neurophysiol 2007;24(1):31–8.

63. Zangen A, Roth Y, Voller B, et al. Transcranial magnetic stimulation of deep brain regions: evidence for efficacy of the H-Coil. Clin Neurophysiol 2005;116(4):775–9.

64. Levkovitz Y, Isserles M, Padberg F, et al. Efficacy and safety of deep transcranial magnetic stimulation for major depression: a prospective multicenter randomized controlled trial. World Psychiatr 2015;14(1):64–73.

65. Filipčić I, Šimunović Filipčić I, Milovac Ž, et al. Efficacy of repetitive transcranial magnetic stimulation using a figure-8-coil or an H1-Coil in treatment of major depressive disorder; A randomized clinical trial. J Psychiatr Res 2019;114:113–9.

66. Tendler A, Roth Y, Harmelech T. Deep repetitive TMS with the H7 coil is sufficient to treat comorbid MDD and OCD. Brain Stimul 2021;14(3):658–61.

67. Blumberger DM, Maller JJ, Thomson L, et al. Unilateral and bilateral MRI-targeted repetitive transcranial magnetic stimulation for treatment-resistant depression: a randomized controlled study. J Psychiatry Neurosci 2016;41(4):E58–66.

68. Fitzgerald PB, Hoy KE, Singh A, et al. Equivalent beneficial effects of unilateral and bilateral prefrontal cortex transcranial magnetic stimulation in a large randomized trial in treatment-resistant major depression. Int J Neuropsychopharmacol 2013;16(9):1975–84.

69. Berlim MT, Van den Eynde F, Daskalakis ZJ. A systematic review and meta-analysis on the efficacy and acceptability of bilateral repetitive transcranial magnetic stimulation (rTMS) for treating major depression. Psychol Med 2013;43(11):2245–54.

70. Diamond D, Dunwiddie T, Rose G. Characteristics of hippocampal primed burst potentiation in vitro and in the awake rat. J Neurosci 1988;8(11):4079–88.

71. Capocchi G, Zampolini M, Larson J. Theta burst stimulation is optimal for induction of LTP at both apical and basal dendritic synapses on hippocampal CA1 neurons. Brain Res 1992;591(2):332–6.
72. Chung SW, Hoy KE, Fitzgerald PB. Theta-burst stimulation: a new form of tms treatment for depression? Depress Anxiety 2015;32(3):182–92.
73. Perera T, George MS, Grammer G, et al. The Clinical TMS Society Consensus Review and Treatment Recommendations for TMS Therapy for Major Depressive Disorder. Brain Stimul 2016;9(3):336–46.
74. McDonald WM, Durkalski V, Ball ER, et al. Improving the antidepressant efficacy of transcranial magnetic stimulation: maximizing the number of stimulations and treatment location in treatment-resistant depression. Depress Anxiety 2011; 28(11):973–80.
75. Voigt J, Carpenter L, Leuchter A. Cost effectiveness analysis comparing repetitive transcranial magnetic stimulation to antidepressant medications after a first treatment failure for major depressive disorder in newly diagnosed patients – A lifetime analysis. In: Yuan T, editor. PLoS One 2017;12(10):e0186950.
76. Simpson KN, Welch MJ, Kozel FA, et al. Cost-effectiveness of transcranial magnetic stimulation in the treatment of major depression: a health economics analysis. Adv Ther 2009;26(3):346–68.
77. Jacobson L, Koslowsky M, Lavidor M. tDCS polarity effects in motor and cognitive domains: a meta-analytical review. Exp Brain Res 2012;216(1):1–10.
78. Rawji V, Ciocca M, Zacharia A, et al. tDCS changes in motor excitability are specific to orientation of current flow. Brain Stimul 2018;11(2):289–98.
79. Nitsche MA, Cohen LG, Wassermann EM, et al. Transcranial direct current stimulation: State of the art 2008. Brain Stimul 2008;1(3):206–23.
80. Reinhart RMG, Xiao W, McClenahan LJ, et al. Electrical Stimulation of Visual Cortex Can Immediately Improve Spatial Vision. Curr Biol 2016;26(14):1867–72.
81. Cambiaghi M, Velikova S, Gonzalez-Rosa JJ, et al. Brain transcranial direct current stimulation modulates motor excitability in mice. Eur J Neurosci 2010;31(4): 704–9.
82. Milighetti S, Sterzi S, Fregni F, et al. Effects of tDCS on spontaneous spike activity in a healthy ambulatory rat model. Brain Stimul 2020;13(6):1566–76.
83. Jonker ZD, Gaiser C, Tulen JHM, et al. No effect of anodal tDCS on motor cortical excitability and no evidence for responders in a large double-blind placebo-controlled trial. Brain Stimul 2021;14(1):100–9.
84. Liu A, Vöröslakos M, Kronberg G, et al. Immediate neurophysiological effects of transcranial electrical stimulation. Nat Commun 2018;9(1):5092.
85. Kronberg G, Bridi M, Abel T, et al. Direct Current Stimulation Modulates LTP and LTD: Activity Dependence and Dendritic Effects. Brain Stimul 2017;10(1):51–8.
86. Lu H, Gallinaro JV, Rotter S. Network remodeling induced by transcranial brain stimulation: A computational model of tDCS-triggered cell assembly formation. Netw Neurosci 2019;3(4):924–43.
87. MayankS Jog, Kim E, Anderson C, et al. In-vivo imaging of targeting and modulation of depression-relevant circuitry by transcranial direct current stimulation: a randomized clinical trial. Transl Psychiatry 2021;11(1):138.
88. Chrysikou EG, Wing EK, van Dam WO. Transcranial Direct Current Stimulation Over the Prefrontal Cortex in Depression Modulates Cortical Excitability in Emotion Regulation Regions as Measured by Concurrent Functional Magnetic Resonance Imaging: An Exploratory Study. Biol Psychiatry Cogn Neurosci Neuroimaging 2022;7(1):85–94.

89. Kalu UG, Sexton CE, Loo CK, et al. Transcranial direct current stimulation in the treatment of major depression: a meta-analysis. Psychol Med 2012;42(9): 1791–800.

90. Brunoni AR, Valiengo L, Baccaro A, et al. The Sertraline vs Electrical Current Therapy for Treating Depression Clinical Study: Results From a Factorial, Randomized, Controlled Trial. JAMA Psychiatr 2013;70(4):383.

91. Brunoni AR, Moffa AH, Sampaio-Junior B, et al. Trial of Electrical Direct-Current Therapy versus Escitalopram for Depression. N Engl J Med 2017;376(26): 2523–33.

92. Brunoni AR, Moffa AH, Fregni F, et al. Transcranial direct current stimulation for acute major depressive episodes: Meta-analysis of individual patient data. Br J Psychiatry 2016;208(6):522–31.

93. Fregni F, El-Hagrassy MM, Pacheco-Barrios K, et al. Evidence-Based Guidelines and Secondary Meta-Analysis for the Use of Transcranial Direct Current Stimulation in Neurological and Psychiatric Disorders. Int J Neuropsychopharmacol 2021;24(4):256–313.

94. Zhang R, Lam CLM, Peng X, et al. Efficacy and acceptability of transcranial direct current stimulation for treating depression: A meta-analysis of randomized controlled trials. Neurosci Biobehav Rev 2021;126:481–90.

95. Wang J, Luo H, Schülke R, et al. Is transcranial direct current stimulation, alone or in combination with antidepressant medications or psychotherapies, effective in treating major depressive disorder? A systematic review and meta-analysis. BMC Med 2021;19(1):319.

96. Razza LB, De Smet S, Moffa A, et al. Follow-up effects of transcranial direct current stimulation (tDCS) for the major depressive episode: A systematic review and meta-analysis. Psychiatry Res 2021;302:114024.

97. Greinacher R, Buhôt L, Möller L, et al. The time course of ineffective sham-blinding during low-intensity (1 mA) transcranial direct current stimulation. Eur J Neurosci 2019;50(8):3380–8.

98. Turi Z, Csifcsák G, Boayue NM, et al. Blinding is compromised for transcranial direct current stimulation at 1 mA for 20 min in young healthy adults. Eur J Neurosci 2019;50(8):3261–8.

99. Binney RJ, Zuckerman BM, Waller HN, et al. Cathodal tDCS of the bilateral anterior temporal lobes facilitates semantically-driven verbal fluency. Neuropsychologia 2018;111:62–71.

100. Karthikeyan R, Smoot MR, Mehta RK. Anodal tDCS augments and preserves working memory beyond time-on-task deficits. Sci Rep 2021;11(1):19134.

101. Friehs MA, Frings C. Pimping inhibition: Anodal tDCS enhances stop-signal reaction time. J Exp Psychol Hum Percept Perform 2018;44(12):1933–45.

102. Segrave RA, Arnold S, Hoy K, et al. Concurrent Cognitive Control Training Augments the Antidepressant Efficacy of tDCS: A Pilot Study. Brain Stimul 2014;7(2): 325–31.

103. Cole L, Dukelow SP, Giuffre A, et al. Sensorimotor Robotic Measures of tDCS- and HD-tDCS-Enhanced Motor Learning in Children. Neural Plast 2018; 2018:1–13.

104. Begemann MJ, Brand BA, Ćurčić-Blake B, et al. Efficacy of non-invasive brain stimulation on cognitive functioning in brain disorders: a meta-analysis. Psychol Med 2020;50(15):2465–86.

105. Antal A, Alekseichuk I, Bikson M, et al. Low intensity transcranial electric stimulation: Safety, ethical, legal regulatory and application guidelines. Clin Neurophysiol 2017;128(9):1774–809.

106. Nikolin S, Huggins C, Martin D, et al. Safety of repeated sessions of transcranial direct current stimulation: A systematic review. Brain Stimul 2018;11(2):278–88.

107. Chew T, Ho KA, Loo CK. Inter- and Intra-individual Variability in Response to Transcranial Direct Current Stimulation (tDCS) at Varying Current Intensities. Brain Stimul 2015;8(6):1130–7.

108. Chung H, Im C, Seo H, et al. Key factors in the cortical response to transcranial electrical Stimulations—A multi-scale modeling study. Comput Biol Med 2022; 144:105328.

109. Esmaeilpour Z, Marangolo P, Hampstead BM, et al. Incomplete evidence that increasing current intensity of tDCS boosts outcomes. Brain Stimul 2018; 11(2):310–21.

110. Vignaud P, Mondino M, Poulet E, et al. Duration but not intensity influences transcranial direct current stimulation (tDCS) after-effects on cortical excitability. Neurophysiol Clin 2018;48(2):89–92.

111. Monte-Silva K, Kuo MF, Liebetanz D, et al. Shaping the Optimal Repetition Interval for Cathodal Transcranial Direct Current Stimulation (tDCS). J Neurophysiol 2010;103(4):1735–40.

112. Klaus J, Schutter DJLG. Electrode montage-dependent intracranial variability in electric fields induced by cerebellar transcranial direct current stimulation. Sci Rep 2021;11(1):22183.

113. Mosayebi-Samani M, Jamil A, Salvador R, et al. The impact of individual electrical fields and anatomical factors on the neurophysiological outcomes of tDCS: A TMS-MEP and MRI study. Brain Stimul 2021;14(2):316–26.

114. Khan A, Antonakakis M, Vogenauer N, et al. Individually optimized multi-channel tDCS for targeting somatosensory cortex. Clin Neurophysiol 2022;134:9–26.

115. Bienenstock E, Cooper L, Munro P. Theory for the development of neuron selectivity: orientation specificity and binocular interaction in visual cortex. J Neurosci 1982;2(1):32–48.

116. Iyer MB, Schleper N, Wassermann EM. Priming Stimulation Enhances the Depressant Effect of Low-Frequency Repetitive Transcranial Magnetic Stimulation. J Neurosci 2003;23(34):10867–72.

117. Fitzgerald PB, Hoy K, McQueen S, et al. Priming Stimulation Enhances the Effectiveness of Low-Frequency Right Prefrontal Cortex Transcranial Magnetic Stimulation in Major Depression. J Clin Psychopharmacol 2008;28(1):52–8.

118. Johnson JS, Hamidi M, Postle BR. Using EEG to Explore How rTMS Produces Its Effects on Behavior. Brain Topogr 2010;22(4):281–93.

119. Fuggetta G, Noh NA. A neurophysiological insight into the potential link between transcranial magnetic stimulation, thalamocortical dysrhythmia and neuropsychiatric disorders. Exp Neurol 2013;245:87–95.

120. Leuchter AF, Cook IA, Feifel D, et al. Efficacy and Safety of Low-field Synchronized Transcranial Magnetic Stimulation (sTMS) for Treatment of Major Depression. Brain Stimul 2015;8(4):787–94.

121. Maeda F, Keenan JP, Tormos JM, et al. Modulation of corticospinal excitability by repetitive transcranial magnetic stimulation. Clin Neurophysiol 2000;111(5):800–5.

122. Jung J, Lambon Ralph MA, Jackson RL. Subregions of DLPFC Display Graded yet Distinct Structural and Functional Connectivity. J Neurosci 2022;42(15):3241–52.

123. Rajkowska G, Goldman-Rakic PS. Cytoarchitectonic Definition of Prefrontal Areas in the Normal Human Cortex: II. Variability in Locations of Areas 9 and

46 and Relationship to the Talairach Coordinate System. Cereb Cortex 1995; 5(4):323–37.

124. Ahdab R, Ayache SS, Brugières P, et al. Comparison of "standard" and "navigated" procedures of TMS coil positioning over motor, premotor and prefrontal targets in patients with chronic pain and depression. Neurophysiol Clin Neurophysiol 2010;40(1):27–36.

125. Herbsman T, Avery D, Ramsey D, et al. More Lateral and Anterior Prefrontal Coil Location Is Associated with Better Repetitive Transcranial Magnetic Stimulation Antidepressant Response. Biol Psychiatry 2009;66(5):509–15.

126. Herwig U, Satrapi P, Schönfeldt-Lecuona C. Using the International 10-20 EEG System for Positioning of Transcranial Magnetic Stimulation. Brain Topogr 2003; 16(2):95–9.

127. Mir-Moghtadaei A, Caballero R, Fried P, et al. Concordance Between BeamF3 and MRI-neuronavigated Target Sites for Repetitive Transcranial Magnetic Stimulation of the Left Dorsolateral Prefrontal Cortex. Brain Stimul 2015;8(5):965–73.

128. Trapp NT, Bruss J, King Johnson M, et al. Reliability of targeting methods in TMS for depression: Beam F3 vs. 5.5 cm. Brain Stimul 2020;13(3):578–81.

129. Fitzgerald PB, Hoy K, McQueen S, et al. A Randomized Trial of rTMS Targeted with MRI Based Neuro-Navigation in Treatment-Resistant Depression. Neuropsychopharmacology 2009;34(5):1255–62.

130. Li CT, Cheng CM, Chen MH, et al. Antidepressant Efficacy of Prolonged Intermittent Theta Burst Stimulation Monotherapy for Recurrent Depression and Comparison of Methods for Coil Positioning: A Randomized, Double-Blind, Sham-Controlled Study. Biol Psychiatry 2020;87(5):443–50.

131. Balderston NL, Beer JC, Seok D, et al. Proof of concept study to develop a novel connectivity-based electric-field modelling approach for individualized targeting of transcranial magnetic stimulation treatment. Neuropsychopharmacology 2022;47(2):588–98.

132. Thielscher A, Opitz A, Windhoff M. Impact of the gyral geometry on the electric field induced by transcranial magnetic stimulation. Neuroimage 2011;54(1): 234–43.

133. Javaheripour N, Li M, Chand T, et al. Altered resting-state functional connectome in major depressive disorder: a mega-analysis from the PsyMRI consortium. Transl Psychiatry 2021;11(1):511.

134. Santarnecchi E, Momi D, Sprugnoli G, et al. Modulation of network-to-network connectivity via spike-timing-dependent noninvasive brain stimulation. Hum Brain Mapp 2018;39(12):4870–83.

135. Rudebeck PH, Putnam PT, Daniels TE, et al. A role for primate subgenual cingulate cortex in sustaining autonomic arousal. Proc Natl Acad Sci U S A 2014; 111(14):5391–6.

136. Mayberg HS, Lozano AM, Voon V, et al. Deep Brain Stimulation for Treatment-Resistant Depression. Neuron 2005;45(5):651–60.

137. Fox MD, Buckner RL, White MP, et al. Efficacy of Transcranial Magnetic Stimulation Targets for Depression Is Related to Intrinsic Functional Connectivity with the Subgenual Cingulate. Biol Psychiatry 2012;72(7):595–603.

138. Cash RFH, Zalesky A, Thomson RH, et al. Subgenual Functional Connectivity Predicts Antidepressant Treatment Response to Transcranial Magnetic Stimulation: Independent Validation and Evaluation of Personalization. Biol Psychiatry 2019;86(2):e5–7.

139. Weigand A, Horn A, Caballero R, et al. Prospective Validation That Subgenual Connectivity Predicts Antidepressant Efficacy of Transcranial Magnetic Stimulation Sites. Biol Psychiatry 2018;84(1):28–37.
140. Barbour T, Lee E, Ellard K, et al. Individualized TMS target selection for MDD: clinical outcomes, mechanisms of action and predictors of response. Brain Stimul 2019;12(2):516.
141. Singh A, Erwin-Grabner T, Sutcliffe G, et al. Personalized repetitive transcranial magnetic stimulation temporarily alters default mode network in healthy subjects. Sci Rep 2019;9(1):5631.
142. Cash RFH, Cocchi L, Lv J, et al. Personalized connectivity-guided DLPFC-TMS for depression: Advancing computational feasibility, precision and reproducibility. Hum Brain Mapp 2021;42(13):4155–72.
143. Cole EJ, Stimpson KH, Bentzley BS, et al. Stanford Accelerated Intelligent Neuromodulation Therapy for Treatment-Resistant Depression. Am J Psychiatry 2020;177(8):716–26.
144. Cole EJ, Phillips AL, Bentzley BS, et al. Stanford Neuromodulation Therapy (SNT): A Double-Blind Randomized Controlled Trial. Am J Psychiatry 2022; 179(2):132–41.

Photobiomodulation
An Emerging Treatment Modality for Depression

Willians Fernando Vieira, PT, MSc, PhD[a,b,c],
Dan V. Iosifescu, MD, MSc[d,e], Kayla Marie McEachern, BS[a],
Maia Gersten, BS[a], Paolo Cassano, MD, PhD[a,b,*]

KEYWORDS

- Photobiomodulation • NIR • Transcranial photobiomodulation • LLLT
- Major depressive disorder • Treatment-resistant depression

KEY POINTS

- Treatment-resistant depression (TRD) is classified as an unsatisfactory response to 2 adequate trials of antidepressants at optimum dosage for a sufficient duration.
- More than one-third of patients in treatment for depression are treatment-resistant.
- Emerging evidence supports the use of transcranial photobiomodulation (t-PBM) for the treatment of depression.
- t-PBM refers to the application of light on the head aiming to enhance neural function, human cognition, and mood.
- The main focus of this review is to revisit such t-PBM effects in individuals with major depressive disorder who do not respond to other more traditional treatment approaches.

INTRODUCTION

Major depressive disorder (MDD) is one of the greatest factors undermining global health and is considered a financial burden for health systems.[1] Depression is the leading cause of suicide and is associated with several medical conditions, such as

[a] Division of Neuropsychiatry and Neuromodulation, Massachusetts General Hospital (MGH), 149 13th Street (2612), Boston, MA 02129, USA; [b] Department of Psychiatry, Harvard Medical School (HMS), 25 Shattuck Street, Boston, MA 02115, USA; [c] Department of Anatomy, Institute of Biomedical Sciences (ICB), University of Sao Paulo (USP), 2415 Prof. Lineu Prestes Avenue, Sao Paulo, SP 05508-000, Brazil; [d] Clinical Research Division, Nathan Kline Institute (NKI) for Psychiatric Research, 140 Old Orangeburg Road, Orangeburg, NY 10962, USA; [e] Department of Psychiatry, New York University (NYU) School of Medicine, 550 First Avenue, New York, NY 10016, USA
* Corresponding author. Division of Neuropsychiatry and Neuromodulation, Massachusetts General Hospital (MGH), 149 13th Street (2612), Boston, MA 02129.
E-mail address: pcassano@mgh.harvard.edu

Psychiatr Clin N Am 46 (2023) 331–348
https://doi.org/10.1016/j.psc.2023.02.013

diabetes, obesity, stroke, Parkinson's disease, multiple sclerosis, Alzheimer's disease, and sudden cardiac death.[2] A plethora of factors have been implicated in the cause of MDD, including neuroinflammation, the overdrive of the hypothalamic-pituitary-adrenal axis, the dysfunction of the neuroanatomic circuits, the imbalance of neurotransmitters, and overall abnormal neuronal activity.[3] Moreover, MDD is heritable with a genetic predisposition accounting for about 35% of the risk, and it is highly influenced by adverse life experiences.[2,4,5] The complexity and heterogeneity of MDD might explain the inconsistent response to many existing antidepressant strategies, thus representing a challenge for patients and their families.

Treatment-resistant depression (TRD) is classified as an unsatisfactory response to 2 adequate trials of antidepressants at optimum dosage for a sufficient duration.[6,7] According to Nierenberg and colleagues,[8] lack of response is defined as an improvement in depression severity of less than 50% (measured with a rating scale such as the Hamilton Rating Scale for Depression, HAM-D). Also, a posttreatment HAM-D score that remains greater than a certain measure at a specified time point, such as an HAM-D > 16 after 6 weeks, can be a criterion for TRD.[8] Treatment resistance can also develop in patients who were previously responsive to treatment; comorbid and progressive illness contribute to the likelihood of chronic MDD with treatment resistance.[9] Not surprisingly, patients with TRD have twice the chance of being hospitalized,[10] representing a 6-fold increase in overall medical costs compared with non-TRD patients.[11]

The main goal of antidepressant treatment is full psychologic/psychosocial recovery with minimal residual symptoms. Unfortunately, according to a meta-analysis performed by Fava and Davidson,[12] more than one-third of patients in treatment for depression are treatment-resistant. Furthermore, 29% to 46% of the patients treated with standard antidepressant doses for at least 6 weeks failed to respond fully. Conversely, only 60% to 70% of patients who tolerate antidepressant medications well will respond to first-line monotherapy.[13] Another meta-analysis performed by Golden and colleagues[14] reviewed 25 double-blind trials involving 4016 depressed patients and found that more than 50% of patients, treated with a single antidepressant medication, failed to reach full remission. The remaining patients experienced either a partial response or no response. Thus, it is well documented that TRD represents a significant clinical challenge, despite the development of numerous antidepressant medications by the pharmaceutical industry.[15] To say more, even pharmacotherapy-responsive patients have a high chance of still experiencing a significant burden of residual symptoms, such as fatigue and insomnia.[16] Besides affecting quality of life, residual symptoms lead to poor prognosis; in fact, Paykel and colleagues[17] observed residual symptoms to be associated with an increased risk of relapse in 76% of patients.

Beyond antidepressant medications and psychotherapies, growing evidence supports the use of neuromodulation techniques to target the corticolimbic pathways, including in individuals suffering from TRD.[18] A study performed by Milev and colleagues[19] pointed to device-based treatments as options for individuals who do not respond, tolerate, or accept medications or psychotherapy. These non-pharmacologic therapies include the Food and Drug Administration (FDA)-approved electroconvulsive therapy (ECT), and repetitive transcranial magnetic stimulation, as well as other, still experimental options: transcranial direct current stimulation, vagus nerve stimulation (VNS), magnetic seizure therapy, and deep brain stimulation. Although a significant percentage of patients with MDD still exhibit resistance to device-based interventions, variable levels of evidence support the use of these devices in MDD.[9] More recently, there has been emerging evidence for the use of transcranial photobiomodulation (t-PBM) for the treatment of depression.[20–22]

t-PBM refers to the application of light on the head aiming to enhance neural function, human cognition, and mood.[23] In this method, near-infrared (NIR) light crosses several tissue layers, including the scalp, periosteum, skull bone, meninges, and dura mater, before reaching the cortical brain surface.[23] A fraction of the NIR light directly increases neuronal metabolism through a photochemical energy transfer.[24,25] The scientific basis for the use of light as a potential therapeutic approach comes from a surplus of published studies, including its application for tissue regeneration[26–28] and pain relief,[29,30] among others.[31] Primarily, the biological mechanisms of t-PBM are due to the NIR and red-light absorption by the cytochrome c oxidase (CCO) essential mitochondrial enzyme, with a consequent increase in CCO activity, nitric oxide release, and adenosine triphosphate (ATP) production.[32,33] Secondarily, cerebral blood flow and brain energy metabolism are enhanced.[23] Given its unique mechanism of action, t-PBM has the potential to benefit depressed patients; the main focus of this review is to revisit such t-PBM effects in individuals with MDD who do not respond to other more traditional treatment approaches.

METHODS
Search Strategy

The authors examined the application of t-PBM for the treatment of TRD. They searched clinical studies on PubMed and ClinicalTrials.gov using the following keywords: ("photobiomodulation" OR "PBM" OR "near-infrared radiation" OR "NIR" OR "low-level light therapy" OR "low-level laser therapy" OR "LLLT" OR "near-infrared light therapy" OR "NILT") AND ("major depressive disorder" OR "MDD") AND ("treatment-resistant depression" OR "TRD"). The search was performed in June, July, and August 2022; there were no restrictions regarding language or date of publication. For the inclusion criteria, the authors considered only clinical studies on the t-PBM modality. Studies on t-PBM for MDD and those on t-PBM for other diagnoses with comorbid depressive symptoms were included, and the presence of TRD participants in those studies was further investigated. References to the t-PBM mechanisms of action were considered for general information. For that, the authors also considered review articles, studies not focused on MDD or TRD, other photobiomodulation (PBM) modalities (eg, systemic PBM) rather than just t-PBM, and preclinical studies of TRD.

RESULTS
Preclinical Evidence of Treatment-Resistant Depression

There is little preclinical evidence about the contributing factors to the development of TRD. One of the reasons is that the use of animal models in MDD research is challenging, as few human behaviors are amenable to study in murine species. Animal models can capture certain features of MDD, such as motivation, anhedonia, negative affect, hypothalamic dysregulation, and homeostasis.[34] However, other key symptoms, such as sadness, guilt, ruminations, or suicidality symptoms, are not easily captured in nonhuman models of depression. Heretofore, several acute and chronic stress models have been used, but it is complicated to distinguish between the adaptative versus maladaptive responses to stress.[2]

One of the most important risk factors for TRD is previous history of depressive episodes, and each episode increases the probability of a subsequent episodes.[35,36] In the same way, each successive episode decreases the severity of stressors needed to precipitate the following episode.[37,38] These recurrent depressive episodes are also more resistant to pharmacotherapy than the first episodes.[39] In the context of stress, as a trigger for a depressive episode, the chronic mild stress (CMS) animal model is the most extensively validated, despite early concerns about its reliability. In the CMS model, rodents are chronically exposed to unpredictable microstressors, resulting in the development of a plethora of behavioral changes, including decreased response to rewards (a behavioral correlate of the clinical core symptom of depression and anhedonia.[40]) A study conducted by Isingrini and colleagues[41] used BALB/c mice, who were submitted to two 7-week periods of CMS separated by a 6-week interval. In comparison to the first period of CMS, the second period showed an increase in stress sensitivity. Mice were maintained on a normal diet, and chronic treatment with fluoxetine decreased all the behavioral impairments. However, in mice fed a high-fat diet, mimicking the vascular risk for depression,[42] and whereas mice treated with fluoxetine showed no behavioral impairment after the first CMS period, fluoxetine had no effect following the second CMS exposure. Thus, the study of Isingrini and colleagues[41] demonstrated increased stress sensitivity in previously stressed animals, and antidepressant resistance was induced by an interaction between a high-fat diet and a history of repeated stress exposure. These experimental aspects of past life experience, including comorbidities, provide clues about the predisposition of individuals with MDD to develop TRD.

Systematic Review of Transcranial Photobiomodulation for Major Depressive Disorder with Focus on Treatment-Resistant Depression

Studies selection

A search in PubMed (https://pubmed.ncbi.nlm.nih.gov/) and ClinicalTrials.gov using the combination of previously described keywords returned 367 records. After a systematic screening aimed to categorize each study, the authors identified that 76 records (20.71%), n = 38 from PubMed and n = 38 from ClinicalTrials.gov, did not have MDD or TRD measures as their first analyzed outcomes. The authors also identified 60 records (16.35%, n = 53 from PubMed; n = 7 from ClinicalTrials.gov) that had MDD as the first outcome, but did not involve PBM (or t-PBM). One hundred twenty-five records (34.06%, n = 107 on PubMed; n = 18 on ClinicalTrials.gov) were studies involving neither MDD or TRD, nor PBM. Furthermore, 53 records (14.44%, n = 28 on PubMed; n = 25 on ClinicalTrials.gov) were studies involving diverse applications of PBM, such as systemic PBM, but not t-PBM. Only 14.44% of all the records (n = 53, n = 43 from PubMed; n = 10 from ClinicalTrials.gov) were fully related to the topic of t-PBM, MDD, and TRD. The records from PubMed included 20 review articles, 10 preclinical/animal models, 2 simulation studies, 2 case reports, and 9 clinical trials, including 1 open-label single arm-study and 4 randomized clinical trials (RCTs) (one of them is a protocol). The statuses from the 10 clinical trials resulting from the search in ClinicalTrials.gov were as follows: n = 3, "not yet recruiting"; n = 1, "recruiting"; n = 6, "completed." Finally, from the 53 records fully related to t-PBM, MDD, and TRD, the authors considered 9 records as "original data." Although related to the topic, preclinical studies (animal models; n = 10) were not considered because it was not possible to identify TRD occurrence among rodents. **Fig. 1** shows a flow diagram summarizing the studies selection, from identification to inclusion.

Clinical Studies

Most of the studies involving the application of t-PBM for MDD present insufficient information about TRD occurrence. In addition, in the same studies, the diagnosis of TRD lacks standardization. Furthermore, there are methodologic limitations and

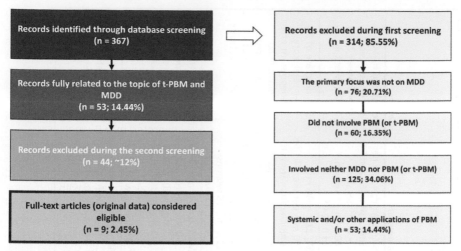

Fig. 1. The studies' selection, from identification to inclusion/exclusion. Rectangles on the left represent all records resulting from the search on PubMed and ClinicalTrials.gov, and the inclusion/exclusion during the first and the second screenings; rectangles on the right specify reasons for records' exclusion. "%" represents the percentage of records regarding the total of studies resulting from the search (X/100 of 367).

heterogeneity of t-PBM regimens across the studies included in this review. The authors present details for the t-PBM regimens in **Table 1**.

An open study performed by Schiffer and colleagues[43] included 10 patients with MDD with a comorbid anxiety disorder under unaltered treatment with serotonin and norepinephrine reuptake inhibitor (SNRI) or selective serotonin reuptake inhibitor (SSRI) (n = 8), benzodiazepine (n = 4), buprenorphine (n = 5), methadone (n = 1), and psychotherapy (n = 4). Four patients were receiving at least 2 antidepressants from different classes. By definition (see Introduction), the participants of the Schiffer and colleagues' study can be considered patients with TRD. They were treated with a t-PBM NIR light-emitting diode (LED) device in a single session, at 2 sites on the forehead, aiming at the dorsolateral prefrontal cortex (DLPFC), bilaterally. At 2- and 4-weeks posttreatment, a significant decrease in depression symptoms was observed (HAM-D$_{21}$, −13.2 and −6.5 points, respectively); anxious symptoms were also reduced. The response rate of MDD in week 2 (decrease in HAM-D$_{21}$ score ≥ 50%) was 40%. On the fourth week posttreatment, depressive symptoms were on the increase, suggesting the short-lasting effect of a single treatment and progressive resistance.

Cassano and colleagues[44] tested the safety and efficacy of multiple sessions of t-PBM in patients with moderate MDD during a double-blind sham-controlled study; 50% (n = 4) of the participants had a lack of response to at least 1 antidepressant medication and psychotherapy course (stable treatment for at least 6 and 8 weeks, respectively) during the current episode. Patients with MDD were treated for 3 weeks with t-PBM or sham and followed by crossover to 3 more weeks of t-PBM or sham after a 1-week interval. The investigators used an 808-nm NIR laser device. Both the device and the specific parameters, such as localization on the forehead, were similar to those of Schiffer and colleagues[43] (see **Table 1**). At baseline, patients presented an average HAM-D$_{17}$ of 19.8 ± 4.35 (thus also qualifying for TRD-based HAM-D severity, for those patients who had been in treatment). The 4 patients with TRD were all randomized to

336   Vieira et al

Table 1
Antidepressant effect of transcranial photobiomodulation in clinical studies

Study	Design (Duration)	Diagnosis and Number of Participants	Concomitant Antidepressant Treatments	Wavelength/Device	Parameters	Results
Schiffer et al,[43] 2009	Open pilot (4 wk)	Treatment-resistant MDD (n_{NIR} = 10)	Pharmacotherapy (8/10) Psychotherapy (4/10)	810 nm LED Marubeni America Corp, Santa Clara, CA, USA	250 mW/cm^2; 4 min per site; 2 sites (F3 and F4); ~1 cm^2 per site; 60 J/cm^2; 1 session of 0.12 kJ	Decrease in HAM-D scores: remission 40% at week 2 and 20% at week 4
Naeser et al,[46] 2014	Open pilot (8 wk)	TBI with comorbid depression ($n_{NIR and Red}$ = 8)	Pharmacotherapy (8/8)	633- and 870-nm LEDs (0.5 W) MedX Health, Model 1100, Toronto, ON, Canada	CW; 22.2 mW/cm^2; 10 min per site; 11 sites (midline from front-to-back hairline; bilaterally on frontal, parietal, and temporal areas); total area of 22.48 cm^2; 3 J/cm^2; 18 sessions (3/wk for 6 wk)	≥50% decrease of BDI-II total score; antidepressant effect was maintained after 8 additional weeks (without t-PBM) in 2 patients
Cassano et al,[44] 2015	Open pilot (8 wk)	MDD (n_{NIR} = 4)	Psychotherapy (1/4) None (3/4)	808-nm laser (5 W) NeuroThera PhotoThera Inc, Carlsbad, CA, USA	CW; 700 mW/cm^2; 2 min per site; 4 sites (2 R- and 2 L-forehead); 7.1 cm^2 per site; 84 J/cm^2; 6 sessions of 2.41 kJ (2/wk for 3 wk)	Decrease in HAM-D scores: response 50% at week 6–7 but no response at week 8
Morries et al,[45] 2015	Retrospective case series (8 wk)	TBI with comorbid depression (n_{NIR} = 10)	Not reported	808- and 980-nm laser (9 and 13 W) LiteCure, Newark, DE, USA, and Diowave, Riviera Beach, FL, USA	PW; 10 min per site; large area of the forehead/frontal cortex; 132 cm^2; 14.8 and 28.3 J/cm^2	Decrease in QIDS total score; 5 patients remitted from depression

Study	Design	Population	Comparison	Device	Parameters	Outcomes
Disner et al,[48] 2016	RCT (2 wk) Parallel design	Elevated depressive symptoms ($n_{NIR \text{ on right}}$ = 18) ($n_{NIR \text{ on left}}$ = 18) ($n_{Sham/controls}$ = 15)	ABM	1064-nm laser (3.4 W) CG-5000 Cell Gen Therapeutics, Dallas, TX, USA	CW; 250 mW/cm², 4 min per site (2 sites at ~Fp2 or at ~Fp1); 13.6 cm² per site; 60 J/cm²; 2 sessions of 1.63 kJ (48 h apart)	Right PBM enhanced the effect of ABM on depression (CES-D) in individuals with strong bias away from negative words. No significant differences in decrease of CES-D across PBM groups when ABM-responsiveness was not factored
Henderson & Morries,[47] 2017	Retrospective case series (from March 2013 to May 2017)	TBI with comorbid depression (n_{NIR} = 39)	Pharmacotherapy (29/39)	810- and 980-nm laser (8–15 W) LT1000 LiteCure, Newark, DE, USA; Diowave 810, Riviera Beach, FL, USA; Aspen Laser, Denver, CO, USA	PW; 30–45 W/cm²; 9–12 min per site (2 sites at forehead and temporal regions); 222–327 cm²; 55–81 J/cm²; 8–34 sessions	Decrease in HAM-D and QIDS-SR scores
Cassano et al,[49] 2018	RCT (8 wk) Double-blind, parallel design	MDD (n_{NIR} = 10) ($n_{Sham/controls}$ = 11)	Pharmacotherapy (6/21) Psychotherapy (5/21) None (12/21)	823-nm LED (~1W × 2, bilateral) Omnilux New U Photomedex Inc, Littleton, CO, USA	CW; 36 mW/cm²; 20–30 min per site (2 sites at F3 and F4); 28.7 cm² per site; up to 65 J/cm²; 16 sessions of 3.4 kJ (2/wk for 8 wk)	Decrease in HAM-D scores significantly greater in the PBM group. Higher rate of response in the PBM group at endpoint: 50% vs 27% in controls. No significant differences at QIDS-SR

(continued on next page)

**Table 1
(continued)**

Study	Design (Duration)	Diagnosis and Number of Participants	Concomitant Antidepressant Treatments	Wavelength/Device	Parameters	Results
Kerppers et al,[50] 2020	Nonrandomized clinical trial (4 wk)	Elevated depressive symptoms and anxiety (n_{NIR} = 11) ($n_{Sham/controls}$ = 11)	Not reported	945-nm LED (0.11 W) RL5-R12008, St. Louis, MO, USA	9.25 J/cm^2; 1 min and 25 s per site; 1 site at the frontal sinus region; 30 daily sessions	Improvement in the brain activity of t-PBM-treated individuals; reduced values for depression in HADS score
Iosifescu et al,[52] 2022	RCT (6 wk)	MDD Phase 1 (n_{NIR} = 18) ($n_{Sham/controls}$ = 31) Phase 2 (n_{NIR} = 10) ($n_{Sham/controls}$ = 7)	Psychotherapy and/or pharmacotherapy (31/49)	830-nm LED (~2 W) LiteCure LLC TPBM-1000, Newark, DE, USA	CW; 54.8 mW/cm^2; 20 min total; 4 spots at the forehead (Fp1, Fp2, F3, and F4); 35.8 cm^2; 65.8 J/cm^2; 12 sessions of 2.35 kJ (2/wk for 6 wk)	Reduction in HAM-D17 scores when comparing pretreatment and posttreatment. However, there was no superior effect of the active treatment over sham

Abbreviations: CGICW, continuous wave; NO, nitric oxide; PFC, prefrontal cortex; PW, pulsed wave; QIDS-SR, quick inventory of depressive symptomatology self-report.

sham first and dropped from the study before crossover to NIR. At weeks 6 and 7, 50% of the non-TRD participants achieved remission with HAM-D$_{17}$ of 4 and 3, respectively. In sum, only 4 non-TRD participants concluded the treatment (main age of 47 ± 14 years [1 woman and 3 men]), with a mean HAM-D$_{17}$ total score of 13 ± 5.35; t-PBM was the only intervention driving the antidepressant effect, and no other antidepressant treatment had been delivered for the last 6 months.

Morries and colleagues[45] reported a case series including 10 patients with traumatic brain injury (TBI) who experienced symptoms of depression, with a Quick Inventory of Depressive Symptomatology (QIDS) mean total score of 12.9 ± 4.6. Out of the 10 patients, 6 were diagnosed with MDD. The investigators applied t-PBM through a class IV laser device (980 nm and 808 nm) over a large area of the forehead/frontal cortex. At the endpoint, all patients presented a significant reduction of depression symptoms (mean QIDS total score 2.2 ± 2.3), and those with MDD showed a decrease of QIDS total score ≥ 50% from baseline; 5 patients remitted from depression (QIDS total score ≤ 5). The investigators did not mention TRD occurrence rates, although no other treatment modalities (medications, exercise regimen, supplements) were added, discontinued, or changed while receiving t-PBM. Moreover, they reported significant clinical improvement with the resolution of many of their symptoms, including headache, insomnia, irritability, anxiety, and suicidal thoughts.

Naeser and colleagues[46] also reported the beneficial effects of t-PBM in patients with TBI with comorbid depression. Eleven patients with mild, moderate, or severe depression (based on Beck Depression Inventory [BDI-II] total score [mean BDI-II total scores were 22 ± 7.4]) were treated with a 3-LED cluster heads device (870 nm and 633 nm). Skull sites of t-PBM involved the midline from front to back, and bilaterally on frontal, parietal, and temporal areas. At the end of the treatment period, 3 patients presented an antidepressant response (≥50% decrease of BDI-II total score from baseline; mean total scores of 14.8 ± 6.5), whereas 2 continued to report severe or moderate depression at 2 months posttreatment. Therefore, these 2 patients can be considered TRD for both pharmacologic and nonpharmacologic therapies (t-PBM).

A study performed by Henderson and Morries[47] included 39 patients with chronic TBI with comorbid depression treated with t-PBM. Of the 39 patients, 27 had a prior diagnosis of depression by an outside clinician and 69% had taken antidepressant medication before their evaluation for t-PBM treatment. In addition, 74% were taking antidepressants during t-PBM treatment. The average duration of treatment with traditional antidepressants exceeded 72 months, and all 39 patients continued to have symptoms of depression. Medications included typical antidepressants (eg, fluoxetine, paroxetine, and sertraline) and atypical antidepressants, such as bupropion. Other medications reported were mood stabilizers (eg, lithium) and those for sleep or pain (eg, gabapentin). According to the investigators, 9 patients had been previously diagnosed with TRD. Henderson and Morries[47] used 3 different NIR laser devices (810 nm and 980 nm), which were applied to the forehead and temporal regions bilaterally. The total duration of each t-PBM session was 30 minutes, and the total number of t-PBM applications ranged from 8 to 34 sessions, based on individual patient improvement. The mean HAM-D score decreased from 21.48 ± 5.24 (at baseline) to 6.0 ± 5.12 (at the endpoint) (P<.001; socioeconomic status [SES] = 2.99), thus demonstrating full remission in most subjects. The QIDS-SR (self-rated before and after finishing the entire t-PBM treatment) decreased from 14.1 ± 3.3 to 3.41 ± 3.3 (P<.001; SES = 3.24). Thirty-six patients (92%) responded to the treatment (decrease of QIDS total score ≥ 50% from baseline).

Disner and colleagues[48] analyzed the effects of t-PBM (1064-nm laser) as a synergist tool for attention bias modification (ABM) technique in patients with elevated levels of depressive symptoms. The investigators used the Center for Epidemiological Studies Depression (CES-D) scale, with a total score of greater than 16 as an inclusion criterion. A total of 51 patients were randomized into 3 groups: 2 sessions of t-PBM on the right forehead, left forehead, or sham. The interval between the 2 sessions was 48 hours, and ABM was performed for all participants before and after each t-PBM session. In those who responded to ABM, the improvement in CES-D total score was enhanced by the right t-PBM, whereas no significant effect was observed for the left and sham t-PBM. As reported by the investigators, participants were permitted to use psychotropic medication, so long as they had been on a stable dose for at least 2 months before study enrollment. Thirty-nine participants (76%) were unmedicated, and no participants adjusted their psychiatric medication during their 2 weeks of follow-up. Among medicated participants (n = 12; 24%), the most prescribed family of medications were SSRIs (eg, fluoxetine; n = 8), followed by mood stabilizers (eg, lamotrigine; n = 4), atypical antidepressants (eg, bupropion; n = 2), and anxiolytics (eg, alprazolam; n = 2).

Cassano and colleagues[49] assessed the efficacy of t-PBM (823-nm LED) in 21 patients with MDD randomized to receive bilateral irradiation on DLPFC (electroencephalogram [EEG] sites F3 and F4) or sham treatment. Only patients who, during the current depressive episode, failed no more than 1 FDA-approved antidepressant medication (for at least 6 weeks) and had no more than 1 course of structured psychotherapy for depression (for at least 8 weeks) were included in the study. Treatment was applied twice a week for 8 weeks (see **Table 1**). In the PBM group, depression severity (as assessed by the HAM-D_{17}) significantly decreased from baseline (>50%) compared with sham (-10.8 ± 7.55 vs -4.4 ± 6.65). A secondary outcome was that the t-PBM–treated patients had improvement in sexual dysfunction independent of the antidepressant effect.

Kerppers and colleagues[50] analyzed the effects of t-PBM on 22 university students (17–25 years old) with symptoms of anxiety and depression, who obtained a score of 8 to 21 points on the Hospital Anxiety and Depression Scale (HADS) (adapted by Botega[51]). One group (n = 11) received t-PBM treatment (device composed of 7 LEDs, 945 nm) on the frontal region (frontal sinus) for 30 consecutive days. The second group (n = 11) received placebo treatment (light off) at the same site. The investigators reported improvement in t-PBM–treated individuals, thus resulting in reduced values for depression (HADS score at baseline = 12.82 ± 3.18 points; HADS score at endpoint = 6.66 ± 2.50 points). No significant differences were observed on the scores of placebo groups. No information regarding TRD and/or subjects' antidepressant medication history was provided.

Iosifescu and colleagues[51,52] included, initially (phase 1), 49 outpatients with MDD randomized (1:2) to receive t-PBM (NIR) or sham for 6 weeks. Exclusion criteria were regarding subjects with active suicidality (Columbia-Suicide Severity Rating Scale, score ≥ 3) and TRD, adopting the definition of ≥ 2 FDA-approved antidepressant medication trials failed during the current depressive episode (as assessed by the Massachusetts General Hospital Antidepressant Treatment Response Questionnaire) or any failed FDA-approved device-based intervention (ie, TMS, ECT, VNS) during the current MDD episode. After the 6-week period, patients who did not respond to sham were rerandomized (1:1) between NIR or sham for an additional 6 weeks (phase 2). This study showed that when comparing the pretreatment and posttreatment scores in participants who received the active treatment, there was a reduction in depression scores on the HAM-D17 of 3.44 ± 5.03 (SES = 0.68) in phase 1 (first 6 weeks) and 2.6 ± 6.52 (SES = 0.40) in phase 2 (additional 6 weeks). However, there was no superior effect of the active treatment over sham (P_{phase1} = .378; SES_{phase1} = 0.17 and P_{phase2} = .302; SES_{phase2} = 0.38).

DISCUSSION

Data presented in this review pointed to a beneficial effect of t-PBM on MDD even in patients showing previous resistance to conventional or complementary treatments. To better understand the mechanistic effects of NIR on biological tissues, one needs to consider the evolutionary aspects of living beings and their relationship to sunlight. In this sense, light, in general, is known to have a wide range of effects on physiologic and behavioral functions, including circadian rhythm, mood, and cognition. Moreover, light, the circadian clock, and sleep may closely interact to allow organisms to adapt to their environments.[53] This interaction can explain why changes in the light environment (eg, shiftwork, shortened day lengths in winter, and transmeridian travel) are associated with general changes in health, including mental health issues, such as seasonal affective disorder, depression, and cognitive dysfunction.[54] In addition, light deprivation can induce depressive-like symptoms, which further indicates that light energy is a powerful modulator of mood-related disorders.[3] Therefore, it is not surprising that recent research studies support the antidepressant effects of light therapy, especially NIR and red light.

Photons in the range of red to NIR spectra (600–1100 nm) can efficiently penetrate biological tissues, including the central nervous system, especially the brain, and produce "photobiomodulatory" effects. It is worth mentioning the capacity of NIR light to penetrate the scalp and skull, thus reaching the brain. Haeussinger and colleagues[55] estimated that the mean penetration depth of NIR light through the scalp and skull is about 23.6 ± 0.7 mm, considering the deepest 5% of light. A study performed by Jagdeo and colleagues[56] used human cadaver heads (skulls with intact soft tissue) to measure penetration of 830-nm light. They observed that NIR light penetration depends on the anatomic region of the skull (0.9% at the temporal region, 2.1% at the frontal region, and 11.7% at the occipital region). The study of Tedford and colleagues[57] found that 808-nm light can reach a depth in the human cadaver brain of 40 to 50 mm. Because the NIR light reaches the brain, it can increase ATP synthesis, neurogenesis, brain perfusion, and modulation of inflammation.[33] Several animal and clinical studies on MDD have shown that t-PBM can induce antidepressant-like effects when the prefrontal cortex is targeted, for example.[3] Moreover, increasing evidence supports the capacity of t-PBM to improve neuromuscular performance, increase brain-derived neurotrophic factor, reduce brain lesion volume in TBI, and enhance of learning and memory. Xu and colleagues[58] showed that t-PBM effectively decreased depression-like behaviors, increased ATP biosynthesis, and increased levels of mitochondrial complex IV expression and activity in 2 depressive-related mice models. In another study using the forced swim test and electrocorticography spectral analysis, t-PBM was shown to successfully ameliorate depressive-related behavior induced by reserpine in rats.[59]

As MDD symptoms are closely related to the monoamine neurotransmitters (eg, dopamine, serotonin, and norepinephrine levels), the pathogenesis of MDD has been hypothesized to be neurotransmitter-dependent.[60] Although speculative, some lines of evidence suggest a possible dopamine-related mechanism in the genesis of TRD. A study performed by Williams and colleagues[61,62] demonstrated that abuse (physical, sexual, or emotional) occurring at ages 4 to 7 years was associated with significantly poorer outcomes following the treatment with sertraline compared with another SSRI, escitalopram, and the SNRI venlafaxine-XR. Participants who were abused at this age showed significantly less improvement in both clinician and self-rated symptoms following 8 weeks of treatment with sertraline. Sertraline, in contrast to other SSRI antidepressants, has an additional relatively specific effect on inhibiting dopamine.[59] There is some evidence that subgroups of patients with MDD are also characterized by dopamine circuit dysfunction, and a number of traumatic events have been associated with higher ventral striatal dopamine response to amphetamine. (Interestingly, in the study of Henderson and Morries,[47] 74% of the participants were taking antidepressants during the course of t-PBM treatment.) This information arouses the possible dopamine-related TRD genesis in those patients with MDD. In this sense, the general improvement of depressive symptoms observed in the studies included in this review could be related to the effects of t-PBM (or PBM) on the levels of serotonin and dopamine in the brain. A preclinical study performed by Xu and colleagues[58] has shown that Ahi1 KO mice present a significant down-regulation of serotonin and dopamine levels and depressive-like behaviors. Moreover, after the treatment with t-PBM, Ahi1 KO mice had depressive-like behaviors attenuated, which was related to the enhancement of serotonin and dopamine levels in the brain. Thus, the therapeutic mechanism of t-PBM in depression seems to be closely associated with the same monoamine neurotransmitters, which are abnormal in TRD individuals.

In consonance with the aspects of TRD genesis mentioned above, Williams and colleagues[61] suggest a critical period for childhood trauma, which has the most significant impact on subsequent poor response to antidepressants in adulthood. Thus, the greater the exposure to trauma during critical neurodevelopmental periods, the less likely these depressed patients were to remit following antidepressant response. Unfortunately, the authors cannot track if there is a history of childhood trauma experienced by the participants in the studies considered in their review, but it is worth considering such possible correlation with TRD.

It is important for psychiatrists to be aware of pseudoresistance occurrence, which mainly includes inadequate antidepressant dosing and/or early discontinuation of treatment before the completion of an adequate trial. Other causes of pseudoresistance can be due to atypical pharmacokinetics, patient noncompliance with treatment, and misdiagnosis of the primary disorder.[15] In this sense, a significant portion of patients with MDD can be undertreated and receive inadequate doses of antidepressants, thus being diagnosed as TRD, despite truly being pseudoresistant.[63] This lack of consensus in the psychiatric community regarding TRD diagnosis contributes to the misidentification of treatment-resistant patients,[15,63] which could explain the underreporting of TRD status in the studies involving MDD and t-PBM that were considered for this review. However, according to a review performed by Greden,[64] the TRD category can be used to broadly identify patients with MDD who are nonresponsive to conventional therapies, such as pharmacotherapy and psychotherapy. Considering that broad definition, all the studies considered, except Kerppers and colleagues,[50] included patients with low, mid, or high TRD.

A rigorous diagnosis of MDD is crucial. In fact, treatment strategies and their effectiveness vary depending upon the diagnosis (eg, psychotic depression, bipolar depression, atypical depression, unipolar depression, and other subtypes). Comorbid illnesses need to be considered, such as organic causes like medications, substance abuse, and metabolic disorders. In this sense, patients with TRD should be thoroughly evaluated for the occurrence of comorbid psychiatric or general medical disorders, as observed in the studies of Morries and colleagues,[45] Naeser and colleagues,[46] and Henderson and Morries[47] about patients with TBIs with comorbid depression. In the same way, all patients with MDD included in the study of Schiffer and colleagues[43] had a comorbid anxiety disorder, and 20% of Morries and colleagues[45] study participants reported substance abuse. In general, anxiety disorders, substance abuse, and personality disorders are frequently associated with nonresponse to antidepressant therapies.[65] As mentioned above, some investigators also consider that a history of early life stress increases treatment resistance.[66,67] For instance, missing the diagnosis of bipolar disorder is also a common cause of apparent treatment resistance,[68] as antidepressants are then mistakenly prescribed to patients with bipolar depression.[69] A study on the relationship between episode duration and antidepressant therapy concluded that little progress has been made in reducing the length of depressive episodes in bipolar disorder.[70]

Regarding comorbid anxiety, the study of Schiffer and colleagues[43] demonstrated that such an associated disorder could adversely affect MDD patients' responsiveness to t-PBM. Nevertheless, the investigators applied a single t-PBM session, leading one to theorize that repeated light-therapy sessions are necessary for achieving MDD remission. However, it is still difficult to predict the efficacy of t-PBM simply based on the number of delivered treatments, as the physiologic capacity of individuals to respond to the therapy might be compromised by chronic anxiety and other comorbid psychiatric illness.

t-PBM effects may be strengthened through combination with other treatments, such as psychotherapy and psychotropic medications. However, as demonstrated by Cassano and colleagues,[44] subjects with MDD achieved remission (HAM-D$_{17}$ scores $\leq$ 7) after t-PBM with no concurrent treatment being administrated during the course of the study. Accordingly, the participants that completed the study of Cassano and colleagues[44] were not considered TRD, thus raising the idea that t-PBM could be applied as the main therapy for MDD rather than a secondary treatment approach administered only after the failure of antidepressants. In the study of Henderson and Morries,[47] the 82% treatment remission rate is considered superior to that described for oral antidepressants[71,72] and to that described by Schiffer and colleagues[43] (60%) in 10 patients and Cassano and colleagues[44] (50%) in 4 patients using NIR.

Prescribing Considerations

t-PBM is a promising new therapy with potential benefits for patients with TRD. Despite evidence demonstrating its mechanisms in the brain and clinical trials showing an antidepressant effect, t-PBM is still a non-FDA–approved treatment for MDD. However, clinical trials have shown that t-PBM can be safely offered to patients who do not respond to, are unable to tolerate, or decline to receive antidepressants or psychotherapy. t-PBM treatment in this context would therefore need to be administered as an off-label treatment or through participation within a clinical trial. In either scenario, it is likely that patients will receive close monitoring by a physician and contribute to the science behind t-PBM applications. If a patient is not interested in participating in research trials, they may want to consider t-PBM devices that may be commercially available.

There are no standardized treatment parameters for t-PBM, as a more personalized approach to treatment may be necessary for each patient. Based on data obtained from clinical trials on t-PBM for TRD, one could consider an average of the following parameters: using laser or LED devices; wavelengths of 810 and 850 nm are typical; location is bilaterally on the forehead (EEG sites F3 and F4) targeting the DLPFC; fluences from 60 to 100 J/cm^2; irradiances from 200 to 300 mW/cm^2; pulsed-wave mode (40 or 10 Hz, and duty cycle of 50%); duration from 5 to 10 minutes; surface of application ranging from 10 to 20 cm^2.

Relative contraindications for the use of t-PBM include patients with brain stents, shunts, and surgical aneurysm clips because infrared light can improve cerebral blood flow and theoretically might dislodge implants. In some cases, after careful consideration from neurologists and neurosurgeons, these patients have received t-PBM, particularly when the site of their implant was distant enough from the light source to consider safe use of t-PBM. Patients with recent hemorrhagic stroke may also not be eligible candidates for t-PBM treatment, owing to the increased chance of bleeding secondary to vasodilation induced by t-PBM. A third concern is the related potential warming, and potential interference on light penetration, owing to brain hematoma subjacent to the source of light. Although there is a lack of evidence regarding the safety of t-PBM during pregnancy and breast-feeding, the authors do not believe it poses a risk to embryos or fetuses, and there is a lack of evidence regarding its safety in this special population; however, risks for the embryo and fetus are not expected from this topical and transcranial intervention. Regarding the use of t-PBM in children, although parents may be more inclined to noninvasive neuromodulation techniques over pharmacologic interventions, the safety of t-PBM in developing brains is still unknown.

SUMMARY

The predominant challenges for ongoing and future studies about the effects of t-PBM in MDD treatment-resistant patients are the accuracy and standardization of diagnoses of MDD and/or TRD as well as the standardization of t-PBM parameters. Comorbidities and the patient's antidepressant medication history are also relevant to the responsiveness to t-PBM.

CLINICS CARE POINTS

- MDD is one of the greatest factors undermining global health and is considered a financial burden for the health systems. Clinicians should be aware of the individual impairment and suffering associated with MDD. Treatment of MDD should not be delayed, and when first-line treatments are not effective or not tolerated or even just declined, other interventions should be promptly considered.

- Resistance to antidepressant treatment can develop, even in patients who were previously responsive; comorbid and progressive illnesses contribute to the likelihood of chronic MDD with treatment resistance. The latter should prompt the clinician to more aggressive treatment regimens, including trials with less proven, but safe, interventions for depression.

- Whenever confronted with treatment-resistance, clinicians should more carefully consider differential diagnoses, such as bipolar depression.- Clinical trials have shown that t-PBM can be safely offered to patients who do not respond to, are unable to tolerate or decline to receive antidepressants or psychotherapy.

- While comorbid anxiety disorders are typically associated with higher chances of TRD, the limited available evidence shows that t-PBM could benefit both depressive and anxiety symptoms in these patients.

- While little is known about t-PBM in combination with antidepressant medications and psychotherapy, these associations are typically well-tolerated and might potentially offset some side effects of antidepressant pharmacotherapy, such as sexual side effects or cognitive side effects.

DISCLOSURE

In the last 5 years, Dr D.V. Iosifescu has received consulting honoraria from Alkermes, Allergan, Axsome, Biogen, Boehringer Ingelheim, Centers for Psychiatric Excellence, Clexio, Global Medical Education, Jazz, Lundbeck, Neumora, Otsuka, Precision

Neuroscience, Relmada, Sage, and Sunovion and research support (through his academic institution) from Alkermes, Ireland, AstraZeneca, United Kingdom, BrainsWay, Burlington, MA, USA; Cresskill, NJ, USA, and Jerusalem, Israel, LiteCure, NeoSync, United States, Otsuka, United States, Roche, Switzerland, and Shire. Dr P. Cassano consulted for Janssen Research and Development and for Niraxx Light Therapeutics Inc; was funded by PhotoThera Inc, LiteCure LLC, and Cerebral Sciences Inc to conduct studies on transcranial photobiomodulation; is a shareholder of Niraxx Light Therapeutics Inc; and has filed several patents related to the use of near-infrared light in psychiatry. The other authors have nothing to disclose.

REFERENCES

1. Murray C, Lopez A. Global mortality, disability, and the contribution of risk factors: global burden of disease study. Lancet 1997;349:1436–42.
2. Akil H, Gordon J, Hen R, et al. Treatment resistant depression: a multi-scale, systems biology approach. Neurosci Biobehav Rev 2018;84:272–88.
3. Khoodoruth MAS, Estudillo-Guerra MA, Pacheco-Barrios K, et al. Glutamatergic system in depression and its role in neuromodulatory techniques optimization. Front Psychiatry 2022;13:886918.
4. Geschwind DH, Flint J. Genetics and genomics of psychiatric disease. Science 2015;349:1489–94.
5. Otte C, Gold SM, Penninx BW, et al. Major depressive disorder. Nat Rev Dis Primers 2016;2:16065.
6. Thase ME, Rush AJ. When at first you don't succeed: sequential strategies for antidepressant nonresponders. J Clin Psychiatry 1997;58:23–9.
7. Souery D. Treatment resistant depression: methodological overview and operational criteria. Eur Psychopharmacol 1999;9:83–91.
8. Nierenberg A, Keck PJ, Samson J, et al. Methodological considerations for the study of treatment-resistant depression. In: Amsterdam J, editor. Advances in neuropsychiatry and psychopharmacology, Vol. 2. New York, NY: Raven Press; 1991.
9. Thase ME, Schwartz TL. Choosing medications for treatment-resistant depression based on mechanism of action. J Clin Psychiatry 2015;76:720–7.
10. Crown WH, Finkelstein S, Berndt ER, et al. The impact of treatment-resistant depression on health care utilization and costs. J Clin Psychiatry 2002;63:963–71.
11. Pandarakalam JP. Challenges of treatment-resistant depression. Psychiatr Danub 2018;30:273–84.
12. Fava M, Davidson KG. Definition and epidemiology of treatment-resistant depression. Psychiatr Clin North Am 1996;19:179–200.
13. Thase ME, Rush JA. Treatment-resistant depression. In: Bloom FE, Kupfer DJ, editors. Psychopharmacology. New York: Raven; 1995. p. 1081–97.
14. Golden RN, Nemeroff CB, McSorley P, et al. Efficacy and tolerability of controlled-release and immediate-release paroxetine in the treatment of depression. J Clin Psychiatry 2002;63:577–84.
15. Souery D, Papakostas GI, Trivedi MH. Treatment-resistant depression. J Clin Psychiatry 2006;67:16–22.
16. Nierenberg AA, Keefe BR, Leslie VC, et al. Residual symptoms in depressed patients who respond acutely to fluoxetine. J Clin Psychiatry 1999;60:221–5.
17. Paykel ES, Ramana R, Cooper Z, et al. Residual symptoms after partial remission: an important outcome in depression. Psychol Med 1995;25:1171–80.

18. Mayberg HS, Lozano AM, Voon V, et al. Deep brain stimulation for treatment-resistant depression. Neuron 2005;45:651–60.

19. Milev RV, Giacobbe P, Kennedy SH, et al. Canadian Network for Mood and Anxiety Treatments (CANMAT) 2016 Clinical Guidelines for the Management of Adults with Major Depressive Disorder: Section 4. Neurostimulation Treatments. Can J Psychiatry 2016;61:561–75.

20. Cassano P, Petrie SR, Hamblin MR, et al. Review of transcranial photobiomodulation for major depressive disorder: targeting brain metabolism, inflammation, oxidative stress, and neurogenesis. Neurophotonics 2016;3:31404.

21. Caldieraro MA, Cassano P. Transcranial and systemic photobiomodulation for major depressive disorder: a systematic review of efficacy, tolerability and biological mechanisms. J Affect Disord 2019;243:262–73.

22. Caldieraro MA, Laufer-Silva T, Cassano P. Dosimetry and clinical efficacy of transcranial photobiomodulation for major depression disorder: could they guide dosimetry for Alzheimer's disease? J Alzheimers Dis 2021;83:1453–69.

23. Salehpour F, Mahmoudi J, Kamari F, et al. Brain photobiomodulation therapy: a narrative review. Mol Neurobiol 2018;55:6601–36.

24. Barrett DW, Gonzalez-Lima F. Transcranial infrared laser stimulation produces beneficial cognitive and emotional effects in humans. Neuroscience 2013;230: 13–23.

25. Lapchak PA. Taking a light approach to treating acute ischemic stroke patients: transcranial near-infrared laser therapy translational science. Ann Med 2010;42: 576–86.

26. Vieira WF, Kenzo-Kagawa B, Cogo JC, et al. Low-level laser therapy (904 nm) counteracts motor deficit of mice hind limb following skeletal muscle injury caused by snakebite-mimicking intramuscular venom injection. PLoS One 2016;11:e0158980.

27. Vieira WF, Kenzo-Kagawa B, Britto MHM, et al. Vibrational spectroscopy of muscular tissue intoxicated by snake venom and exposed to photobiomodulation therapy. Lasers Med Sci 2018;33:503–12.

28. Vieira WF, Kenzo-Kagawa B, Alvares LE, et al. Exploring the ability of low-level laser irradiation to reduce myonecrosis and increase Myogenin transcription after Bothrops jararacussu envenomation. Photochem Photobiol Sci 2021;20:571–83.

29. Vieira WF, de Magalhães SF, Farias FH, et al. Raman spectroscopy of dorsal root ganglia from streptozotocin-induced diabetic neuropathic rats submitted to photobiomodulation therapy. J Biophotonics 2019;12:e201900135.

30. Vieira WF, Malange KF, de Magalhães SF, et al. Anti-hyperalgesic effects of photobiomodulation therapy (904 nm) on streptozotocin-induced diabetic neuropathy imply MAPK pathway and calcium dynamics modulation. Sci Rep 2022;12: 16730.

31. Rochkind S. Photobiomodulation in neuroscience: a summary of personal experience. Photomed Laser Surg 2017;35:604–15.

32. Chung H, Dai T, Sharma SK, et al. The nuts and bolts of low-level laser (light) therapy. Ann Biomed Eng 2012;40:516–33.

33. De Freitas LF, Hamblin MR. Proposed mechanisms of photobiomodulation or low-level light therapy. IEEE J Sel Top Quantum Electron 2016;22:348–64.

34. Nestler EJ, Hyman SE. Animal models of neuropsychiatric disorders. Nat Neurosci 2010;13:1161–9.

35. American Psychiatric Association. Diagnostic and statistical manual of mental disorders. 4th edn. Washington: American Psychiatric Association; 2000.

36. Solomon DA, Keller MB, Leon AC, et al. Multiple recurrences of major depressive disorder. Am J Psychiatry 2000;157:229–33.
37. Slavich GM, Monroe SM, Gotlib IH. Early parental loss and de- pression history: associations with recent life stress in major depressive disorder. J Psychiatr Res 2011;45:1146–52.
38. Morris MC, Ciesla JA, Garber J. A prospective study of stress autonomy versus stress sensitization in adolescents at varied risk for depression. J Abnorm Psychol 2010;119:341–54.
39. Rush AJ, Wisniewski SR, Zisook S, et al. Is prior course of illness relevant to acute or longer-term outcomes in depressed out-patients? A STAR*D report. Psychol Med 2011;19:1–19.
40. Willner P, Belzung C. Treatment-resistant depression: are animal models of depression fit for purpose? Psychopharmacology (Berl) 2015;232:3473–95.
41. Isingrini E, Camus V, Le Guisquet AM, et al. Association between repeated unpredictable chronic mild stress (UCMS) procedures with a high fat diet: a model of fluoxetine resistance in mice. PLoS One 2010;5:e10404.
42. Camus V, Kraehenbuhl H, Preisig M, et al. Geriatric depression and vascular diseases: what are the links? J Affect Disord 2004;81:1–16.
43. Schiffer F, Johnston AL, Ravichandran C, et al. Psychological benefits 2 and 4 weeks after a single treatment with near infrared light to the forehead: a pilot study of 10 patients with major depression and anxiety. Behav Brain Funct 2009;5:46.
44. Cassano P, Cusin C, Mischoulon D, et al. Near-Infrared transcranial radiation for major depressive disorder: proof of concept study. Psychiatry J 2015;2015: 352979.
45. Morries LD, Cassano P, Henderson TA. Treatments for traumatic brain injury with emphasis on transcranial near infrared laser phototherapy. Neuropsychiatr Dis Treat 2015;11:2159–75.
46. Naeser MA, Zafonte R, Krengel MH, et al. Significant improvements in cognitive performance post-transcranial, red/near-infrared light-emitting diode treatments in chronic, mild traumatic brain injury: open-protocol study. J Neurotrauma 2014;31:1008–17.
47. Henderson TA, Morries LD. Multi-watt near-infrared phototherapy for the treatment of comorbid depression: an open-label single-arm study. Front Psychiatry 2017;8:187.
48. Disner S, Beevers CG, Gonzalez-Lima F. Transcranial laser stimulation as neuroenhancement for attention bias modification in adults with elevated depression symptoms. Brain Stimul 2016;9:780–7.
49. Cassano P, Petrie SR, Mischoulon D, et al. Transcranial photobiomodulation for the treatment of major depressive disorder. The ELATED-2 pilot trial. Photomed Laser Surg 2018;36:634–46.
50. Kerppers FK, Dos Santos KMMG, Cordeiro MER, et al. Study of transcranial photobiomodulation at 945-nm wavelength: anxiety and depression. Lasers Med Sci 2020;35:1945–54.
51. Botega NJ. Mood disorders among medical in-patients: a validation study of the hospital anxiety and depression scale (HAD). Rev Saude Publica 1995;29:55–63.
52. Iosifescu DV, Norton RJ, Tural U, et al. Very low-level transcranial photobiomodulation for major depressive disorder: The ELATED-3 multicenter, randomized, sham-controlled trial. J Clin Psychiatry 2022;83:21m14226.
53. LeGates TA, Fernandez DC, Hattar S. Light as a central modulator of circadian rhythms, sleep and affect. Nature Reviews Neurosci 2014;15:443–54.

54. Zelinski EL, Deibel SH, McDonald RJ. The trouble with circadian clock dysfunction: Multiple deleterious effects on the brain and body. Neurosci Biobehav Rev 2014;40C:80–101.
55. Haeussinger FB, Heinzel S, Hahn T, et al. Simulation of near-infrared light absorption considering individual head and prefrontal cortex anatomy: implications for optical neuroimaging. PLoS One 2011;6:e26377.
56. Jagdeo JR, Adams LE, Brody NI, et al. Transcranial red and near infrared light transmission in a cadaveric model. PLoS One 2012;7:e47460.
57. Tedford CE, DeLapp S, Jacques S, et al. Quantitative analysis of transcranial and intraparenchymal light penetration in human cadaver brain tissue. Lasers Surg Med 2015;47:312–22.
58. Xu Z, Guo X, Yang Y, et al. Low-level laser irradiation improves depression-like behaviors in mice. Mol Neurobiol 2017;54:4551–9.
59. Mohammed HS. Transcranial low-level infrared laser irradiation ameliorates depression induced by reserpine in rats. Lasers Med Sci 2016;31:1651–6.
60. Nutt DJ. Relationship of neurotransmitters to the symptoms of major depressive disorder. J Clin Psychiatry 2008;69:4–7.
61. Williams LM, Debattista C, Duchemin AM, et al. Childhood trauma predicts antidepressant response in adults with major depression: data from the randomized international study to predict optimized treatment for depression. Transl Psychiatry 2016;6:e799.
62. Gatt JM, Nemeroff CB, Dobson-Stone C, et al. Interactions between BDNF Val66-Met polymorphisms and early life stress predict brain and arousal pathways to syndromal depression and anxiety. Mol Psychiatry 2009;14:681–95.
63. Sackeim HA. The definition and meaning of treatment-resistant depression. J Clin Psychiatry 2001;62:10–7.
64. Greden JF. The burden of disease for treatment-resistant depression. J Clin Psychiatry 2001;62:26–31.
65. Kornstein SG, Schneider RK. Clinical features of treatment-resistant depression. J Clin Psychiatry 2001;62:18–25.
66. Bernet CZ, Stein MB. Relationship of childhood maltreatment to the onset and course of major depression in adulthood. Depress Anxiety 1999;9:169–74.
67. Nanni V, Uher R, Danese A. Childhood maltreatment predicts unfavorable course of illness and treatment outcome in depression: a meta-analysis. Am J Psychiatry 2012;169:141–51.
68. Fagiolini A, Kupfer DJ. Is treatment-resistant depression a unique subtype of depression? Biol Psychiatry 2003;53:640–8.
69. Ghaemi SN, Sachs GS, Chiou AM, et al. Is bipolar disorder still underdiagnosed? Are antidepressants overutilized? J Affect Disord 1999;52:135–44.
70. Frankle WG, Perlis RH, Deckersbach T, et al. Bipolar depression: relationship between episode length and antidepressant treatment. Psychol Med 2002;32:1417–23.
71. Thase ME, Entsuah AR, Rudolph RL. Remission rates during treatment with venlafaxine or selective serotonin reuptake inhibitors. Br J Psychiatry 2001;178:234–41.
72. Connolly KR, Thase ME. If at first you don't succeed: a review of the evidence for antidepressant augmentation, combination and switching strategies. Drugs 2011;71:43–64.

The Role of Psychotherapy in the Management of Treatment-Resistant Depression

Taylor Rogan, BS, Samuel T. Wilkinson, MD*

KEYWORDS

- Major depressive disorder • Treatment-resistant depression • Psychotherapy
- Cognitive behavioral therapy • Electroconvulsive therapy
- Transcranial magnetic stimulation • Ketamine • Neuroplasticity

KEY POINTS

- Question - Can psychotherapy improve outcomes for patients with treatment-resistant depression?
- Findings - Evidence shows that psychotherapy is more likely to lead to response or remission compared with control conditions.
- Combining psychotherapy with powerful somatic/medical therapies that enhance plasticity may improve long-term outcomes.
- Future Directions - More research is needed on the combination of psychotherapy with somatic/medical therapies to improve long-term outcomes. Digital therapeutics also is a new avenue that may allow for substantially more funding into the development of tools based on psychotherapeutic principles to ameliorate the burden of treatment-resident depression.

INTRODUCTION

Major depressive disorder (MDD) is among the leading causes of disability worldwide. According to the National Institute of Mental Health, an estimated 14.8 million US adults had at least one major depressive episode leading to impairment in the year 2020.[1] As of 2010, the economic burden associated with MDD was estimated to be $210.5 billion in the United States alone.[2,3]

In the aftermath of the COVID-19 pandemic, the public health burden of depression is expected to worsen. The National Institute of Mental Health predicts that in the wake of the COVID-19 pandemic, mental health burden (most notably in the form of depression) is expected to increase substantially.[4] This highlights the need for increased understanding and more effective and accessible treatments for this devasting and increasingly prevalent disorder.

The Department of Psychiatry, Yale School of Medicine, New Haven, CT 06511, USA
* Corresponding author. 100 York Street, STE 2J, New Haven, CT 06511.
E-mail address: Samuel.wilkinson@yale.edu

Psychiatr Clin N Am 46 (2023) 349–358
https://doi.org/10.1016/j.psc.2023.02.006
0193-953X/23/© 2023 Elsevier Inc. All rights reserved.

A significant proportion of patients diagnosed with MDD do not respond to standard early line treatments, despite that there are many treatments available (>20). The diagnosis/categorization of treatment-resistant depression (TRD) is generally given after two antidepressant therapies fail to produce an adequate response for a patient. Most estimates suggest TRD comprises a substantial portion (12%–40%) of all patients with depression.[5,6]

Episodes of TRD are associated with prolonged patient suffering, significant burdens to caregivers, and great costs to health care systems. Compared with patients with treatment-responsive depression, patients with TRD have been found to have a greater risk of attempting suicide,[7] significantly higher rates of hospitalization,[8–10] spend longer time periods in depressed states, and be more likely to experience job loss.[8] Additionally, there are dramatic increases in health care resource utilization among TRD patients, including higher numbers of emergency department visits, outpatient visits, and prescriptions filled.[9] A recent study of 48,440 individuals with depression found that those with TRD had an average depression duration of 571 days and total medical costs to be 164% higher than non-TRD patients with depression. In sum, TRD yields a substantial burden to patients, caregivers, and health care systems. This review focuses on the role that psychotherapy has in the management of TRD.

PSYCHOTHERAPY ALONE FOR TREATMENT-RESISTANT DEPRESSION

More than a dozen clinical trials have examined the efficacy of some modality of psychotherapy (mostly some form of cognitive therapy) as a therapeutic approach for TRD. A 2018 meta-analysis included six clinical trials (total n = 924) that examined the efficacy of cognitive behavioral therapy (CBT) (k = 2 trials of mindfulness-based cognitive therapy, k = 3 trials of traditional CBT, k = 1 trial of CBT delivered via smartphone) in adults.[11] Immediately following the therapy period, patients assigned to cognitive therapy interventions were more likely to achieve response (risk ratio = 2.09; 95% confidence interval [CI], 1.49–2.92; Z = 4.30; $P < 0.00001$) and remission (risk ratio = 1.82; 95% CI, 1.17–2.83; Z = 2.65; $P = 0.008$) compared with the control condition. At a 6-month posttreatment follow-up, patients assigned to cognitive therapy interventions achieved response (risk ratio = 1.95; 95% CI, 1.26–3.02; Z = 3.01; $P = 0.02$), and remission (risk ratio = 1.91; 95% CI, 1.45–2.53; Z = 4.54; $P < 0.00001$). At 12-month follow-up, patients assigned to cognitive therapy were more likely to achieve response (risk ratio = 1.73; 95% CI, 1.42–2.11; Z = 5.40; $P < 0.00001$) and remission (risk ratio = 2.01; 95% CI, 1.54–2.62; Z = 5.14; $P < 0.00001$) compared with control condition. This meta-analysis did not find any evidence of publication bias using formal statistical testing. Although the rate of response or remission to CBT was greater than that of the control condition in this meta-analysis, response and remission rates were generally lower than in studies of uncomplicated MDD.

A more recent (2020) meta-analysis investigated psychotherapy approaches for the treatment of TRD. In 18 randomized trials (total n = 1734), the effect of various types of psychotherapy (cognitive-based therapy approach [k = 10], psychodynamic/psychoanalytic [k = 2], third-wave therapies [ie, mindfulness-based cognitive therapy, k = 5], and interpersonal psychotherapy [k = 1]) were investigated. The overall meta-analysis had a high heterogeneity between studies but showed an overall positive effect (based on symptom severity, a continuous measure) of therapy in the management of TRD (standardized mean difference of 0.818; 95% CI, 0.556–1.081; $P < 0.001$). There was significant evidence of publication bias. After imputation of potential missing studies, there was still a positive effect of psychotherapy, albeit with a lower effect size (standardized mean difference = 0.452; 95% CI, 0.157–0.748). In a subgroup analysis, there was no difference between different modalities of psychotherapy (cognitive-based therapy vs interpersonal psychotherapy); however, the meta-analysis had a small number of studies (k = 18) such that these comparisons may have been underpowered.[12]

PSYCHOTHERAPY IN COMBINATION WITH OTHER APPROACHES

Increasingly, mood disorders can be conceptualized as disorders of impaired plasticity, resulting in an inability to adapt to life events and stressors. There is now evidence that many treatments affect plasticity to some degree, which may be related to their therapeutic effects. Traditional pharmacologic approaches (ie, oral antidepressants) achieve enhanced plasticity to some degree.[13] However, novel and more powerful therapies (ie, ketamine, electroconvulsive therapy [ECT]) may induce clinical and neuroplastic effects more robustly and more rapidly.[14–16] Although these therapies can induce clinical improvements initially, their effects often dissipate once the treatment is tapered. Given the nature of these therapies, indefinite treatment in an intensive pattern is unstable or may have unacceptable side effects. In this line of therapy, one potential approach is to combine these therapies with psychotherapy to improve the longer-term outcomes of TRD. This approach may even have the potential to produce a synergistic combination of therapies to achieve better and more enduring clinical effects. Here, we review psychotherapy in combination with ECT, ketamine/esketamine, and transcranial magnetic stimulation (TMS).

Electroconvulsive Therapy

Historically, ECT has been considered the most effective therapy for TRD. ECT has been shown to decrease the risk of hospital readmission,[17] has shown superiority compared with pharmacology for unipolar major depression,[18] has been linked to a strong reduction in risk of all-cause mortality,[19] and may even reduce the risk of suicide.[20]

However, one of the key clinical problems is ECT's high relapse rate following cessation of the treatment. For instance, relapse rates of 84% have been seen within 6 months if no form of continuation/maintenance therapy is implemented.[21] With combination lithium/nortriptyline therapy, this relapse rate is reduced to 39%, but this remains unacceptably high. In elderly patients, continuation/maintenance of ECT can improve longer-term outcomes.[22] However, even some patients who clearly derive clinical benefits from ECT still experience bothersome side effects leading to a desire to discontinue treatment. Furthermore, ECT is not widely available, and such factors as transportation and lack of availability can limit the ability to receive a course of continuation/maintenance therapy in the outpatient setting.[23,24] This means that there is still a need to find other ways to improve long-term outcomes besides more ECT.

Even when the full mechanism of action of ECT's therapeutic effects are not understood, much evidence suggests that an enhancement in neuroplastic changes may be a critical driver. In rodent models of ECT (electroconvulsive stimulation), an enhancement in cognitive flexibility is seen.[25] There is also some evidence in humans that this may be the case, including changes in default mode network connectivity,[26] peripheral brain-derived neurotrophic factor,[27] and changes in amygdala/hippocampal volumes.[28–30] These findings, along with recent developments in ECT techniques that minimize cognitive burden of the treatment,[31] make attractive the potential combination of ECT with forms of cognitive and behavioral interventions to help address the relapse problem.

Three early phase pilot studies have combined ECT in series with CBT (either traditional in-person, a computer-simulated approach, or in groups).[4,32,33] These studies suggest promise to this approach. The only randomized clinical trial (n = 60) of this approach to date demonstrated that group CBT was more efficacious in maintaining response (77%) compared with either ECT alone (40%) or pharmacotherapy alone (44%).[34] The CBT arm received additional pharmacotherapy adjustment but not additional ECT.

Ketamine

Ketamine has been approved as an anesthetic since 1970. In the last 20 years, several studies have shown that subanesthetic doses of ketamine can have powerful and rapid-onset antidepressant effects.[35–38]

The S-enantiomer of ketamine, esketamine (delivered via intranasal spray), has now received regulatory approval in the United States as a therapy for TRD and depression with suicidal ideation. Nonetheless, it seems that racemic ketamine (primarily delivered via intravenous route) will still be used as a therapeutic for the foreseeable future for various reasons.[39]

Considerable controversy exists as to the primary mechanism of action that underlies ketamine's antidepressant effect. Nonetheless, it is likely that because of some common final pathway, there is an increase in synaptogenesis, which may also lead to an enhancement in cognitive flexibility.[15] Several clinical studies have shown that cognition may improve in patients with severe depression following exposure to ketamine.[40–42] Whether this is independent of ketamine's antidepressant effects has not been definitively shown.

In the early days of ketamine, there was concern about long-term cognitive deterioration from repeated exposure. This concern was founded on the literature of observational studies of ketamine abusers, which showed worrisome trends in spatial memory and hippocampal activation for people who used more than three times per week for a year or longer.[43] Even ex-ketamine and infrequent ketamine users have demonstrated concerning cognitive and psychiatric patterns (greater tendency for delusions) compared with healthy control subjects.[44] Fortunately, long-term studies of esketamine have suggested no or minimal cognitive changes. However, there are still reasons that limiting long-term exposure is a worthwhile therapeutic goal. Among these reasons, the treatment is inconvenient to patients (requiring approximately missing a half day of work or other activity; patients cannot drive on treatment days) and it is expensive. For this reason, finding ways to prolong the antidepressant effect while minimizing repeated treatments has been a goal of several research programs.

Studies examining lithium or riluzole as approaches to extend ketamine's antidepressant effects have not been successful.[45–47] The most successful approach so far has involved pairing ketamine with cognitive and behavioral restructuring approaches (ie, CBT). An early pilot study (open-label) showed a relapse rate of 25% (2/8) in the 8 weeks following cessation of ketamine (among responders) as long as CBT continued.[42] This was much lower than historical relapse rates, which ranged from 50% to 70% when ketamine was discontinued without any relapse prevention strategy.[37,48] A follow-up, randomized trial wherein ketamine responders were randomized to receive CBT plus treatment as usual or treatment as usual alone also suggests this is a promising approach. In this proof-of-concept trial (n = 28), there was a significant treatment-by-time interaction of self-reported depression severity measures, suggesting CBT resulted in a lower depression burden after 17 weeks.[49] However, clinician-reported measures (Montgomery-Asberg Depression Rating Scale) were not significant. In this study, in a partial sample, patients who responded to ketamine showed significantly improved cognitive control compared with ketamine nonresponders. This suggests a potential interactive effect between ketamine treatment and CBT, whereby ketamine renders patients better able to engage in cognitive restructuring and CBT locks down these effects to improve longer-term outcomes.

The largest study to date involves a fully automated cognitive training approach applied after a single dose of ketamine. In this study, participants (n = 154 total) were randomized (1:1:1 ratio) to ketamine infusion plus cognitive training, ketamine infusion plus sham intervention, or placebo infusion plus cognitive training. One month following ketamine infusion, the ketamine plus cognitive training group had significantly lower depression severity than the other groups.[50]

An ongoing study is assessing this approach in participants with depression and some level of suicidal ideation among psychiatric inpatients and outpatients. This study, the CBT-ENDURE study (NCT04760652), will recruit approximately 100 participants who will be followed for up to 6 months; preliminary results will read out at the end of 2024.

Transcranial Magnetic Stimulation

TMS involves the stimulation of cortical neurons via externally applied magnetic pulses that induce motor stimulations. When the magnetic pulses are applied in rapid succession (several pulses per second), this is repeated TMS (rTMS). rTMS was developed to mimic the efficacy but minimize the side effects of ECT. rTMS is Food and Drug Administration (FDA)-indicated for patients with MDD who have failed to achieve satisfactory improvement from prior antidepressant therapy. In at least three large, multisite trials, adults with MDD who failed one to four antidepressant trials showed more improvement following rTMS therapy compared with a sham condition.[51–53] The FDA-approved treatment protocols involve 20 to 30 sessions of 10-Hz rTMS applied to the left dorsolateral prefrontal cortex. Additional evidence exists for other protocols (notably, low-frequency rTMS delivered to the right dorsolateral prefrontal cortex[54] and bilateral rTMS[55]).

As is the case with other somatic treatments, there is a high relapse rate following a successful course of rTMS.[56] There are few studies that have attempted to pair rTMS with cognitive and behavioral strategies to improve longer-term outcomes. One large (n = 196) but nonrandomized study treated patients with depression for 10 weeks with simultaneous rTMS and CBT (in fact, CBT sessions were conducted during TMS) and showed a response rate of 66% and a remission rate of 56%. Most did not relapse (65% of responders retained response and 60% of remitters retained remission).[57] Further validation of this study in a randomized design is still lacking. Although the current review focuses on TRD, it is worth pointing out that rTMS combined with CBT in posttraumatic stress disorder has shown superior clinical outcomes in one comparatively large (n = 103)[58] and two small (n = 9; n = 30)[59,60] sham-controlled studies. An ongoing clinical trial is testing the efficacy of combining rTMS with an Internet-delivered CBT approach. This study aims to recruit 100 participants, randomizing them (1:1 ratio) to either rTMS alone or rTMS plus CBT. The primary outcome will be depression severity measured at 6 months (NCT04329651); results should be forthcoming soon.[61]

FUTURE DIRECTIONS

Historically, the development of medical products to treat depression has received the most research funding compared with psychotherapeutic approaches. This is primarily because there has been no way to regulate and commercialize psychotherapies; hence, companies that develop new therapies had no interest or stake in the development of psychotherapies.

In recent years, there has been a huge surge of interest in digital therapeutics. As of December 2022, there are more than 600 clinical trials of a digital therapeutic being tested in some form of depression that are registered on the US Clinical Trials Registry. A digital therapeutic platform makes it possible for patients to learn and practice principles of psychotherapy by use of a digital app that can be downloaded onto a smartphone, tablet, or similar device. In the United States, there is at least one instance of regulatory authorities authorizing the marketing of such a device through FDA clearance (the equivalent of FDA approval for device regulation). This approach may have significant promise to allow for significantly more funding to develop and test psychotherapeutic approaches compared with historical patterns. Up until now, most funding for the research and development of therapies for depression has been devoted to pharmaceutical products through industry sponsors. Only a small fraction of total funding has supported the development, refinement, and implementation of psychotherapy approaches, primarily through the National Institutes of Health. The primary reason for this imbalance in funding approaches is because of the inability to market and commercialize psychotherapy approaches; hence, industry sponsors have not historically had interest in funding psychotherapy trials. The advent of digital therapeutics has the potential to change this and provide better balance to funding of a variety of treatment approaches. This is critical to the field because most psychiatric disorders, including TRD, have component causes that come from a combination of biologic, psychological, and social factors. Hence, it is unlikely that there will be a magic bullet pharmacotherapy approach that will lead to high remission rates in large groups of patients.[62] Further development and refinement of reimbursement codes for psychotherapies and collaboration with third-party payers will likely be necessary to fully allow for adequate research and development of these approaches.

SUMMARY

Psychotherapeutic approaches, most commonly cognitive-based therapies, can play an important role in the management of TRD. At least a dozen randomized trials in patients with TRD have shown evidence of efficacy. Cognitive-based approaches also show promise in combination with medication or somatic therapies (ie, ketamine) to harness a state of enhanced neural plasticity and therefore improve longer-term outcomes of refractory mood disorders.

CLINICS CARE POINTS

- Psychotherapy can be of benefit to patients with treatment-resistant depression
- There is not sufficient evidence to indicate that one form of psychotherapy is superior to another (i.e., cognitive behavioral therapy v. interpersonal psychotherapy)
- The most clinical evidence of benefit is for cognitive behavioral therapy

DISCLOSURES

S.T. Wilkinson has received contract funding from Janssen, United State, Sage Therapeutics, United State, and Oui Therapeutics for the conduct of clinical trials administered through Yale University. He has received consulting fees from Janssen, Biohaven, and Oui Therapeutics.

FUNDING

None.

REFERENCES

1. Mathew SJ, Wilkinson ST, Altinay M, et al. ELEctroconvulsive therapy (ECT) vs. Ketamine in patients with treatment-resistant depression: the ELEKT-D study protocol. Contemp Clin Trials 2019;77:19–26.
2. Greenberg PE, Fournier AA, Sisitsky T, et al. The economic burden of adults with major depressive disorder in the United States (2005 and 2010). J Clin Psychiatry 2015;76(2):155–62.
3. Gordon, J.A., One Year In: COVID-19 and Mental Health. National Institute of Mental Health blog, 2021. Available at: https://www.nimh.nih.gov/about/director/messages/2021/one-year-in-covid-19-and-mental-health.
4. Wilkinson ST, Ostroff RB, Sanacora G. Computer-assisted cognitive behavior therapy to prevent relapse following electroconvulsive therapy. J ECT 2017; 33(1):52–7.
5. Rush AJ, Trivedi MH, Wisniewski SR, et al. Acute and longer-term outcomes in depressed outpatients requiring one or several treatment steps: a STAR*D report. Am J Psychiatry 2006;163(11):1905–17.
6. Corey-Lisle PK, Birnbaum HG, Greenberg PE, et al. Identification of a claims data "signature" and economic consequences for treatment-resistant depression. J Clin Psychiatry 2002;63(8):717–26.
7. Conway CR, Gebara MA, Walker MC, et al. Clinical characteristics and management of treatment-resistant depression. J Clin Psychiatry 2015;76(11):1569–70.
8. Amital D, Fostick L, Silberman A, et al. Serious life events among resistant and non-resistant MDD patients. J Affect Disord 2008;110(3):260–4.
9. Crown WH, Finkelstein S, Berndt ER, et al. The impact of treatment-resistant depression on health care utilization and costs. J Clin Psychiatry 2002;63(11):963–71.
10. Lin J, Szukis H, Sheehan JJ, et al. Economic burden of treatment-resistant depression among patients hospitalized for major depressive disorder in the United States. Psychiatric Research and Clinical Practice 2019;1(2):68–76.
11. Li J-M, Zhang Y, Su W-J, et al. Cognitive behavioral therapy for treatment-resistant depression: a systematic review and meta-analysis. Psychiatry Res 2018;268:243–50.
12. Gloster AT, Rinner MT, Ioannou M, et al. Treating treatment non-responders: a meta-analysis of randomized controlled psychotherapy trials. Clin Psychol Rev 2020;75:101810.
13. Castren E, Hen R. Neuronal plasticity and antidepressant actions. Trends Neurosci 2013;36(5):259–67.
14. Cornwell BR, Salvadore G, Furey M, et al. Synaptic potentiation is critical for rapid antidepressant response to ketamine in treatment-resistant major depression. Biol Psychiatry 2012;72(7):555–61.
15. Li N, Lee B, Liu RJ, et al. mTOR-dependent synapse formation underlies the rapid antidepressant effects of NMDA antagonists. Science (New York, N.Y.). 2010; 329(5994):959–64.

16. Takamiya A, Kishimoto T, Hirano J, et al. Association of electroconvulsive therapy-induced structural plasticity with clinical remission. Progress in Neuropsychopharmacology & Biological Psychiatry 2021;110:110286.

17. Slade EP, Jahn DR, Regenold WT, et al. Association of electroconvulsive therapy with psychiatric readmissions in US hospitals. JAMA Psychiatr 2017;74(8): 798–804.

18. Kverno KS, Mangano E. Treatment-resistant depression: approaches to treatment. J Psychosoc Nurs Ment Health Serv 2021;59(9):7–11.

19. Rhee TG, Sint K, Olfson M, et al. Association of ECT With risks of all-cause mortality and suicide in older Medicare patients. Am J Psychiatry 2021;178(12): 1089–97.

20. Wilkinson ST, Trujillo Diaz D, Rupp ZW, et al. Pharmacological and somatic treatment effects on suicide in adults: a systematic review and meta-analysis. Depress Anxiety 2021;39(2):100–12.

21. Sackeim HA, Haskett RF, Mulsant BH, et al. Continuation pharmacotherapy in the prevention of relapse following electroconvulsive therapy: a randomized controlled trial. JAMA 2001;285(10):1299–307.

22. Kellner CH, Husain MM, Knapp RG, et al. A novel strategy for continuation ECT in geriatric depression: phase 2 of the PRIDE study. Am J Psychiatry 2016;173(11): 1110–8.

23. Wilkinson ST, Agbese E, Leslie DL, et al. Identifying recipients of electroconvulsive therapy: data from privately insured Americans. Psychiatr Serv 2018;69(5): 542–8.

24. Wilkinson ST, Kitay BM, Harper A, et al. Barriers to the implementation of electroconvulsive therapy (ECT): results from a nationwide survey of ECT practitioners. Psychiatr Serv 2021;72(7):752–7.

25. Svensson M, Grahm M, Ekstrand J, et al. Effect of electroconvulsive seizures on cognitive flexibility. Hippocampus 2016;26(7):899–910.

26. Mulders PC, van Eijndhoven PF, Pluijmen J, et al. Default mode network coherence in treatment-resistant major depressive disorder during electroconvulsive therapy. J Affect Disord 2016;205:130–7.

27. Rocha RB, Dondossola ER, Grande AJ, et al. Increased BDNF levels after electroconvulsive therapy in patients with major depressive disorder: a meta-analysis study. J Psychiatry Res 2016;83:47–53.

28. Dukart J, Regen F, Kherif F, et al. Electroconvulsive therapy-induced brain plasticity determines therapeutic outcome in mood disorders. Proc Natl Acad Sci U S A 2014;111(3):1156–61.

29. Joshi SH, Espinoza RT, Pirnia T, et al. Structural plasticity of the hippocampus and amygdala induced by electroconvulsive therapy in major depression. Biol Psychiatry 2016;79(4):282–92.

30. Nordanskog P, Larsson MR, Larsson EM, et al. Hippocampal volume in relation to clinical and cognitive outcome after electroconvulsive therapy in depression. Acta Psychiatr Scand 2014;129(4):303–11.

31. Sackeim HA, Prudic J, Nobler MS, et al. Effects of pulse width and electrode placement on the efficacy and cognitive effects of electroconvulsive therapy. Brain Stimul 2008;1(2):71–83.

32. Carstens L, Hartling C, Aust S, et al. EffECTively treating depression: a pilot study examining manualized group CBT as follow-up treatment after ECT. Front Psychol 2021;12:723977.

33. Fenton L, Fasula M, Ostroff R, et al. Can cognitive behavioral therapy reduce relapse rates of depression after ECT? A preliminary study. J ECT 2006;22(3): 196–8.

34. Brakemeier EL, Merkl A, Wilbertz G, et al. Cognitive-behavioral therapy as continuation treatment to sustain response after electroconvulsive therapy in depression: a randomized controlled trial. Biol Psychiatry 2014;76(3):194–202.

35. Berman RM, Cappiello A, Anand A, et al. Antidepressant effects of ketamine in depressed patients. Biol Psychiatry 2000;47(4):351–4.

36. Murrough JW, Iosifescu DV, Chang LC, et al. Antidepressant efficacy of ketamine in treatment-resistant major depression: a two-site randomized controlled trial. Am J Psychiatry 2013;170(10):1134–42.

37. Murrough JW, Perez AM, Pillemer S, et al. Rapid and longer-term antidepressant effects of repeated ketamine infusions in treatment-resistant major depression. Biol Psychiatry 2013;74(4):250–6.

38. Murrough JW, Soleimani L, DeWilde KE, et al. Ketamine for rapid reduction of suicidal ideation: a randomized controlled trial. Psychol Med 2015;45(16):3571–80.

39. O'Brien B, Wilkinson ST, Mathew SJ. An update on community ketamine practices. Am J Psychiatr 2022;179(5):393–4.

40. Murrough JW, Wan LB, Iacoviello B, et al. Neurocognitive effects of ketamine in treatment-resistant major depression: association with antidepressant response, [published online ahead of print, 2013 Sep.]. Psychopharmacology 2013. https://doi.org/10.1007/s00213-013-3255-x.

41. Shiroma PR, Albott CS, Johns B, et al. Neurocognitive performance and serial intravenous subanesthetic ketamine in treatment-resistant depression. Int J Neuropsychopharmacol 2014;17(11):1805–13.

42. Wilkinson ST, Wright D, Fasula MK, et al. Cognitive behavior therapy may sustain antidepressant effects of intravenous ketamine in treatment-resistant depression. Psychother Psychosom 2017;86(3):162–7.

43. Morgan CJ, Dodds CM, Furby H, et al. Long-term heavy ketamine use is associated with spatial memory impairment and altered hippocampal activation. Front Psychiatry 2014;5:149.

44. Morgan CJ, Muetzelfeldt L, Curran HV. Consequences of chronic ketamine self-administration upon neurocognitive function and psychological wellbeing: a 1-year longitudinal study. Addiction 2010;105(1):121–33.

45. Ibrahim L, Diazgranados N, Franco-Chaves J, et al. Course of improvement in depressive symptoms to a single intravenous infusion of ketamine vs add-on riluzole: results from a 4-week, double-blind, placebo-controlled study. Neuropsychopharmacology 2012;37(6):1526–33.

46. Mathew SJ, Murrough JW, aan het Rot M, et al. Riluzole for relapse prevention following intravenous ketamine in treatment-resistant depression: a pilot randomized, placebo-controlled continuation trial. Int J Neuropsychopharmacol 2010; 13(1):71–82.

47. Costi S, Soleimani L, Glasgow A, et al. Lithium continuation therapy following ketamine in patients with treatment resistant unipolar depression: a randomized controlled trial. Neuropsychopharmacology 2019;44(10):1812–9.

48. Shiroma PR, Johns B, Kuskowski M, et al. Augmentation of response and remission to serial intravenous subanesthetic ketamine in treatment resistant depression. J Affect Disord 2014;155:123–9.

49. Wilkinson ST, Rhee TG, Joormann J, et al. Cognitive behavioral therapy to sustain the antidepressant effects of ketamine in treatment-resistant depression: a randomized clinical trial. Psychother Psychosom 2021;90(5):318–27.

50. Price RB, Spotts C, Panny B, et al. A novel, brief, fully automated intervention to extend the antidepressant effect of a single ketamine infusion: a randomized clinical trial. Am J Psychiatry 2022;179(12):959–68.
51. George MS, Lisanby SH, Avery D, et al. Daily left prefrontal transcranial magnetic stimulation therapy for major depressive disorder: a sham-controlled randomized trial. Arch Gen Psychiatry 2010;67(5):507–16.
52. Levkovitz Y, Isserles M, Padberg F, et al. Efficacy and safety of deep transcranial magnetic stimulation for major depression: a prospective multicenter randomized controlled trial. World Psychiatr 2015;14(1):64–73.
53. O'Reardon JP, Solvason HB, Janicak PG, et al. Efficacy and safety of transcranial magnetic stimulation in the acute treatment of major depression: a multisite randomized controlled trial. Biol Psychiatry 2007;62(11):1208–16.
54. Berlim MT, Van den Eynde F, Jeff Daskalakis Z. Clinically meaningful efficacy and acceptability of low-frequency repetitive transcranial magnetic stimulation (rTMS) for treating primary major depression: a meta-analysis of randomized, double-blind and sham-controlled trials. Neuropsychopharmacology 2013;38(4):543–51.
55. Brunoni AR, Chaimani A, Moffa AH, et al. Repetitive transcranial magnetic stimulation for the acute treatment of major depressive episodes: a systematic review with network meta-analysis. JAMA Psychiatr 2017;74(2):143–52.
56. Dunner DL, Aaronson ST, Sackeim HA, et al. A multisite, naturalistic, observational study of transcranial magnetic stimulation for patients with pharmacoresistant major depressive disorder: durability of benefit over a 1-year follow-up period. J Clin Psychiatry 2014;75(12):1394–401.
57. Donse L, Padberg F, Sack AT, et al. Simultaneous rTMS and psychotherapy in major depressive disorder: clinical outcomes and predictors from a large naturalistic study. Brain Stimul 2018;11(2):337–45.
58. Kozel FA, Motes MA, Didehbani N, et al. Repetitive TMS to augment cognitive processing therapy in combat veterans of recent conflicts with PTSD: a randomized clinical trial. J Affect Disord 2018;229:506–14.
59. Osuch EA, Benson BE, Luckenbaugh DA, et al. Repetitive TMS combined with exposure therapy for PTSD: a preliminary study. J Anxiety Disord 2009;23(1):54–9.
60. Isserles M, Shalev AY, Roth Y, et al. Effectiveness of deep transcranial magnetic stimulation combined with a brief exposure procedure in post-traumatic stress disorder: a pilot study. Brain Stimul 2013;6(3):377–83.
61. Abou El-Magd RM, Obuobi-Donkor G, Adu MK, et al. Repetitive transcranial magnetic stimulation with and without internet-delivered cognitive-behavioral therapy for the treatment of resistant depression: protocol for patient-centered randomized controlled pilot trial. JMIR Res Protoc 2020;9(10):e18843.
62. Narayan VA, Mohwinckel M, Pisano G, et al. Beyond magic bullets: true innovation in health care. Nat Rev Drug Discov 2013;12(2):85–6.

Special Populations
Treatment-Resistant Depression in Children and Adolescents

Check for updates

Emine Rabia Ayvaci, MD[a], Paul E. Croarkin, DO, MS[b],*

KEYWORDS

- Treatment-resistant depression • Children • Adolescents
- Major depressive disorder • Antidepressants • Novel treatments

KEY POINTS

- As many as 20% of adolescents will have a major depressive episode before adulthood.
- The evidence-based treatments will fail to improve symptoms in approximately 30% of adolescents.
- Treatment-resistant depression in adolescents is broadly defined as a depressive disorder that does not respond to an adequate dose of psychotherapeutic treatment or antidepressant medications.
- Staging classifications and interventional research for treatment-resistant depression in adolescents are emerging.

INTRODUCTION

Depressive disorders are common in adolescents, and the estimated lifetime prevalence of major depressive disorder (MDD) in adolescents is 11.0% in the United States.[1] The average duration of a major depressive episode in children is around 6 to 9 months[2] and symptoms of depression impact multiple areas of adolescents' life including emotional well-being, academic functioning, peer relationships, and family interactions across developmental stages. The adverse consequences of developing MDD in adolescence persist into adulthood with recurrent episodes of depression, substance use, occupational impairment, and suicidal behavior.

The initial treatment of MDD in adolescents involves psychotherapy, pharmacotherapy, or a combination of both. Both the American Academy of Child and Adolescent Psychiatry (AACAP) Depression practice parameters[3] and the Texas Children's

[a] Department of Psychiatry, UT Southwestern Medical Center, 6300 Harry Hines Boulevard, Dallas, TX 75235, USA; [b] Department of Psychiatry and Psychology, Mayo Clinic, 200 First Street Southwest, Rochester, MN 55905, USA
* Corresponding author.
E-mail address: croarkin.paul@mayo.edu
Twitter: @AyvaciRabia (E.R.A.); @DrPaulCroarkin (P.E.C.)

Psychiatr Clin N Am 46 (2023) 359–370
https://doi.org/10.1016/j.psc.2023.02.007
0193-953X/23/© 2023 Elsevier Inc. All rights reserved.

Medication Algorithm Project[4] recommend pharmacotherapy for moderate to severe cases of MDD. The initial pharmacotherapy approach often starts with a selective serotonin reuptake inhibitor (SSRI). If the initial trial with an SSRI does not achieve an adequate response, guidelines recommend a second SSRI with the addition of therapy.[3,4] To date, fluoxetine (age 8 and above) and escitalopram (age 12 and above) are two Food and Drug Administration (FDA)-approved medications for the treatment of depression in children and adolescents.

Despite the efficacy of antidepressants as shown in controlled trials, evidence-based treatments fail to improve symptoms in approximately 30% of adolescents.[5–8] The Treatment for Adolescents with Depression Study (TADS)[5] showed among adolescents treated with fluoxetine, 40% failed to respond to initial pharmacotherapy. The largest study looking beyond initial pharmacotherapy to date, the Treatment of Resistant Depression in Adolescents (TORDIA) study, also showed similar results.[6] In TORDIA, adolescents with resistance to initial SSRI treatment were randomized into either medication switch (another SSRI or venlafaxine) or medication switch plus cognitive behavioral therapy (CBT). Of the 334 adolescents enrolled in the study, approximately 60% failed to achieve remission by 24 weeks regardless of the initial treatment choice.[9] Although TORDIA provided insights about treatment resistance in adolescent populations, the data are limited for further treatment strategies. Treatment guidelines suggest augmentation strategies for those who fail to respond to initial treatment options; however, those recommendations are largely extrapolated from adult studies. Therefore, strategies for nonresponse to acute treatment or subsequent treatment strategies need to be examined in larger studies.

DEFINITION OF TREATMENT-RESISTANT DEPRESSION

Treatment-resistant depression (TRD) in adolescents is broadly defined as a depressive disorder that does not respond to a 2-month course of an antidepressant medication at a dose equivalent of 40 mg of fluoxetine daily or 8 to 16 sessions of a cognitive behavioral or interpersonal therapy. Response to treatment is defined by at least a 50% reduction in depressive symptoms within the treatment period.[10,11]

The AACAP Practice Parameters recommend treatment with an adequate dose of an antidepressant for at least 4 weeks and clinical response needs to be assessed at 4-week intervals.[3] The dose can be increased based on the response and tolerability with the goal of remission within 12 weeks. However, the exact definition of adequate dosing for adolescents with is not well-defined in current guidelines. As a result, the dose of antidepressant medications prescribed for adolescents is similar to adults.[3] For prepubertal children, antidepressants are usually started at lower doses and titrated up slower than adolescent dosing to prevent intolerance and side effects. Children are also more susceptible to activation symptoms such as irritability, mood lability, and restlessness which complicates the adequacy of treatment strategies. Thus, finding a well-established definition for treatment resistance is still difficult to achieve.

RISK FACTORS AND PREDICTORS OF POOR OUTCOME

When a clinician encounters an inadequate response to an antidepressant, further assessment should focus on adherence and tolerability. Although it is difficult to determine what percentage of nonresponse accounts for treatment nonadherence, studies have demonstrated up to 50% nonadherence rates.[12] Even after establishing adherence, children and adolescents may experience medication side effects. The variability of cytochrome P450 enzyme affects the metabolism of antidepressant medications; some children can be more susceptible to side effects of the medication regimen. Starting from a below therapeutic dose can be a strategy to prevent unwanted effects, but this can also delay the time to response to the medication. The rate of improvement of symptoms in early phases of treatment identifies remission status in clinical trials.[13] Therefore, finding the appropriate antidepressant dosing with adequate titration within an adequate time interval remains essential yet challenging.

Risk factors of treatment resistance can be grouped into three major categories: clinical characteristics, comorbid diagnoses, and environmental influences. Studies in adolescents with MDD demonstrated that depression severity, chronicity of symptoms, and the number of previous episodes predict poor response to acute treatment.[14,15] In addition, feeling hopelessness, anhedonia, and suicidal ideations are associated with poor response to treatment.[14,16] The presence of comorbid disorders such as diagnosis of dysthymia, attention-deficit hyperactive disorder (ADHD), anxiety disorders, substance use disorders, and a history of trauma has been associated with poor response to treatment.[17,18] Environmental factors such as a history of trauma, peer victimization, parental depression, and family conflict are associated with poor treatment responses in adolescents.[13,19,20]

DIFFERENTIAL DIAGNOSIS

The diagnosis of depression in children is challenging for the following reasons. Many symptoms of depression overlap with symptoms of other psychiatric disorders during childhood and adolescence. For example, irritability is the core symptom of a major depressive episode in children and adolescents, but it can also be a symptom for other psychiatric conditions such as anxiety disorders, trauma, and autism spectrum disorder. Therefore, the delineation of symptomatology in common psychiatric conditions can be particularly difficult in children and adolescents. One way to overcome this challenge is to establish the timeline of depressive symptoms and to identify the key symptoms. Depressive symptoms may overlap with other psychiatric diagnoses and normative behavioral changes in adolescence can make the differential diagnosis even more difficult.

When depression co-occurs with other psychiatric disorders, identifying treatment resistance and managing multiple diseases may require more advanced approaches. For example, symptoms of ADHD resulting in academic failure may precipitate a depressive episode. The Children's Medication Algorithm Project consensus[4] recommended that clinicians should assess the severity of the comorbid ADHD and MDD and treat the most severe disorder first. Similarly, consideration of other psychiatric disorders such as anxiety disorder, post-traumatic stress disorder, or substance use disorders needs to be incorporated into treatment planning.

Another consideration for diagnostic challenges is the emergence of bipolarity.[21] Studies of adult bipolar disorder revealed that 25% of patients experience their first episode of mania or depression before age 13 and 65% experience it before age 19.[22,23] In an observational study of adults, the rate of bipolar spectrum disorders reached more than 50% in treatment-resistant patients diagnosed with unipolar MDD.[24] The data regarding the relationship between bipolarity and treatment resistance are insufficient and current guidelines recommend diagnostic reevaluation after the failure of augmentation strategies.[3] A latent class analysis of the TORDIA study reported that the group of adolescents with resistance to treatment had higher scores of sub-syndromal manic symptoms without meeting the full criteria of bipolar disease.[25] Identifying bipolar spectrum disorder in treatment-resistant children can guide treatment planning.

STAGING EFFORTS

Several staging strategies exist primarily focusing on TRD in adults. Some of the adult-staging models are designed for research purposes and others are designed for clinical practice. The Thase and Rush Staging Model[26] proposed a staging model which included the response to antidepressants and electroconvulsive therapy (ECT). This staging model did not include augmentation strategies. Another staging model, the European Staging Model[27] divided patients into three different groups: (1) the nonresponder group: nonresponse to antidepressant medication for 6 to 8 weeks of treatment duration; (2) the treatment-resistant group: failure to respond two antidepressants from different classes, subdivided into five categories based on treatment duration; (3) chronic depression: duration of depression lasting more than a year despite using augmentation strategies. These two models primarily focused on medication trials. The Antidepressant Treatment History Form[28] proposed a model questioning the adequate dosing and duration of treatment.

To advance staging models, the Massachusetts General Hospital Staging method[11] was developed by using the Antidepressant Treatment Response Questionnaire (ATRQ).[29] ATRQ is a clinician-rated questionnaire for depression treatment history. This staging method used detailed characteristics of treatment history including different levels of treatment response (>25%, 25%–49%, 50%–74%, and <75%) and minimum dose and duration criteria based on the specific antidepressant medication. Another advanced model named Maudsley Staging Method[30] included symptom severity and duration of symptoms for staging efforts. The Dutch Measure for Quantification of Treatment Resistance in Depression[31] was developed as an extension of the Maudsley method. This method added items for functional impairment, comorbid anxiety, personality disorders, and psychosocial stressors. The augmentation section was expanded by several augmentation strategies used, evidence-based psychotherapy trials, and intensive treatment history such as day treatment.

Despite extensive efforts for the staging of TRD in adults, none of these models mentioned how to approach treatment resistance in children. Dwyer and colleagues[32] proposed a 10-stage model to identify treatment resistance in childhood depression. The model defined TRD as significant depressive symptoms despite two adequate medication trials and one adequate psychotherapy trial. The model pointed out the scarcity of evidence for advanced pharmacologic and psychotherapeutic modalities, thus identifying treatment resistance versus lack of evidence-based options continues to be an issue.

INITIAL TREATMENT STRATEGIES

Initial treatment strategies include antidepressant monotherapy and/or psychotherapy. Fluoxetine and escitalopram are two FDA-approved antidepressant medications for treatment of depression in adolescents. The data are scarce regarding which antidepressant is superior to another in terms of efficacy. Treatment selection is usually based on individual characteristics such as comorbid psychiatric conditions, previous medication history, family history, and medical history. For those with symptoms that do not respond favorably to initial treatment for 4 to 6 weeks, the recommendation is to increase the dose of the medication.[3] Although there is limited evidence for the dose–response relationship of antidepressants in studies of children and adolescents, some patients may respond to higher doses. In a previous clinical trial, examining children who did not respond to 20 mg of fluoxetine has shown that increasing the dose of fluoxetine was more effective than maintaining the dose.[33]

When initial treatment fails to achieve an adequate response, there can be several strategies: (1) combining with evidence-based psychotherapy if not included in the treatment plan, (2) switching to another antidepressant from a similar class or different class, (3) augmentation strategies, and (4) interventional treatment options.

Combining with Evidence-Based Psychotherapy

Psychotherapy can be used as an initial treatment strategy for mild depression, or it can be incorporated into psychopharmacological treatment.[3] When initial treatment with either antidepressants or psychotherapy alone do not improve depressive symptoms, combining these two modalities can result in a better outcome.[5] In clinical practice, different types of psychotherapy are being used for depression treatment. These therapy modalities are CBT, interpersonal psychotherapy (IPT), family intervention, dialectical behavioral therapy, motivational interviewing, and play therapy. Data from systematic reviews suggest that CBT and IPT should be considered as main options for treating adolescent depression.[34]

To date, CBT has the most data for either monotherapy or combination with antidepressant medications.[5] Similarly, the addition of relapse prevention CBT to acute response to medication management had a continued effect on reducing the risk of relapse.[35] In the TORDIA sample, among nonresponders, augmentation with psychotherapy resulted in eventual remission.[9] The effect of CBT after the initial treatment phase was not replicated in some other studies. In the ADAPT trial, 208 individuals between the ages of 11 and 17 years were randomized to either SRRI alone or SSRI plus CBT. The results of the study did not show a difference in response rates between the two groups.[36] A reanalysis of the TADS study also supported these findings and showed that the combination treatment (SSRI plus CBT) did not increase effectiveness significantly at high severity of depressive illness.[15] These trials point out that more studies are needed to establish clinical subgroups responsive to different treatment modalities.

IPT focuses on psychosocial and interpersonal events associated with depression, and it was designed for the treatment of the acute MDD.[37] IPT has shown improvement of depressive symptoms in adult studies,[38] and this result was replicated in studies with adolescents.[39,40] Although the use of CBT and IPT is established in studies with children and adolescents, the comparative effectiveness of those modalities is unknown due to the lack of randomized clinical trials.

Switching to Another Anti-depressant from a Similar Class or Different Class

Evidence-based treatment strategies after initial antidepressant treatment are limited in studies of children and adolescents. TORDIA still remains the largest study for SSRI-resistant depression in adolescents. The TORDIA[6] examined several strategies for treatment-resistant adolescents: (1) switching to a different SSRI, (2) switching to a different SSRI plus CBT, (3) switching to venlafaxine, or (4) switching to venlafaxine plus CBT. The results of this study did not show a differential effect between switching to another SSRI or venlafaxine. However, venlafaxine was associated with more side effects. Switching to another antidepressant plus CBT resulted in a higher rate of response. Given these findings, the standard clinical practice of antidepressant failure is to switch to a second SSRI with a combination of CBT. After the inadequate response to switching to another SSRI and the addition of CBT, there is little guidance for the next step. In parallel to adult studies, switching to SNRI or augmentation is recommended in child and adolescent guidelines.[3,4]

Studies investigating other classes of antidepressants for child and adolescent depression have limited evidence of efficacy compared with SSRIs. A 36-week randomized controlled trial (RCT) that examined the effects of duloxetine (30 and 60 mg), fluoxetine, and placebo reported that duloxetine was not superior to the placebo.[41] Desvenlafaxine was studied in open-label studies for its safety and tolerability, and long-term treatment with desvenlafaxine was well tolerated.[42] However, two recent RCT studies examined desvenlafaxine, fluoxetine, and placebo arms did not demonstrate efficacy of treatment of depression.[43,44] A relatively newer antidepressant, vortioxetine, was approved for the treatment of MDD in adults; however, a recent 12-week placebo-controlled RCT of vortioxetine 10 mg, vortioxetine 20 mg, fluoxetine 20 mg, or placebo in adolescents with MDD did not show statistical difference between vortioxetine and placebo.[45] Similarly, an RCT of 473 adolescents examined the use of vilazodone for the treatment of depression. Vilazodone 15 to 30 mg/d was well tolerated in the study; however, it was not significantly superior to the placebo in terms of reducing depressive symptoms.[46] Other antidepressants bupropion, buspirone, and mirtazapine do not have RCTs, yet, thus they should be considered after inadequate response to first-line treatment options.

Paroxetine, an SSRI with a relatively shorter half-life, is not FDA-approved for the treatment of depression in children and adolescents. A multicenter, double-blind RCT of paroxetine study examined 206 adolescents with MDD and showed that paroxetine was not more efficacious than the placebo.[47] This was in contrast to a previous paroxetine study[48] which showed paroxetine had significantly greater improvement compared with placebo. A reanalysis of the data of this study concluded that the efficacy of paroxetine was not statistically or clinically significantly different from the placebo. The study also reported an increased risk of suicidal ideation and behavior in the paroxetine group.[49] Therefore, paroxetine is not recommended for the treatment of depression in children and adolescents.

Tricyclic antidepressants (TCAs) are historically used for the treatment of depression in adults and children. RCTs of TCAs demonstrated that they are effective in treating several conditions including depression, obsessive-compulsive disorders, ADHD, and enuresis. However, a systematic review including 14 trials and 590 participants examined the use of TCAs for childhood depression and endorsed only a small reduction in depression symptoms.[50] TCAs are typically not recommended in children and adolescent depression due to their side effect profile and the lethality in cases of overdose. Another nontraditional option for depression in adolescents is monoamine oxidase inhibitors (MAOIs); however, their use is also limited due to dietary restrictions. The MAOIs have not been extensively studied in adolescent populations. A double-blind RCT of selegiline treatment in depressed adolescents did not show a statistically significant treatment response compared with the placebo.[51]

Augmentation/Combination

Augmentation with lithium, especially in cases of suicidality, is a common strategy for TRD in adults. Previous case studies showed favorable responses when lithium was used as an adjunctive treatment for adolescent depression.[52,53] Lithium can be an effective treatment strategy, especially for patients with subsyndromal bipolarity, mixed features, or patients with a family history of bipolar disease.[54] A recent retrospective chart review[55] suggested that the use of lithium is overall safe and tolerable for children and adolescents with and without bipolar disease. However, there is little evidence for the efficacy of lithium as an adjunct treatment for treatment-resistant patients.

Another classic augmentation strategy in adult depression is augmentation with antipsychotic medications. In a meta-analysis of antipsychotic augmentation in adult depression showed efficacy with increased rates of adverse events.[56] However, no

RCTs have been published investigating the use of antipsychotics in treatment-resistant child and adolescent populations. Despite limited evidence, antipsychotics are often prescribed in child and adolescent populations and specifically in foster care patients.[57] Augmentation with antipsychotics can be a strategy after failing initial treatment strategies, and clinicians should inform patients and guardians about the evidence base, potential risks, and side effects.

Interventional Options and Novel Treatments

When a patient continues to experience severe symptoms despite multiple medication trials and adequate psychotherapy, consideration of novel interventional treatment options might be an option. In clinical practice, interventional strategies are commonly used as an off-label treatment option for children and adolescents. Thus, more research is needed to establish their efficacy and tolerability.

Ketamine is an N-methyl D-aspartate glutamate receptor antagonist and is approved by FDA as an anesthetic at higher doses. Ketamine is commonly used in children for nonpsychiatric indications due to its tolerability and safety. RCTs for adult depression have been done almost a decade ago[58,59]; it is being increasingly used as an off-label treatment for refractory depression in adults. The first RCT of ketamine versus midazolam in 17 adolescents with TRD demonstrated a greater reduction in depressive symptoms 24 hours after infusion with a single dose of ketamine compared with midazolam. Seventy-six percent of adolescents responded to ketamine, compared with 35% of midazolam ($P = .046$). Treatment gains associated with ketamine remained 14 days after treatment.[60] Further studies are needed in children with TRD to understand the effects of repeated dosing, safety, feasibility, and sustenance of symptomatic improvement.

Esketamine is the S-enantiomer of ketamine, and the intranasal form of esketamine gained FDA approval in 2019 for TRD in adults.[59] Esketamine is used in conjunction with antidepressant medications, and it was also found to be effective in reducing suicidal thoughts or actions in adult literature.[61] An industry-sponsored trial examining the efficacy of esketamine (NCT03185819) in children and adolescent depression populations is currently ongoing.

Non-pharmacological options can be considered for TRD in children and adolescents. ECT is a well-established treatment of TRD in adults; however, it can have a significant side-effect burden. The use of ECT for depression in adolescents is limited.[62] No RCTs have been published for TRD in children; most studies in the literature are open-label trials or case series.[62] A recent systematic review that included 154 children treated for various psychiatric diagnoses has suggested that ECT is safe and effective for treatment of mood disorders.[62] The AACAP guidelines recommend that ECT can be considered after two medication trials with those experiencing severe depressive symptoms.[3]

Transcranial magnetic stimulation (TMS) has been used increasingly for the treatment of adolescent depression who do not respond to initial treatment strategies. Several TMS protocols have been investigated in the literature. Repetitive TMS (rTMS) has been approved by FDA for TRD in adults, and controlled studies in adults supported its effectiveness. The only RCT that examined the use of rTMS in adolescents with TRD was published recently. Adolescents with TRD (aged 12–21 years) were enrolled in a randomized, sham-controlled trial of bilateral rTMS across 13 sites. Although patients experienced an improvement in depressive symptoms, there was no statistically significant difference from the sham treatment group.[63] More recently, a novel type of rTMS known as intermittent theta-burst stimulation (iTBS) was approved by the FDA for the treatment of adult depression. iTBS delivers bursts of high-frequency pulses within a shortened duration.Protocols of TBS with adolescents may have more tolerability than standard TMS as treatments are delivered over brief sessions.[64] iTBS has not been evaluated in an RCT in the treatment of adolescent depression. More studies are needed to explore interventional treatment strategies in children and adolescents.

SUMMARY

This review highlights existing challenges and the limited evidence base for TRD in children and adolescents. Although this is a common and impairing condition in childhood, the related research base and clinical guidelines are underdeveloped. As many as 30% of all adolescents treated for depression will have recalcitrant symptoms. Data regarding TRD in children are even more limited. Future work should focus on the underlying neurophysiology and related biomarkers. Ideal future staging classifications will have translation utility for both clinical practice and research. Novel intervention development for the population is critical and this research should diverge from the standard approach of adapting adult treatment protocols for children and adolescents.

CLINICS CARE POINTS

- Treatment-resistant depression is common in children and adolescents in treatment.
- Treatment-resistant depression is broadly defined as a depressive disorder that does not respond to a 2-month course of an antidepressant medication at a dose equivalent of 40 mg of fluoxetine daily or 8 to 16 sessions of a cognitive behavioral or interpersonal therapy.
- Adherence, tolerability, differential diagnosis, and psychosocial factors should be reassessed and addressed first. Reassessing for symptoms or risk of bipolar disorder is particularly important.
- Treatment considerations include the addition of an evidence-based psychotherapy if not included in the treatment plan, switching to another antidepressant from a similar or different class, augmentation strategies, or interventional treatment options.
- Research focused on treatment-resistant depression in children and adolescents is underdeveloped.

DISCLOSURE

Dr P.E. Croarkin has received research support from the Brain and Behavior Research Foundation, Mayo Clinic Foundation, National Institute of Mental Health, National Science Foundation, United States, Pfizer, United States, Neuronetics Inc., and NeoSync, United States. He has received equipment support from Neuronetics Inc, and MagVenture, United States, Inc for investigator-initiated research. He has received material support from Myriad Genetics for investigator-initiated research. He has consulted for Engrail Therapeutics, Myriad Genetics, Procter & Gamble Company, and Sunovion. Dr R. Ayvaci has no disclosures.

REFERENCES

1. Avenevoli S, Swendsen J, He J-P, et al. Major depression in the national comorbidity survey–adolescent supplement: Prevalence, correlates, and treatment. J Am Acad Child Adolesc Psychiatry 2015;54(1):37–44. e2.

2. Lewinsohn PM, Clarke GN, Seeley JR, et al. Major depression in community adolescents: age at onset, episode duration, and time to recurrence. J Am Acad Child Adolesc Psychiatry 1994;33(6):809–18.

3. Birmaher B, Brent D, Issues AWGoQ. Practice parameter for the assessment and treatment of children and adolescents with depressive disorders. J Am Acad Child Adolesc Psychiatry 2007;46(11):1503–26.

4. Hughes CW, Emslie GJ, Crismon ML, et al. Texas children's medication algorithm project: update from Texas consensus conference panel on medication treatment of childhood major depressive disorder. J Am Acad Child Adolesc Psychiatry 2007;46(6):667–86.

5. March JS, Silva S, Petrycki S, et al. The Treatment for Adolescents With Depression Study (TADS): long-term effectiveness and safety outcomes. Arch Gen Psychiatry 2007;64(10):1132–44.

6. Brent D, Emslie G, Clarke G, et al. Switching to another SSRI or to venlafaxine with or without cognitive behavioral therapy for adolescents with SSRI-resistant depression: the TORDIA randomized controlled trial. Jama 2008;299(8):901–13.

7. Cipriani A, Zhou X, Del Giovane C, et al. Comparative efficacy and tolerability of antidepressants for major depressive disorder in children and adolescents: a network meta-analysis. Lancet 2016;388(10047):881–90.

8. Zhou X, Teng T, Zhang Y, et al. Comparative efficacy and acceptability of antidepressants, psychotherapies, and their combination for acute treatment of children and adolescents with depressive disorder: a systematic review and network meta-analysis. Lancet Psychiatry 2020;7(7):581–601.

9. Emslie GJ, Mayes T, Porta G, et al. Treatment of Resistant Depression in Adolescents (TORDIA): week 24 outcomes. Am J Psychiatry 2010;167(7):782–91.

10. Nemeroff CB. Prevalence and management of treatment-resistant depression. J Clin Psychiatry 2007;68(8):17.

11. Fava M. Diagnosis and definition of treatment-resistant depression. Biol Psychiatry 2003;53(8):649–59.

12. Fontanella CA, Bridge JA, Marcus SC, et al. Factors associated with antidepressant adherence for Medicaid-enrolled children and adolescents. Ann Pharmacother 2011;45(7–8):898–909.

13. Tao R, Emslie G, Mayes T, et al. Early prediction of acute antidepressant treatment response and remission in pediatric major depressive disorder. J Am Acad Child Adolesc Psychiatry 2009;48(1):71–8.

14. Wilkinson P, Dubicka B, Kelvin R, et al. Treated depression in adolescents: predictors of outcome at 28 weeks. Br J Psychiatry 2009;194(4):334–41.

15. Curry J, Rohde P, Simons A, et al. Predictors and moderators of acute outcome in the Treatment for Adolescents with Depression Study (TADS). J Am Acad Child Adolesc Psychiatry 2006;45(12):1427–39.

16. McMakin DL, Olino TM, Porta G, et al. Anhedonia predicts poorer recovery among youth with selective serotonin reuptake inhibitor treatment–resistant depression. J Am Acad Child Adolesc Psychiatry 2012;51(4):404–11.

17. Melton TH, Croarkin PE, Strawn JR, et al. Comorbid anxiety and depressive symptoms in children and adolescents: a systematic review and analysis. J Psychiatr Pract 2016;22(2):84.

18. Goldstein BI, Shamseddeen W, Spirito A, et al. Substance use and the treatment of resistant depression in adolescents. J Am Acad Child Adolesc Psychiatry 2009;48(12):1182–92.

19. Asarnow JR, Scott CV, Mintz J. A combined cognitive–behavioral family education intervention for depression in children: A treatment development study. Cogn Ther Res 2002;26(2):221–9.

20. Feeny NC, Silva SG, Reinecke MA, et al. An exploratory analysis of the impact of family functioning on treatment for depression in adolescents. J Clin Child Adolesc Psychol 2009;38(6):814–25.

21. Dudek D, Rybakowski JK, Siwek M, et al. Risk factors of treatment resistance in major depression: association with bipolarity. J affective Disord 2010;126(1–2): 268–71.

22. Etain B, Lajnef M, Bellivier F, et al. Clinical expression of bipolar disorder type I as a function of age and polarity at onset: convergent findings in samples from France and the United States. J Clin Psychiatry 2012;73(4):2757.

23. Perlis RH, Miyahara S, Marangell LB, et al. Long-term implications of early onset in bipolar disorder: data from the first 1000 participants in the systematic treatment enhancement program for bipolar disorder (STEP-BD). Biol Psychiatry 2004;55(9):875–81.

24. Sharma V, Khan M, Smith A. A closer look at treatment resistant depression: is it due to a bipolar diathesis? J affective Disord 2005;84(2–3):251–7.

25. Maalouf FT, Porta G, Vitiello B, et al. Do sub-syndromal manic symptoms influence outcome in treatment resistant depression in adolescents? A latent class analysis from the TORDIA study. J affective Disord 2012;138(1–2):86–95.

26. Thase ME, Rush AJ. When at first you don't succeed: sequential strategies for antidepressant nonresponders. J Clin Psychiatry 1997;58(13):23–9.

27. Souery D, Amsterdam J, De Montigny C, et al. Treatment resistant depression: methodological overview and operational criteria. Eur Neuropsychopharmacol 1999;9(1–2):83–91.

28. Sackeim HA. The definition and meaning of treatment-resistant depression. J Clin Psychiatry 2001;62:10–7.

29. Fava M, Davidson KG. Definition and epidemiology of treatment-resistant depression. Psychiatr Clin North Am 1996;19(2):179–200.

30. Donaldson AFSWC, Poon KMBML, Cleare AJ. A multidimensional tool to quantify treatment resistance in depression: the Maudsley staging method. J Clin Psychiatry 2009;70(2):12363.

31. Peeters FP, Ruhe HG, Wichers M, et al. The Dutch measure for quantification of treatment resistance in depression (DM-TRD): an extension of the Maudsley staging method. J affective Disord 2016;205:365–71.

32. Dwyer JB, Stringaris A, Brent DA, et al. Annual Research Review: Defining and treating pediatric treatment-resistant depression. J Child Psychol Psychiatry 2020;61(3):312–32.

33. Heiligenstein JH, Hoog SL, Wagner KD, et al. Fluoxetine 40–60 mg versus fluoxetine 20 mg in the treatment of children and adolescents with a less-than-complete response to nine-week treatment with fluoxetine 10–20 mg: APilot study. J Child Adolesc Psychopharmacol 2006;16(1–2):207–17.

34. Zhou X, Hetrick SE, Cuijpers P, et al. Comparative efficacy and acceptability of psychotherapies for depression in children and adolescents: A systematic review and network meta-analysis. World psychiatry 2015;14(2):207–22.

35. Emslie GJ, Kennard BD, Mayes TL, et al. Continued Effectiveness of Relapse Prevention Cognitive-Behavioral Therapy Following Fluoxetine Treatment in Youth With Major Depressive Disorder. J Am Acad Child Adolesc Psychiatry 2015; 54(12):991–8.

36. Goodyer I, Dubicka B, Wilkinson P, et al. A randomised controlled trial of cognitive behaviour therapy in adolescents with major depression treated by selective serotonin reuptake inhibitors. The ADAPT trial. Health Technol Assess 2008; 12(14):1–80.

37. Weissman MM, Markowitz JC, Klerman GL. The guide to interpersonal psychotherapy: updated and expanded edition. New York, NY: Oxford University Press; 2017.

38. Markowitz JC. The cutting edge: IPT and PTSD. Depress Anxiety 2010; 27(10):879.

39. Rosselló J, Bernal G, Rivera-Medina C. Individual and group CBT and IPT for Puerto Rican adolescents with depressive symptoms. Cultur Divers Ethnic Minor Psychol 2012;14(3):234–45.

40. Mufson L, Sills R. Interpersonal psychotherapy for depressed adolescents (IPT-A): An overview. Nord J Psychiatry 2006;60(6):431–7.

41. Emslie GJ, Prakash A, Zhang Q, et al. A double-blind efficacy and safety study of duloxetine fixed doses in children and adolescents with major depressive disorder. J child Adolesc Psychopharmacol 2014;24(4):170–9.

42. Findling RL, Groark J, Chiles D, et al. Safety and tolerability of desvenlafaxine in children and adolescents with major depressive disorder. J child Adolesc Psychopharmacol 2014;24(4):201–9.

43. Atkinson S, Lubaczewski S, Ramaker S, et al. Desvenlafaxine versus placebo in the treatment of children and adolescents with major depressive disorder. J child Adolesc Psychopharmacol 2018;28(1):55–65.

44. Weihs KL, Murphy W, Abbas R, et al. Desvenlafaxine versus placebo in a fluoxetine-referenced study of children and adolescents with major depressive disorder. J child Adolesc Psychopharmacol 2018;28(1):36–46.

45. Findling RL, DelBello MP, Zuddas A, et al. Vortioxetine for Major Depressive Disorder in Adolescents: 12-Week Randomized, Placebo-Controlled, Fluoxetine-Referenced, Fixed-Dose Study. J Am Acad Child Adolesc Psychiatry 2022; 61(9):1106–18.e2.

46. Findling RL, McCusker E, Strawn JR. A randomized, double-blind, placebo-controlled trial of vilazodone in children and adolescents with major depressive disorder with twenty-six-week open-label follow-up. J Child Adolesc Psychopharmacol 2020;30(6):355–65.

47. Emslie GJ, Wagner KD, Kutcher S, et al. Paroxetine treatment in children and adolescents with major depressive disorder: a randomized, multicenter, double-blind, placebo-controlled trial. J Am Acad Child Adolesc Psychiatry 2006;45(6): 709–19.

48. Keller MB, Ryan ND, Strober M, et al. Efficacy of paroxetine in the treatment of adolescent major depression: a randomized, controlled trial. J Am Acad Child Adolesc Psychiatry 2001;40(7):762–72.

49. Le Noury J, Nardo JM, Healy D, et al. Restoring Study 329: efficacy and harms of paroxetine and imipramine in treatment of major depression in adolescence. BMJ 2015;351.

50. Hazell P, Mirzaie M. Tricyclic drugs for depression in children and adolescents. Cochrane Database Syst Rev 2013;6.

51. DelBello MP, Hochadel TJ, Portland KB, et al. A double-blind, placebo-controlled study of selegiline transdermal system in depressed adolescents. J child Adolesc Psychopharmacol 2014;24(6):311–7.

52. Ryan ND, Meyer V, Dachille S, et al. Lithium antidepressant augmentation in TCA-refractory depression in adolescents. J Am Acad Child Adolesc Psychiatry 1988; 27(3):371–6.

53. Walter G, Lyndon B, Kubb R. Lithium augmentation of venlafaxine in adolescent major depression. Aust N Z J Psychiatry 1998;32(3):457–9.

54. Sugawara H, Sakamoto K, Harada T, et al. Predictors of efficacy in lithium augmentation for treatment-resistant depression. J affective Disord 2010; 125(1–3):165–8.

55. Güneş H, Tanıdır C, Doktur H, et al. Long-Term Effects of Lithium Use on Children and Adolescents: A Retrospective Study from Turkey. J Child Adolesc Psychopharmacol 2022;32(3):162–70.

56. Nelson JC, Papakostas GI. Atypical antipsychotic augmentation in major depressive disorder: a meta-analysis of placebo-controlled randomized trials. Am J Psychiatry 2009;166(9):980–91.

57. DosReis S, Yoon Y, Rubin DM, et al. Antipsychotic treatment among youth in foster care. Pediatrics 2011;128(6):e1459–66.

58. Murrough JW, Perez AM, Pillemer S, et al. Rapid and longer-term antidepressant effects of repeated ketamine infusions in treatment-resistant major depression. Biol Psychiatry 2013;74(4):250–6.

59. Singh JB, Fedgchin M, Daly EJ, et al. A double-blind, randomized, placebo-controlled, dose-frequency study of intravenous ketamine in patients with treatment-resistant depression. Am J Psychiatry 2016;173(8):816–26.

60. Dwyer JB, Landeros-Weisenberger A, Johnson JA, et al. Efficacy of intravenous ketamine in adolescent treatment-resistant depression: a randomized midazolam-controlled trial. Focus 2022;20(2):241–51.

61. Surjan J, Grossi JD, Del Porto JA, et al. Efficacy and safety of subcutaneous esketamine in the treatment of suicidality in major depressive disorder and bipolar depression. Clin Drug Invest 2022;1–9.

62. Castaneda-Ramirez S, Becker TD, Bruges-Boude A, et al. Systematic review: Electroconvulsive therapy for treatment-resistant mood disorders in children and adolescents. Eur Child Adolesc Psychiatry 2022. https://doi.org/10.1007/s00787-022-01942-7.

63. Croarkin PE, Elmaadawi AZ, Aaronson ST, et al. Left prefrontal transcranial magnetic stimulation for treatment-resistant depression in adolescents: a double-blind, randomized, sham-controlled trial. Neuropsychopharmacology 2021; 46(2):462–9.

64. Elmaghraby R, Sun Q, Ozger C, et al. A Systematic Review of the Safety and Tolerability of Theta Burst Stimulation in Children and Adolescents. Neuromodulation: Technology Neural Interf 2022;25(4):494–503.

Treatment-Resistant Late-Life Depression
A Review of Clinical Features, Neuropsychology, Neurobiology, and Treatment

Subha Subramanian, MD[a,b],*, Hanadi A. Oughli, MD[c],
Marie Anne Gebara, MD[d],
Ben Julian A. Palanca, MD, PhD, MSc[e,f,g,h,i,j], Eric J. Lenze, MD[f]

KEYWORDS

- Treatment-resistant depression • Older adults • Presentation • Diagnosis
- Neuropsychological factors • Treatment • Neuromodulation

KEY POINTS

- Treatment-resistant late-life depression (TRLLD) is defined as major depression in older adults, which persists despite two adequate antidepressant trials.
- Etiologic factors that could contribute to treatment resistance include several syndromes of aging: Alzheimer's disease, vascular insufficiency, medical comorbidities, and inflammation.
- Depressed older adults with treatment-resistant symptoms tend to have more cognitive impairment, apathy, functional impairment, and risk for dementia.
- Augmentation with oral antidepressants, electroconvulsive therapy, repetitive transcranial magnetic stimulation, ketamine/esketamine, and vagal nerve stimulation are potential solutions for TRLLD.

[a] Department of Neurology, Berenson-Allen Center for Noninvasive Brain Stimulation, Beth Israel Deaconess Medical Center, Boston, MA, USA; [b] Department of Psychiatry, Beth Israel Deaconess Medical Center and Harvard Medical School, Boston, MA, USA; [c] Department of Psychiatry, Semel Institute for Neuroscience, University of California Los Angeles, Los Angeles, CA, USA; [d] Department of Psychiatry, University of Pittsburgh School of Medicine, Pittsburgh, PA, USA; [e] Department of Anesthesiology, Washington University School of Medicine in St. Louis, St Louis, MO, USA; [f] Department of Psychiatry, Washington University School of Medicine in St. Louis, St Louis, MO, USA; [g] Division of Biology and Biomedical Sciences, Washington University School of Medicine in St. Louis; [h] Department of Biomedical Engineering, Washington University in St. Louis, St Louis, MO, USA; [i] Center on Biological Rhythms and Sleep, Washington University School of Medicine in St. Louis, USA; [j] Neuroimaging Labs Research Center, Washington University School of Medicine in St. Louis, St Louis, MO, USA
* Corresponding author. Department of Neurology, Berenson-Allen Center for Noninvasive Brain Stimulation, Beth Israel Deaconess Medical Center, Boston, MA.
E-mail address: ssubram5@bidmc.harvard.edu

Psychiatr Clin N Am 46 (2023) 371–389
https://doi.org/10.1016/j.psc.2023.02.008

CASE PRESENTATION

Ms. S is a 78-year-old single retired woman with no prior history of depression who was evaluated for 6 months of low mood, decreased pleasure in hobbies (anhedonia), decreased energy, and somatic complaints such as headaches. Her medical comorbidities included a transient ischemic attack that occurred 1 year ago, hypertension, and coronary artery disease. Medical conditions were adequately managed by primary care physician. Her children noted that over the past 6 months, Ms. S was increasingly unable to conduct her regular household tasks and coordinate finances due to a combination of cognitive difficulties and loss of interest. Ms. S endorsed feeling sad. She was no longer partaking in weekly card games and was isolating herself from friends. Six months ago, she was able to manage her finances independently, drive to and from the supermarket, and host dinners at her house. Given her decline, Ms. S's children flew across the country to live with her to ensure she was compliant with medications and assist with activities of daily living.

Questions to Consider

1. What diagnoses should be considered in the differential?
2. What medical and neuropsychological workup would you order to refine the diagnosis?
3. How does Mrs S's presentation of depression differ from younger adults?

Mrs S's primary care physician ordered the following: complete blood cell count, electrolytes, vitamin B12, vitamin D, thyroid-stimulating hormone (TSH), and head computerized tomography (CT) without contrast; all laboratory results were unremarkable. She conducted a Montreal Cognitive Assessment (MoCA) and gathered extensive medical and psychiatric history. MoCA was 23/30, with deficits in attention and recall. On further questioning, Mrs S reported that she lost four close friends in the past 18 months due to the COVID-19 pandemic. Her physician determined that the most likely diagnosis was major depression; therefore, Mrs S was treated with sertraline, which was titrated to 200 mg over 10 weeks with limited response. Given treatment failure, she was prescribed duloxetine 60 mg daily. Duloxetine only partially improved her symptoms after 8 weeks of treatment, and family confirmed adherence.

Questions to Consider

1. What treatment alternatives should be considered at this point?
2. Of the treatment options, identify risks and benefits.

BACKGROUND

Late-life depression (LLD), defined as major depression in adults ≥60 years of age, is common. Its prevalence in the community is estimated to be up to 5%, and the number of older adults with depression is expected to almost double before 2050.[1–3] LLD is associated with increased disability, functional decline, and premature mortality from medical conditions or suicide.[4–8]

Some depressed older adults have had recurrent depressive episodes from young adulthood or adolescence (termed "early-onset"); others have the first onset of depression after age 60 (termed "late-onset depression"), when changes in the brain and body related to aging have begun to occur (**Fig. 1**). These features of aging—such as executive dysfunction described below—are associated with poorer treatment response. Older adults experiencing depression often have a poor and/or brittle response to antidepressants.[9,10] For instance, the rate of non-remission to a trial of

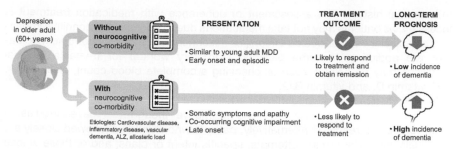

Fig. 1. Treatment-relevant subtypes in late-life depression.

a first-line antidepressant medication such as selective serotonin reuptake inhibitors (SSRIs) or serotonin and norepinephrine reuptake inhibitors (SNRIs) in LLD ranges from 55% to 81%.[11–13] When not adequately treated, LLD follows a chronic and/or relapsing course with increased functional disability and accelerated cognitive decline.[14,15] Persistent depressive illness leads to increased health care utilization, caregiver burden, and decreased quality of life.[16–18]

A subgroup of depressed older adults meets criteria for treatment-resistant depression (TRD). TRD is often defined as the failure to respond to two or more adequate trials of antidepressant medications. An adequate antidepressant trial is defined by dose and duration; it should be at least 4 weeks in duration at a dose known to be efficacious. Treatment resistance should be distinguished from "pseudoresistance," which is failure to receive an adequate trial of at least 4 weeks at an adequate dose, possibly due to poor adherence or side effects.[19] Treatment-resistant LLD (TRLLD) occurs in up to 30% of older adults with depression[20, 21]

TRLLD is a major challenge for clinicians. First, TRLLD tends to co-occur with neurocognitive problems, including cognitive impairment from vascular disease, and Alzheimer's disease (AD) and related neurodegenerative conditions (see **Fig. 1**). This means that TRLLDs presentation and functional impairments tend to be more complex than other cases of depression. Second, the treatment of TRLLD is difficult because patients who have failed two trials are highly unlikely to remit with a third trial of an SSRI/SNRI (especially if one of the two trials was an SNRI)[22]; "next-step" antidepressant options in TRLLD are more complicated to use than these first-line drugs. Because such patients are often seen in primary care settings due to limited access to geriatric psychiatrists, TRLLD is frustrating for patients and practitioners.[23]

Clinical Evaluation

LLD is defined as major depression; thus, it shares similar symptoms with major depression in younger adults. Nevertheless, LLD may present differently than depression in younger adults. Symptoms may be more predominantly somatic complaints and apathy as opposed to feeling sad or blue. Factors that may contribute to depression in older adults include social isolation, medical illness, cognitive decline, lower income, and grief or bereavement.[24] This was illustrated in the case presented earlier in this review: Ms. S had presented with headaches, in addition to feelings of depression and low mood. Her cognitive decline (MoCA score of 23/30), and the loss of her friends were both contributing factors to her depression. Ms. S had not achieved remission of her depressive symptoms despite two adequate trials of antidepressant.

A thorough evaluation covers the current symptoms, suicide risk assessment (see paragraph below), family history, past psychiatric history, past medication trials, and medical history. The assessment of adherence with medication treatment is necessary, as patients may not take medications due to poor insight, cognitive impairment, ambivalence, fear of side effects, or misconception that psychotropic medications are addictive. In some patients, laboratory workup for treatable medical conditions may be helpful, such as checking a complete blood count, electrolytes, TSH, vitamin D, and vitamin B12.

Regarding suicide assessment, older adults have thoughts of death that may occur outside of the scope of depression. These "normative" thoughts can be reported as: "if death comes, I'm ready."[25] Alternatively, patients who should be followed closely are individuals with prior suicide attempts, specific intent or plans, and/or those whose reasons for dying are out of context for reasons of living. Such patients necessitate regularly scheduled appointments and assessment of suicidality, access to weapons or stockpiling medications, reasons for living, and plans for the future.

There are several validated scales or tools that can be used to measure depression severity. The serial assessment of depression severity over the course of treatment can help guide decision-making, especially if a measurement-based care approach is implemented, in which depression scores are reviewed together by the clinician and patient as part of a shared decision-making process. A variety of validated self-administered assessments of depression severity can track treatment response in both mental health and primary care settings. One commonly used tool is the Patient Health Questionnaire (PHQ-9). PHQ-9 scores range between 0 and 27, with higher scores indicating greater depression severity. If a patient scores four or less, this suggests minimal depression and may not necessitate treatment. Scores between 5 and 9, 10 and 14, or greater than 15 points indicate mild, moderate, or severe depression, respectively. A score of 10+ (combined with a proper diagnosis) suggests that depression is sufficiently severe to require initiation or adjustment of treatment.

NEUROPSYCHOLOGICAL EXAMINATION FINDINGS

LLD is associated with distinct cognitive deficits that differentiate it from normal aging processes and might even link it to dementias such as AD.[26] LLD has been associated with deficits in verbal learning, general executive functioning, attention, episodic memory, information processing speed, visuospatial and language skills, learning, and the ability to perform verbal fluency tasks. In particular, episodic memory deficits in LLD have been linked to the progression of mild cognitive impairment (MCI), AD, and other forms of dementia.[27,28] Furthermore, the severity of LLD symptoms is closely related to the development of AD, as more severe and persistent depression increases the risk of AD almost threefold.[29]

The role of LLD in the pathophysiological brain matter changes is best demonstrated by structural neuroimaging research studies. Such studies illustrate that LLD is associated with reduced gray matter volume in the prefrontal cortex, hippocampus, amygdala, and basal ganglia.[30–35] MRI studies have shown that the hippocampus is one of the areas most associated with gray matter volume reduction, with early- and late-onset depression having demonstrated differences in the reduction of gray matter.[36] The hippocampus in late-onset LLD has been implicated with greater volume loss (lower gray matter volume) than early-onset LLD.[37,38] Functional neuroimaging studies have also found reduced activation in the medial temporal lobe and anterior cingulate cortex in LLD patients with cognitive impairment, a pattern similar to that found in non-depressed patient with cognitive impairment and AD. Overall, these studies suggest some overlap between LLD and neurodegenerative disorders such as AD.[39]

Despite this overlay, LLD has its own defining characteristics. Impairment in executive functions—cognitive processes involved in goal-directed behavior including activities in everyday function, medical, and self-care—often coexist with LLD.[19,40] A "depression executive dysfunction" (DED) syndrome has been described in around 30% of depressed older adults exhibiting abnormal performance in tests of verbal fluency, response inhibition, novel problem-solving, cognitive flexibility, working memory, and/or ideomotor planning.[41–43] This executive impairment, often in the absence of broader cognitive impairment, is different than what is seen in AD and is similar to what is typically seen in cerebrovascular disease. The clinical presentation of DED is characterized by anhedonia, psychomotor retardation, disability, poor insight, and increased suspiciousness.[41,43] Apathy is closely associated with executive dysfunction, disability, and poor response to antidepressant treatment.[44] One hypothesis is that the impairment in executive function tests of DED patients could be due to the motivational disturbance associated with apathy.[41]

The circuit mechanisms underlying DED are mostly related to a disruption of frontal-subcortical networks. Diffusion tensor neuroimaging exhibited microstructural abnormalities and hyperintensities in white matter tracts (ie, tracts connecting the prefrontal cortex to subcortical and posterior cortical regions) are associated with executive dysfunction.[41,45] Furthermore, decreased metabolic activity in both the dorsal anterior cingulate cortex and the dorsolateral prefrontal cortex (DLPFC), coupled with diminished resting-state functional connectivity between both regions, have been noted during depressive episodes in older adults.[41,46]

Executive dysfunction in LLD is associated with poor outcomes of oral antidepressant treatment (eg, aripiprazole augmentation), treatment discontinuation, symptom recurrence, and early relapse.[19] However, there remains conflicting evidence as to which executive function deficits are associated with poorer antidepressant response. A meta-analysis showed the domains of planning and organization to be meaningfully associated with poor antidepressant response in LLD.[47] Other studies have showed that among executive dysfunction measures, those of verbal fluency, set shifting, and response inhibition particularly predict the poor response of LLD to antidepressants.[48] Weaker resting-state functional connectivity within the networks supporting executive dysfunction predicted persistence of depressive symptoms, apathy, and dysexecutive behavior after treatment with escitalopram.[48] Comparably, lower activation in the DLPFC and other brain regions during in-scanner performance of the Wisconsin Card Sorting Test (measure of executive function) predicted less positive response to cognitive behavioral therapy in LLD.[49] Thus, the poor response of DED to treatment with antidepressant and the understanding of its mechanisms may guide the development of targeted interventions in the future.[41]

One challenge of neuropsychological testing in LLD is that it has not been able to guide treatment decisions. Said another way, although many studies have found a relationship of treatment resistance with neuropsychological impairments, others have not and none has led to any treatment-specific recommendations (ie, to use treatment A rather than treatment B). This is likely because neuropsychological testing is an incomplete probe of brain function; it is hoped that direct measures of brain function will, in the future, lead to treatment decision-making.[50]

CONTRIBUTORS TO TREATMENT RESISTANCE

The following are factors that have received extensive study as biological or psychological contributors to treatment resistance (see **Fig. 1**). These represent important and influential areas of LLD research over the past 20+ years, which together have shaped our conceptualization of LLD as a heterogeneous condition with treatment-relevant subtypes (see **Fig. 1**).

Medical Comorbidities and Somatic Symptoms

Older adults with greater medical burden have slower and lower rates of treatment response[51,52] and greater relapse rates after achieving remission.[53] The relationship between medical comorbidities and depression is bidirectional, as physical disability predicts occurrence of depression[54,55] and adults with depression have an increased risk of being disabled compared with healthy adults.[7,56] Many severe and chronic conditions co-occur with depressive symptoms. However, it remains unclear exactly what underlies this relationship between medical burden and treatment resistance; it may be multifactorial.

Some conditions strongly correlated with depression and treatment resistance. These include coronary heart disease,[57,58] diabetes,[59] and neurologic conditions.[27,60,61] These conditions affecting cardiovascular health, coupled with advanced age—contribute to vascular dysregulation. Vascular disease contributes to LLD in that it often affects the subcortical structures, including the white matter pathways connecting mood regulatory centers to the frontal cortex.[62] Disruption in these white matter tracks can therefore lead to low mood, executive dysfunction, and amotivation.

Somatic symptoms commonly occur in older adults, and older adults with high degrees of somatization may have higher levels of physiologic distress.[63] Compared with the general population, those with functional symptoms are more likely to have higher severity of depression, particularly chronic pain.[64,65]

Alzheimer's Disease

Depression often precedes dementia onset or accompanies dementia. In fact, the prevalence of major depression was about 15% in a recent meta-analysis of individuals with AD.[66,67] This review has already described some features and distinguishing factors of LLD and AD. Although there may be similar neurobiological mechanisms (eg, microvascular insufficiency) underlying depression and AD,[68,69] there is still incomplete understanding of how depression is a prodromal symptom, etiologic factor, or a result of dementia.[70]

Inflammation

One theory (sometimes called "inflammaging") posits that over a lifespan, certain inflammation cascades become excessive and maladaptive with aging. Such inflammatory changes, including peripheral immune stimulation and cytokine release, disrupt neurobiological pathways and correlate with severity of depressive symptoms. Inflammatory cytokines that reach the brain may activate transcription factors and enzymes (ie, indoleamine 2,3-dioxygenase) that increase the metabolism of tryptophan and decreased serotonin synthesis.[71,72] Cytokines also trigger glutamate release from astrocytes, thus reducing glutamate receptor expression and glutamatergic uptake.[73] Chronic exposure to excess glutamate reduces expression of the N-methyl D-aspartate (NMDA) receptor, leading to decreased brain-derived neurotrophic factor (BDNF) expression.[74,75] A decrease in BDNF expression leads to less neurotropic support, leading to increased neuronal susceptibility to oxidative stress.

Anxiety

Although anxiety may occur across the lifespan, anxiety that co-occurs with LLD is associated with lower remission rates and a longer time to remission. In late-life, anxiety is multidimensional and includes personality, worry, panic, and somatization—symptoms that overlap with depression. Non-responders to typical antidepressants, augmentation strategies, and electroconvulsive therapy (ECT) were more anxious at baseline compared with responders.[76–79] More specifically, worrying was a symptom that predicted poor short-term and long-term remission outcomes.[80] However, one of the largest studies to examine the relationship between comorbid anxiety and remission of depression did not find a relationship between antidepressant response and anxiety symptoms.[81] Instead, this study demonstrated that concurrent anxious symptoms with depression often have a more severe initial presentation, but that anxiety and depressive symptoms resolved in parallel with medication.

Sleep Disturbances

The aging process is associated with known sleep architectural changes. Older adults often experience a reduction in total sleep time and slow wave sleep, an increase in duration of wakefulness after sleep onset, a prolongation in sleep latency, and an increase in number of arousals. Insomnia is defined as having difficulties falling asleep, staying asleep, or waking up too early for at least 3 nights per week for 3 or more months, with resulting distress or daytime impairments. [82]

Insomnia occurs in over half of the population above the ages of 60 years,[83] and is associated with a twofold increased risk of major depression.[84,85] There are bidirectional relationships between depression and poor sleep, such that the treatment of sleep disturbances may improve depression outcomes.[86] Psychoeducation on sleep hygiene, behavioral treatments for insomnia, and appropriate pharmacologic methods are effective adjunctive treatments for TRLLD.[87]

Evaluation for obstructive sleep apnea (OSA) is also encouraged, given the high prevalence of undiagnosed OSA in the TRLLD population.[88] Left untreated, OSA is associated with higher baseline system inflammation and reductions in amount of slow wave sleep and poor sleep efficiency. OSA is associated with poor response in individuals with depression.[89,90] OSA symptoms may overlap with those of depression including low energy, difficulty with concentration, and poor sleep quality. In patients at high risk of having OSA (body habitus, snoring, and so forth), an initial screen using the STOP-Bang questionnaire[91] followed by the polysomnography to confirm the diagnosis is needed to start treatment.

Given the bidirectional relationship between depression and sleep disturbances and the negative impact of both on cognition, the treatment of sleep disturbances should be more actively pursued as a research direction in LLD.

Neural Substrate Changes

Studies have determined how total cerebral white matter density relates to LLD and its treatment course. Increased total cerebral white matter hyperintensity has been found in older individuals with depression and associated with poor antidepressant response, though these findings have not always been replicated.[92–98] In a study of over 200 older adults who received sertraline and were followed for 12 weeks, a poor response to sertraline was associated with greater white matter hyperintensity.[99] Similarly, individuals unable to obtain remission with escitalopram were found to have microstructural white matter abnormalities in frontolimbic areas.[100] White matter hyperintensities in specific tracts, such as the superior longitudinal fasciculi and uncinate, are associated with higher depression severity.[101] White matter volume rate of change may better predict non-remission (compared with a single timepoint measure of white matter hyperintensity).[102,103]

Aging also reduces blood flow velocity and decreases vasomotor reactivity, resulting in perfusion changes.[104] Low blood flow areas are associated with co-localized white matter hyperintensities. Compared with healthy controls, adults with LLD demonstrate low cerebral blood flow in the front-cingulate-striatal areas, temporal, occipital, parietal, precuneus, and cuneus regions, as detected by through pulsed arterial spin labeling. Conversely, high cerebral flow occurs in the frontal and cingulate gyrus area.[41] After antidepressant treatment, some studies have associated improved blood flow in the regions of precuneus and parietal cortex with remission.[105–107]

Although the above findings suggest that greater amounts of vascular dysfunction are implicated in LLD and poor antidepressant response, there are no diagnostic vascular biomarkers established to identify who is more likely to obtain response or remission from specific treatments.

TREATMENT

Currently, our conceptualization and application of TRLLD treatment options are like those of younger adults. This is because many treatment options were developed from young adult research and applied to older adults. The etiologic factors of TRLLD described above (eg, inflammaging, decreased slow wave sleep, vascular insufficiency) were seldom considered in creating solutions for TRLLD.

Approach to Treatment

Personalized treatment requires an evaluation of an individual patient's potential factors to treatment resistance, past medication trials (and their adequacy in terms of dose and duration), stage of treatment resistance, and risk of drug interactions. For example, those who fail two trials of antidepressants from different classes or psychotherapy may require less-invasive measures (namely medication augmentation with oral medications), and those whose depression persists after oral antidepressant augmentation may be considered for ketamine or repetitive transcranial magnetic stimulation (rTMS). The next level of resistance is characterized by failure of one or more of these next-line treatments. These individuals may require ECT, vagus nerve stimulation, or deep brain stimulation.[108] The main goal of treatment is to achieve remission of depressive symptoms. Here, we present treatment options starting with geriatric psychiatry standard-of- care and FDA-approved methods to options that have emerging evidence.

Second-Line Pharmacotherapy

For patients with TRLLD who had partial but not full response to first-line antidepressants (SSRIs and SNRIs), augmentation with a low dose antipsychotic, bupropion, or lithium can be initiated. FDA-approved antipsychotics for augmentation include aripiprazole, olanzapine (when combined with fluoxetine), quetiapine, and brexpiprazole. Of the antipsychotics, aripiprazole augmentation has shown to have the most data supporting its efficacy and safety in older adults, with a multisite trial finding showing 44% experiencing remission with first-line aripiprazole compared with 29% with placebo.[109] can be initiated at 2 mg daily and increased every 2 weeks up to a maximum of 10 to 15 mg daily as tolerated. Of note, greater depression severity may predict treatment-emergent akathisia with aripiprazole augmentation pharmacotherapy, though this is generally mild in severity and responds to dose reduction.[110] If akathisia remains a concern after dose reduction, the antipsychotic brexpiprazole is an antipsychotic less likely to cause akathisia compared with aripiprazole. Another treatment option is quetiapine, with initial doses starting at 25 to 50 mg nightly and increasing in 50-mg intervals upwards to a maximum of 300 mg total daily as tolerated.

Other medications that are recommended as augmentation strategies include bupropion, mirtazapine, and lithium. The choice of which to use may benefit from a consideration of the patient's symptoms and the medication's known side effects. For example, for an older adult who presents with fatigue, weight gain, or sexual dysfunction, a trial of bupropion may be a good option. A recent multisite randomized comparative effectiveness trial demonstrated that in $n = 619$ TRLLD patients, bupropion augmentation had similar efficacy to aripiprazole augmentation and both were more effective than switching to bupropion.[111] Bupropion can be initiated at 150 mg daily and increased up to 300 to 450 mg daily as tolerated. For individuals who are experiencing insomnia, anxiety, or weight loss, mirtazapine would be suitable. Augmenting with a low dose of lithium targeting blood levels from 0.3 to 0.6 mEQ is another strategy.[112] When using lithium, long-term monitoring for chronic kidney disease and hypothyroidism is necessary. Additional considerations might be switching to a tricyclic antidepressant with relatively low anticholinergic burden such as nortriptyline, or a monoamine oxidase inhibitor.

Electroconvulsive Therapy

ECT is one of the most effective interventions for TRLLD across the adult lifespan. ECT is a procedure done under anesthesia, in which a small electric current is passed through the brain to elicit a well-controlled, therapeutic seizure. Reported TRLLD response rates to ECT are 70% and remission rates are 60% in TRLLD.[113] In fact, ECT has been shown to be more effective in older versus younger adults[114] and is associated with lower rates of rehospitalization.[115]

In general, ECT is well-tolerated and considered a safe treatment in older adults, even those with comorbid conditions.[116] Adverse cardiovascular effects for those with arrhythmias or coronary artery disease may occur, but the rates of such potential side effects are low and can be managed medically before and during treatment. Cardiovascular complications are limited but serious adverse effects of ECT.[117] A common side effect is post-ECT delirium, which lasts about an hour and likely secondary due to the anesthesia and induced seizure.[118,119] Cognitive impairments such as retrograde and anterograde amnesia generally resolve within the first few weeks of ECT conclusion.[120]

Over half of those who completed an index course of ECT will relapse within 6 months, even while on maintenance antidepressants.[121,122] Research has shown that in older adults, continuation of ECT after index course (eg, one treatment weekly for 4 weeks) better maintained remission compared with immediately discontinuing ECT after index course and managing with medications alone.[123,124]

Repetitive Transcranial Magnetic Stimulation

rTMS is a noninvasive neuromodulation technique in which a magnetic field is targeted to the external scalp and induces an electrical current to targeted areas, such as the DLPFC in depression. In adults, rTMS has been well tolerated and effective in many randomized controlled trials. Specific to older adults, rTMS has additional advantages, such as decreased side effects, compared with many antidepressant medications or ECT.

Randomized controlled trials focused on the use of rTMS in older adults have shown that rTMS has a better effect compared with sham treatment[125] and that the efficacy in the geriatric population is similar to the younger population.[126] Of note, brain atrophy (higher prevalence in older adults) may increase the distance between the magnetic coil and the intracranial target, leading to a decrease in efficacy. To resolve this, studies have found that an increase in number of pules and stimulus intensity can improve response and remission rates.[127]

Esketamine/ketamine

Esketamine, the s-enantiomer of ketamine (an NMDA receptor antagonist), was FDA-approved for TRD in 2019. The first long-term clinical trial of esketamine in older adults found that the efficacy of esketamine induction and maintenance was no different in younger and older adults. Adults who had a longer time to recurrence received maintenance treatment. In addition, adverse effects on cognitive function were no different between the two groups.[128] A second study (Transform-3) found improvement in the younger group of older adults who received esketamine plus an antidepressant versus placebo plus and antidepressant; however, there were no statistically significant differences in outcomes between the two groups of older adults. [129]

Although intravenous (IV) ketamine is not FDA-approved, preliminary studies suggest that it may be an effective and safe treatment for TRLLD.[130,131] In a pilot trial of 25 older adults receiving IV ketamine twice a week for 4 weeks, we found that (1) IV ketamine was tolerated; (2) the response rate was 48%; and (3) executive function measured via National Institutes of Health (NIH) Toolbox Cognitive Battery improved acutely and was sustained. More randomized clinical trials testing ketamine and esketamine's efficacy and tolerability in TRLLD are necessary.

Vagal Nerve Stimulation

Vagal nerve stimulation (VNS) involves implanting a permanent pulse generator in the chest wall which then stimulates a bipolar electrode on the left vagal nerve. VNS is used as adjunctive long-term treatment for TRD in the adult population; studies researching its efficacy have included adults' ages 18 to 80 years.[132] In a 5-year prospective study including 795 adults over 60 sites, adjunctive VNS had better 5-year outcomes than the treatment-as-usual groups (including those who received ECT).[133]

Despite the promise VNS offers, it remains to be studied in larger groups of older adults. Moreover, insurance coverage for VNS remains a barrier, given that the Centers of Medicare and Medicaid Services retracted their original approval to cover the procedure, and many older adults depend on Medicare for treatment reimbursement.

Summary

TRLLD is the failure to respond to at least two adequate antidepressant trials, and it is a disabling condition associated with disability, cognitive decline, health care utilization, and caregiver burden. Adults with TRLLD are often seen in primary care settings. Here, we have presented an approach to its diagnosis and treatment. Many factors contribute to treatment resistance, such as neurologic and medical comorbidities, anxiety, and sleep disturbance. Although studies comparing and evaluating various options for TRLLD are limited, current standard of care involves an evaluation of level of resistance and initiation of augmentation psychotropic or neurostimulation modalities. More work is needed to identifying treatments with higher remission rates, decreased time to remission, and limited side effects.

CLINICS CARE POINTS

- The clinical presentation of LLD may present differently from its presentation in younger adults.

- LLD has unique cognitive deficits that differentiate it from some forms of dementia, such as impairment in executive function.
- Treatment resistance in LLD can occur due to co-occuring medical comorbidites, inflammation, anxiety, sleep disturbance.
- The step-wise approach to treating TRLLD involves: first, careful assessment to ensure two drugs were adequately trialed; second, medication augmentation with oral agents; third, consideration of rTMS, ketamine or ECT.

FINANCIAL DISCLOSURES

S. Subramanian, M.A. Gebara, B.J.A. Palanca, and H.A. Oughli have no conflicts of interest to disclose. M.A Gebara receives support from Janssen and has received compensation from Otsuka for developing and presenting a disease-state webinar (not product-focused). E.J. Lenze reports consulting fees from Merck, Boehringer-Ingelheim, Pritikin ICR, IngenioRx, and Prodeo. E.J. Lenze also receives grant funding from Janssen, the COVID Early Treatment Fund, and FastGrants. E.J. Lenze has a patent pending on sigma-1 receptor agonists for COVID-19.

REFERENCES

1. Organization WH. Mental Health of Older Adults. Secondary Mental Health of Older Adults. 2017. Available at: https://www.who.int/news-room/fact-sheets/detail/mental-health-of-older-adults.
2. Gottfries CG. Late-life depression. Eur Arch Psychiatry Clin Neurosci 2001; 251(Suppl 2):II57–61.
3. Hall CA, Reynolds-Iii CF. Late-life depression in the primary care setting: challenges, collaborative care, and prevention. Maturitas 2014;79(2):147–52.
4. Lenze EJ, Rogers JC, Martire LM, et al. The association of late-life depression and anxiety with physical disability: a review of the literature and prospectus for future research. Am J Geriatr Psychiatry 2001;9(2):113–35.
5. Nemeroff CB. The curiously strong relationship between cardiovascular disease and depression in the elderly. Am J Geriatr Psychiatry 2008;16(11):857–60.
6. Noel PH, Williams JW Jr, Unutzer J, et al. Depression and comorbid illness in elderly primary care patients: impact on multiple domains of health status and well-being. Ann Fam Med 2004;2(6):555–62.
7. Rovner BW, German PS, Brant LJ, et al. Depression and mortality in nursing homes. JAMA 1991;265(8):993–6.
8. Bruce ML, Ten Have TR, Reynolds CF 3rd, et al. Reducing suicidal ideation and depressive symptoms in depressed older primary care patients: a randomized controlled trial. JAMA 2004;291(9):1081–91.
9. Reynolds CF 3rd, Kupfer DJ. Depression and aging: a look to the future. Psychiatr Serv 1999;50(9):1167–72.
10. Charney DS, Nemeroff CB, Lewis L, et al. National Depressive and Manic-Depressive Association consensus statement on the use of placebo in clinical trials of mood disorders. Arch Gen Psychiatry 2002;59(3):262–70.
11. Allard P, Gram L, Timdahl K, et al. Efficacy and tolerability of venlafaxine in geriatric outpatients with major depression: a double-blind, randomised 6-month comparative trial with citalopram. Int J Geriatr Psychiatry 2004;19(12):1123–30.
12. Raskin J, Wiltse CG, Siegal A, et al. Efficacy of duloxetine on cognition, depression, and pain in elderly patients with major depressive disorder: an

8-week, double-blind, placebo-controlled trial. Am J Psychiatry 2007;164(6): 900–9.

13. Schatzberg A, Roose S. A double-blind, placebo-controlled study of venlafaxine and fluoxetine in geriatric outpatients with major depression. Am J Geriatr Psychiatry 2006;14(4):361–70.

14. Deng Y, McQuoid DR, Potter GG, et al. Predictors of recurrence in remitted late-life depression. Depress Anxiety 2018;35(7):658–67.

15. Unutzer J. Clinical practice. Late-life depression. N Engl J Med 2007;357(22): 2269–76.

16. Snow CE, Abrams RC. The Indirect Costs of Late-Life Depression in the United States: A Literature Review and Perspective. Geriatrics (Basel) 2016;1(4).

17. Zivin K, Wharton T, Rostant O. The economic, public health, and caregiver burden of late-life depression. Psychiatr Clin North Am 2013;36(4):631–49.

18. Benson C, Szukis H, Sheehan JJ, et al. An Evaluation of the Clinical and Economic Burden Among Older Adult Medicare-Covered Beneficiaries With Treatment-Resistant Depression. Am J Geriatr Psychiatry 2020;28(3):350–62.

19. Cristancho P, Lenze EJ, Dixon D, et al. Executive Function Predicts Antidepressant Treatment Noncompletion in Late-Life Depression. J Clin Psychiatry 2018; 79(3). https://doi.org/10.4088/JCP.16m11371.

20. Lenze EJ, Sheffrin M, Driscoll HC, et al. Incomplete response in late-life depression: getting to remission. Dialogues Clin Neurosci 2008;10(4):419–30.

21. Mulsant BH, Pollock BG. Treatment-resistant depression in late-life. J Geriatr Psychiatry Neurol 1998;11(4):186–93.

22. Buchalter ELF, Oughli HA, Lenze EJ, et al. Predicting Remission in Late-Life Major Depression: A Clinical Algorithm Based Upon Past Treatment History. J Clin Psychiatry 2019;80(6). https://doi.org/10.4088/JCP.18m12483.

23. Hamm ME, Karp JF, Lenard E, et al. What else can we do?"-Provider perspectives on treatment-resistant depression in late-life. J Am Geriatr Soc 2022;70(4): 1190–7.

24. Fiske A, Wetherell JL, Gatz M. Depression in older adults. Annu Rev Clin Psychol 2009;5:363–89.

25. Szanto K, Lenze EJ, Waern M, et al. Research to reduce the suicide rate among older adults: methodology roadblocks and promising paradigms. Psychiatr Serv 2013;64(6):586–9.

26. Vu NQ, Aizenstein HJ. Depression in the elderly: brain correlates, neuropsychological findings, and role of vascular lesion load. Curr Opin Neurol 2013;26(6): 656–61.

27. Panza F, Frisardi V, Capurso C, et al. Late-life depression, mild cognitive impairment, and dementia: possible continuum? Am J Geriatr Psychiatry 2010;18(2): 98–116.

28. Potter GG, Wagner HR, Burke JR, et al. Neuropsychological predictors of dementia in late-life major depressive disorder. Am J Geriatr Psychiatry 2013; 21(3):297–306.

29. Chen R, Hu Z, Wei L, et al. Severity of depression and risk for subsequent dementia: cohort studies in China and the UK. Br J Psychiatry 2008;193(5):373–7.

30. Alexopoulos GS. Frontostriatal and limbic dysfunction in late-life depression. Am J Geriatr Psychiatry 2002;10(6):687–95.

31. Chang CC, Yu SC, McQuoid DR, et al. Reduction of dorsolateral prefrontal cortex gray matter in late-life depression. Psychiatry Res 2011;193(1):1–6.

32. Gerritsen L, Comijs HC, van der Graaf Y, et al. Depression, hypothalamic pituitary adrenal axis, and hippocampal and entorhinal cortex volumes–the SMART Medea study. Biol Psychiatry 2011;70(4):373–80.

33. Burke J, McQuoid DR, Payne ME, et al. Amygdala volume in late-life depression: relationship with age of onset. Am J Geriatr Psychiatry 2011;19(9):771–6.

34. Janssen J, Hulshoff Pol HE, de Leeuw FE, et al. Hippocampal volume and subcortical white matter lesions in late-life depression: comparison of early and late onset depression. J Neurol Neurosurg Psychiatry 2007;78(6):638–40.

35. Sawyer K, Corsentino E, Sachs-Ericsson N, et al. Depression, hippocampal volume changes, and cognitive decline in a clinical sample of older depressed outpatients and non-depressed controls. Aging Ment Health 2012;16(6):753–62.

36. Andreescu C, Butters MA, Begley A, et al. Gray matter changes in late-life depression–a structural MRI analysis. Neuropsychopharmacology 2008; 33(11):2566–72.

37. Hickie I, Naismith S, Ward PB, et al. Reduced hippocampal volumes and memory loss in patients with early- and late-onset depression. Br J Psychiatry 2005; 186:197–202.

38. Lloyd AJ, Ferrier IN, Barber R, et al. Hippocampal volume change in depression: late- and early-onset illness compared. Br J Psychiatry 2004;184:488–95.

39. Wang L, Potter GG, Krishnan RK, et al. Neural correlates associated with cognitive decline in late-life depression. Am J Geriatr Psychiatry 2012;20(8):653–63.

40. Snyder HR. Major depressive disorder is associated with broad impairments on neuropsychological measures of executive function: a meta-analysis and review. Psychol Bull 2013;139(1):81–132.

41. Alexopoulos GS. Mechanisms and treatment of late-life depression. Transl Psychiatry 2019;9(1):188.

42. Manning KJ, Steffens DC. State of the Science of Neural Systems in Late-Life Depression: Impact on Clinical Presentation and Treatment Outcome. J Am Geriatr Soc 2018;66(Suppl 1):S17–23.

43. Alexopoulos GS, Kiosses DN, Klimstra S, et al. Clinical presentation of the "depression-executive dysfunction syndrome" of late-life. Am J Geriatr Psychiatry 2002;10(1):98–106.

44. Yuen GS, Bhutani S, Lucas BJ, et al. Apathy in late-life depression: common, persistent, and disabling. Am J Geriatr Psychiatry 2015;23(5):488–94.

45. Bae JN, MacFall JR, Krishnan KR, et al. Dorsolateral prefrontal cortex and anterior cingulate cortex white matter alterations in late-life depression. Biol Psychiatry 2006;60(12):1356–63.

46. Aizenstein HJ, Butters MA, Wu M, et al. Altered functioning of the executive control circuit in late-life depression: episodic and persistent phenomena. Am J Geriatr Psychiatry 2009;17(1):30–42.

47. Pimontel MA, Rindskopf D, Rutherford BR, et al. A Meta-Analysis of Executive Dysfunction and Antidepressant Treatment Response in Late-Life Depression. Am J Geriatr Psychiatry 2016;24(1):31–41.

48. Alexopoulos GS, Hoptman MJ, Yuen G, et al. Functional connectivity in apathy of late-life depression: a preliminary study. J Affect Disord 2013;149(1–3): 398–405.

49. Thompson DG, Kesler SR, Sudheimer K, et al. FMRI activation during executive function predicts response to cognitive behavioral therapy in older, depressed adults. Am J Geriatr Psychiatry 2015;23(1):13–22.

50. Gerlach AR, Karim HT, Pecina M, et al. MRI predictors of pharmacotherapy response in major depressive disorder. Neuroimage Clin 2022;36:103157 [published Online First: Epub Date]|.

51. Katon W, Russo J, Frank E, et al. Predictors of nonresponse to treatment in primary care patients with dysthymia. Gen Hosp Psychiatry 2002;24(1):20–7.

52. Oslin DW, Datto CJ, Kallan MJ, et al. Association between medical comorbidity and treatment outcomes in late-life depression. J Am Geriatr Soc 2002;50(5): 823–8.

53. Reynolds CF 3rd, Dew MA, Pollock BG, et al. Maintenance treatment of major depression in old age. N Engl J Med 2006;354(11):1130–8.

54. McKnight PE, Kashdan TB. The importance of functional impairment to mental health outcomes: a case for reassessing our goals in depression treatment research. Clin Psychol Rev 2009;29(3):243–59.

55. Zeiss AM, Lewinsohn PM, Rohde P, et al. Relationship of physical disease and functional impairment to depression in older people. Psychol Aging 1996;11(4): 572–81.

56. Penninx BW, Guralnik JM, Ferrucci L, et al. Depressive symptoms and physical decline in community-dwelling older persons. JAMA 1998;279(21):1720–6.

57. Carney RM, Freedland KE. Treatment-resistant depression and mortality after acute coronary syndrome. Am J Psychiatry 2009;166(4):410–7.

58. de Guevara MS, Schauffele SI, Nicola-Siri LC, et al. Worsening of depressive symptoms 6 months after an acute coronary event in older adults is associated with impairment of cardiac autonomic function. J Affect Disord 2004;80(2–3): 257–62 [published Online First: Epub Date]|.

59. Park M, Reynolds CF. Depression Among Older Adults with Diabetes Mellitus. Clin Geriatr Med 2015;31(1):117.

60. Ehrt U, Bronnick K, Leentjens AF, et al. Depressive symptom profile in Parkinson's disease: a comparison with depression in elderly patients without Parkinson's disease. Int J Geriatr Psychiatry 2006;21(3):252–8.

61. McDonald WM, Richard IH, DeLong MR. Prevalence, etiology, and treatment of depression in Parkinson's disease. Biol Psychiatry 2003;54(3):363–75.

62. Alexander GE, DeLong MR, Strick PL. Parallel organization of functionally segregated circuits linking basal ganglia and cortex. Annu Rev Neurosci 1986;9: 357–81.

63. Sheehan B, Banerjee S. Review: Somatization in the elderly. Int J Geriatr Psychiatry 1999;14(12):1044–9.

64. Chakraborty K, Avasthi A, Kumar S, et al. Psychological and clinical correlates of functional somatic complaints in depression. Int J Soc Psychiatry 2012;58(1): 87–95 [published Online First: Epub Date]|.

65. Fishbain DA. The association of chronic pain and suicide. Semin Clin Neuropsychiatry 1999;4(3):221–7 [published Online First: Epub Date]|.

66. Asmer MS, Kirkham J, Newton H, et al. Meta-Analysis of the Prevalence of Major Depressive Disorder Among Older Adults With Dementia. J Clin Psychiatry 2018;79(5). https://doi.org/10.4088/JCP.17r11772.

67. Ismail Z, Elbayoumi H, Fischer CE, et al. Prevalence of Depression in Patients With Mild Cognitive Impairment: A Systematic Review and Meta-analysis. JAMA Psychiatry 2017;74(1):58–67.

68. Enache D, Winblad B, Aarsland D. Depression in dementia: epidemiology, mechanisms, and treatment. Curr Opin Psychiatry 2011;24(6):461–72 [published Online First: Epub Date]|.

69. Linnemann C, Lang UE. Pathways Connecting Late-Life Depression and Dementia. Front Pharmacol 2020;11:279 [published Online First: Epub Date]|.

70. Wiels W, Baeken C, Engelborghs S. Depressive Symptoms in the Elderly-An Early Symptom of Dementia? A Systematic Review. Front Pharmacol 2020;11: 34 [published Online First: Epub Date]|.

71. Dantzer R, O'Connor JC, Lawson MA, et al. Inflammation-associated depression: from serotonin to kynurenine. Psychoneuroendocrinology 2011;36(3): 426–36.

72. Miller AH, Maletic V, Raison CL. Inflammation and its discontents: the role of cytokines in the pathophysiology of major depression. Biol Psychiatry 2009;65(9): 732–41 [published Online First: Epub Date]|.

73. Hu S, Sheng WS, Ehrlich LC, et al. Cytokine effects on glutamate uptake by human astrocytes. Neuroimmunomodulation 2000;7(3):153–9 [published Online First: Epub Date]|.

74. Calabrese F, Rossetti AC, Racagni G, et al. Brain-derived neurotrophic factor: a bridge between inflammation and neuroplasticity. Front Cell Neurosci 2014;8: 430 [published Online First: Epub Date]|.

75. Jin Y, Sun LH, Yang W, et al. The Role of BDNF in the Neuroimmune Axis Regulation of Mood Disorders. Front Neurol 2019;10:515 [published Online First: Epub Date]|.

76. Alexopoulos GS, Katz IR, Bruce ML, et al. Remission in depressed geriatric primary care patients: a report from the PROSPECT study. Am J Psychiatry 2005; 162(4):718–24 [published Online First: Epub Date]|.

77. Dombrovski AY, Mulsant BH, Haskett RF, et al. Predictors of remission after electroconvulsive therapy in unipolar major depression. J Clin Psychiatry 2005; 66(8):1043–9 [published Online First: Epub Date]|.

78. Flint AJ, Rifat SL. A prospective study of lithium augmentation in antidepressant-resistant geriatric depression. J Clin Psychopharmacol 1994;14(5):353–6.

79. Saghafi R, Brown C, Butters MA, et al. Predicting 6-week treatment response to escitalopram pharmacotherapy in late-life major depressive disorder. Int J Geriatr Psychiatry 2007;22(11):1141–6 [published Online First: Epub Date]|.

80. Andreescu C, Lenze EJ, Dew MA, et al. Effect of comorbid anxiety on treatment response and relapse risk in late-life depression: controlled study. Br J Psychiatry 2007;190:344–9 [published Online First: Epub Date]|.

81. Saade YM, Nicol G, Lenze EJ, et al. Comorbid anxiety in late-life depression: Relationship with remission and suicidal ideation on venlafaxine treatment. Depress Anxiety 2019;36(12):1125–34 [published Online First: Epub Date]|.

82. Association AP. Diagnostic and statistical Manual of mental disorders Fifth ed, 2013.

83. Foley D, Ancoli-Israel S, Britz P, et al. Sleep disturbances and chronic disease in older adults: results of the 2003 National Sleep Foundation Sleep in America Survey. J Psychosom Res 2004;56(5):497–502 [published Online First: Epub Date]|.

84. Baglioni C, Battagliese G, Feige B, et al. Insomnia as a predictor of depression: a meta-analytic evaluation of longitudinal epidemiological studies. J Affect Disord 2011;135(1–3):10–9 [published Online First: Epub Date]|.

85. Cho HJ, Lavretsky H, Olmstead R, et al. Sleep disturbance and depression recurrence in community-dwelling older adults: a prospective study. Am J Psychiatry 2008;165(12):1543–50 [published Online First: Epub Date]|.

86. Gebara MA, Siripong N, DiNapoli EA, et al. Effect of insomnia treatments on depression: A systematic review and meta-analysis. Depress Anxiety 2018; 35(8):717–31 [published Online First: Epub Date]|.

87. Gebara MA, DiNapoli EA, Lederer LG, et al. Brief behavioral treatment for insomnia in older adults with late-life treatment-resistant depression and insomnia: a pilot study. Sleep Biol Rhythms 2019;17(3):287–95 [published Online First: Epub Date]|.

88. McCall WV, Benca RM, Rumble ME, et al. Prevalence of obstructive sleep apnea in suicidal patients with major depressive disorder. J Psychiatr Res 2019;116: 147–50 [published Online First: Epub Date]|.

89. Waterman L, Stahl ST, Buysse DJ, et al. Self-reported obstructive sleep apnea is associated with nonresponse to antidepressant pharmacotherapy in late-life depression. Depress Anxiety 2016;33(12):1107–13 [published Online First: Epub Date]|.

90. Reddy A, Mansuri Z, Vadukapuram R, et al. Increased Suicidality and Worse Outcomes in MDD Patients With OSA: A Nationwide Inpatient Analysis of 11 Years From 2006 to 2017. J Acad Consult Liaison Psychiatry 2022;63(1): 46–52 [published Online First: Epub Date]|.

91. Nagappa M, Liao P, Wong J, et al. Validation of the STOP-Bang Questionnaire as a Screening Tool for Obstructive Sleep Apnea among Different Populations: A Systematic Review and Meta-Analysis. PLoS One 2015;10(12):e0143697 [published Online First: Epub Date]|.

92. Coffey CE, Figiel GS, Djang WT, et al. Leukoencephalopathy in elderly depressed patients referred for ECT. Biol Psychiatry 1988;24(2):143–61 [published Online First: Epub Date]|.

93. Krishnan KR, Goli V, Ellinwood EH, et al. Leukoencephalopathy in patients diagnosed as major depressive. Biol Psychiatry 1988;23(5):519–22 [published Online First: Epub Date]|.

94. Steffens DC, Helms MJ, Krishnan KR, et al. Cerebrovascular disease and depression symptoms in the cardiovascular health study. Stroke 1999;30(10): 2159–66 [published Online First: Epub Date]|.

95. Taylor WD, MacFall JR, Payne ME, et al. Greater MRI lesion volumes in elderly depressed subjects than in control subjects. Psychiatry Res 2005;139(1):1–7 [published Online First: Epub Date]|.

96. Sneed JR, Culang-Reinlieb ME, Brickman AM, et al. MRI signal hyperintensities and failure to remit following antidepressant treatment. J Affect Disord 2011; 135(1–3):315–20 [published Online First: Epub Date]|.

97. Gunning-Dixon FM, Walton M, Cheng J, et al. MRI signal hyperintensities and treatment remission of geriatric depression. J Affect Disord 2010;126(3): 395–401 [published Online First: Epub Date]|.

98. Salloway S, Boyle PA, Correia S, et al. The relationship of MRI subcortical hyperintensities to treatment response in a trial of sertraline in geriatric depressed outpatients. Am J Geriatr Psychiatry 2002;10(1):107–11.

99. Sheline YI, Pieper CF, Barch DM, et al. Support for the vascular depression hypothesis in late-life depression: results of a 2-site, prospective, antidepressant treatment trial. Arch Gen Psychiatry 2010;67(3):277–85. https://doi.org/10.1001/archgenpsychiatry.2009.204 [published Online First: Epub Date]|.

100. Alexopoulos GS, Murphy CF, Gunning-Dixon FM, et al. Microstructural white matter abnormalities and remission of geriatric depression. Am J Psychiatry 2008;165(2):238–44. https://doi.org/10.1176/appi.ajp.2007.07050744 [published Online First: Epub Date]|.

101. Dalby RB, Frandsen J, Chakravarty MM, et al. Depression severity is correlated to the integrity of white matter fiber tracts in late-onset major depression. Psychiat Res-Neuroim 2010;184(1):38–48. https://doi.org/10.1016/j.pscychresns. 2010.06.008 [published Online First: Epub Date]].

102. Chen PS, McQuoid DR, Payne ME, et al. White matter and subcortical gray matter lesion volume changes and late-life depression outcome: a 4-year magnetic resonance imaging study. Int Psychogeriatr 2006;18(3):445–56. https://doi.org/10.1017/S1041610205002796 [published Online First: Epub Date]].

103. Taylor WD, Steffens DC, MacFall JR, et al. White matter hyperintensity progression and late-life depression outcomes. Arch Gen Psychiatry 2003;60(11): 1090–6. https://doi.org/10.1001/archpsyc.60.11.1090 [published Online First: Epub Date]].

104. Direk N, Koudstaal PJ, Hofman A, et al. Cerebral hemodynamics and incident depression: the Rotterdam Study. Biol Psychiatry 2012;72(4):318–23. https://doi.org/10.1016/j.biopsych.2012.01.019 [published Online First: Epub Date]].

105. Ishizaki J, Yamamoto H, Takahashi T, et al. Changes in regional cerebral blood flow following antidepressant treatment in late-life depression. Int J Geriatr Psychiatry 2008;23(8):805–11. https://doi.org/10.1002/gps.1980 [published Online First: Epub Date]].

106. Ogura A, Morinobu S, Kawakatsu S, et al. Changes in regional brain activity in major depression after successful treatment with antidepressant drugs. Acta Psychiatr Scand 1998;98(1):54–9. https://doi.org/10.1111/j.1600-0447.1998. tb10042.x [published Online First: Epub Date]].

107. Wei W, Karim HT, Lin C, et al. Trajectories in Cerebral Blood Flow Following Antidepressant Treatment in Late-Life Depression: Support for the Vascular Depression Hypothesis. J Clin Psychiatry 2018;79(6). https://doi.org/10.4088/JCP.18m12106 [published Online First: Epub Date]].

108. Conway CR, George MS, Sackeim HA. Toward an Evidence-Based, Operational Definition of Treatment-Resistant Depression: When Enough Is Enough. JAMA Psychiatry 2017;74(1):9–10. https://doi.org/10.1001/jamapsychiatry.2016.2586 [published Online First: Epub Date]].

109. Lenze EJ, Mulsant BH, Blumberger DM, et al. Efficacy, safety, and tolerability of augmentation pharmacotherapy with aripiprazole for treatment-resistant depression in late-life: a randomised, double-blind, placebo-controlled trial. Lancet 2015;386(10011):2404–12 [published Online First: Epub Date]].

110. Hsu JH, Mulsant BH, Lenze EJ, et al. Clinical Predictors of Extrapyramidal Symptoms Associated With Aripiprazole Augmentation for the Treatment of Late-Life Depression in a Randomized Controlled Trial. J Clin Psychiatry 2018; 79(4). https://doi.org/10.4088/JCP.17m11764 [published Online First: Epub Date]].

111. Lenze E.J., Mulsant B.H., Roose S.P., et al., Antidepressant Augmentation versus Switch in Treatment-Resistant Geriatric Depression [published online ahead of print, 2023 Mar 3]. N Engl J Med. 2023;10.1056/NEJMoa2204462. doi:10.1056/NEJMoa2204462.

112. Kok RM, Vink D, Heeren TJ, et al. Lithium augmentation compared with phenelzine in treatment-resistant depression in the elderly: an open, randomized, controlled trial. J Clin Psychiatry 2007;68(8):1177–85 [published Online First: Epub Date]].

113. Kellner CH, Husain MM, Knapp RG, et al. Right Unilateral Ultrabrief Pulse ECT in Geriatric Depression: Phase 1 of the PRIDE Study. Am J Psychiatry 2016; 173(11):1101–9 [published Online First: Epub Date]].

114. Rhebergen D, Huisman A, Bouckaert F, et al. Older age is associated with rapid remission of depression after electroconvulsive therapy: a latent class growth analysis. Am J Geriatr Psychiatry 2015;23(3):274–82 [published Online First: Epub Date]|.

115. Rosen BH, Kung S, Lapid MI. Effect of Age on Psychiatric Rehospitalization Rates After Electroconvulsive Therapy for Patients With Depression. J ECT 2016;32(2):93–8 [published Online First: Epub Date]|.

116. Riva-Posse P, Hermida AP, McDonald WM. The role of electroconvulsive and neuromodulation therapies in the treatment of geriatric depression. Psychiatr Clin North Am 2013;36(4):607–30 [published Online First: Epub Date]|.

117. Andrade C, Arumugham SS, Thirthalli J. Adverse Effects of Electroconvulsive Therapy. Psychiatr Clin North Am 2016;39(3):513–30 [published Online First: Epub Date]|.

118. Fink M. Post-ECT Delirium. Convuls Ther 1993;9(4):326–30.

119. Sackeim HA, Decina P, Malitz S, et al. Postictal excitement following bilateral and right-unilateral ECT. Am J Psychiatry 1983;140(10):1367–8 [published Online First: Epub Date]|.

120. Greenberg RM, Kellner CH. Electroconvulsive therapy: a selected review. Am J Geriatr Psychiatry 2005;13(4):268–81 [published Online First: Epub Date]|.

121. Prudic J, Haskett RF, McCall WV, et al. Pharmacological strategies in the prevention of relapse after electroconvulsive therapy. J ECT 2013;29(1):3–12 [published Online First: Epub Date]|.

122. Sackeim HA, Haskett RF, Mulsant BH, et al. Continuation pharmacotherapy in the prevention of relapse following electroconvulsive therapy: a randomized controlled trial. JAMA 2001;285(10):1299–307 [published Online First: Epub Date]|.

123. Kellner CH, Knapp RG, Petrides G, et al. Continuation electroconvulsive therapy vs pharmacotherapy for relapse prevention in major depression: a multisite study from the Consortium for Research in Electroconvulsive Therapy (CORE). Arch Gen Psychiatry 2006;63(12):1337–44 [published Online First: Epub Date]|.

124. Lisanby SH, McClintock SM, Alexopoulos G, et al. Neurocognitive Effects of Combined Electroconvulsive Therapy (ECT) and Venlafaxine in Geriatric Depression: Phase 1 of the PRIDE Study. Am J Geriatr Psychiatry 2020;28(3):304–16 [published Online First: Epub Date]|.

125. Iriarte IG, George MS. Transcranial Magnetic Stimulation (TMS) in the Elderly. Curr Psychiatry Rep 2018;20(1):6 [published Online First: Epub Date]|.

126. Conelea CA, Philip NS, Yip AG, et al. Transcranial magnetic stimulation for treatment-resistant depression: Naturalistic treatment outcomes for younger versus older patients. J Affect Disord 2017;217:42–7 [published Online First: Epub Date]|.

127. Cappon D, den Boer T, Jordan C, et al. Transcranial magnetic stimulation (TMS) for geriatric depression. Ageing Res Rev 2022;74:101531 [published Online First: Epub Date]|.

128. Ochs-Ross R, Wajs E, Daly EJ, et al. Comparison of Long-Term Efficacy and Safety of Esketamine Nasal Spray Plus Oral Antidepressant in Younger Versus Older Patients With Treatment-Resistant Depression: Post-Hoc Analysis of SUSTAIN-2, a Long-Term Open-Label Phase 3 Safety and Efficacy Study. Am J Geriatr Psychiatry 2022;30(5):541–56 [published Online First: Epub Date]|.

129. Ochs-Ross R, Daly EJ, Zhang Y, et al. Efficacy and Safety of Esketamine Nasal Spray Plus an Oral Antidepressant in Elderly Patients With Treatment-Resistant

Depression-TRANSFORM-3. Am J Geriatr Psychiatry 2020;28(2):121–41 [published Online First: Epub Date]].

130. Lipsitz O, Di Vincenzo JD, Rodrigues NB, et al. Safety, Tolerability, and Real-World Effectiveness of Intravenous Ketamine in Older Adults With Treatment-Resistant Depression: A Case Series. Am J Geriatr Psychiatry 2021;29(9): 899–913 [published Online First: Epub Date]].

131. Oughli HA, Gebara MA, Ciarleglio A, et al. Intravenous Ketamine for Late-Life Treatment-Resistant Depression: A Pilot Study of Tolerability, Safety, Clinical Benefits, and Effect on Cognition [published online ahead of print, 2022 Dec 5]. Am J Geriatr Psychiatry 2022. S1064-S7481(22)00573-00575.

132. George MS, Rush AJ, Marangell LB, et al. A one-year comparison of vagus nerve stimulation with treatment as usual for treatment-resistant depression. Biol Psychiatry 2005;58(5):364–73 [published Online First: Epub Date]].

133. Aaronson ST, Sears P, Ruvuna F, et al. A 5-Year Observational Study of Patients With Treatment-Resistant Depression Treated With Vagus Nerve Stimulation or Treatment as Usual: Comparison of Response, Remission, and Suicidality. Am J Psychiatry 2017;174(7):640–8 [published Online First: Epub Date]].

Brain Features of Treatment-Resistant Depression

A Review of Structural and Functional Connectivity Magnetic Resonance Imaging Studies

Mora M. Grehl, MA[a],*, Sara Hameed, BA[b],
James W. Murrough, MD, PhD[b],*

KEYWORDS

- Neuroimaging • Depression • Treatment-resistant depression
- Anterior cingulate cortex • Resting-state functional connectivity
- Magnetic resonance imaging

KEY POINTS

- Awareness of the increasing disease burden of treatment resistant depression (TRD), in combination with technological advances in structural and functional neuroimaging, affords the unique opportunity to research biomarkers that characterize such individuals.
- Herein, magnetic resonance imaging (MRI) literature concerning structural and functional brain features that associate with treatment-resistance in individuals with MDD and the small literature of predictive brain features of treatment outcome in individuals with TRD are reviewed.
- Despite heterogeneity in findings, features that distinguish TRD from non-TRD samples include: 1) reduced grey matter volume (GMV) within cortical brain regions, particularly in the anterior cingulate cortex (ACC); 2) reduced structural integrity within white matter; and 3) alterations in the resting state functional connectivity (RSFC) of the default mode network (DMN).
- The most common brain features that associate with treatment outcome include the prefrontal cortex (PFC), ACC, and hippocampus.
- While varied research designs, small sample sizes and inconsistent findings call in into question the near-term clinical utility in the prediction or diagnosis of TRD, we aim to underscore notable findings that have the potential to spur future avenues of research.

[a] Department of Psychology and Neuroscience, 1701 North 13th Street, Temple University, Philadelphia, PA 19122, USA; [b] Depression and Anxiety Center for Discovery and Treatment, 1399 Park Avenue, 2nd Floor, New York, NY 10029
* Corresponding authors. Depression and Anxiety Center for Discovery and Treatment, Department of Psychiatry, Icahn School of Medicine at Mount Sinai, One Gustave L. Levy Place, Box 1230, New York, NY 10029.
E-mail addresses: mora.grehl@temple.edu (M.M.G.); james.murrough@mssm.edu (J.W.M.)

Psychiatr Clin N Am 46 (2023) 391–401
https://doi.org/10.1016/j.psc.2023.02.009
0193-953X/23/© 2023 Elsevier Inc. All rights reserved.

INTRODUCTION

Major depressive disorder (MDD) is a debilitating mental health condition character-ized by decreased mood, anhedonia, changes in sleep and appetite, fatigue, restless-ness, and concentration difficulties.[1] MDD is also one of the leading causes of global morbidity, burden and disability, and available treatments often fall short of addressing this large public health burden.[2] Traditional antidepressant medications are ineffective in about a third of patients with MDD and those that do not achieve remission after 2 or more adequate trials of antidepressants, sometimes from different pharmacologic classes, are often characterized as having treatment-resistant depression (TRD).[3,4] Given the high rates of nonresponse to available treatments and the societal burden this portends, it is critical to gain an improved understanding of the underlying brain mechanisms contributing to TRD. There is an increasing interest in elucidating the neurobiological substrates of TRD to develop more targeted treatments based on an understanding of the underlying pathophysiology of the disease.[5]

The continued development and refinement of neuroimaging techniques have pro-vided researchers with the tools to examine both structural and functional neural changes associated with neuropsychiatric disease, including TRD. Advances in MRI methodologies in particular allow for the investigation of structural features associated with disease, including gray matter volume (GMV) and integrity of white matter fiber tracts using diffusion tensor imaging (DTI), as well as functional features associated with disease, including resting state functional connectivity (RSFC). Herein, we pro-vide a critical review of the current literature concerning MRI studies of TRD. Based on the volume of studies and popularity of the techniques, we restrict our review spe-cifically to studies of TRD that utilize structural or RSFC MRI approaches to provide a more focused review.

Herein, we review 2 types of MRI studies related to TRD. In the first case, we consider retrospective case-control studies of TRD samples compared with non-TRD MDD samples and/or unaffected healthy control (HC) samples. In the second case, we consider MRI studies that utilize a prospective design to investigate brain features that associated with treatment outcome among individuals who are TRD. Of note, we do not consider the large topic of brain features that associate treatment response in individuals with MDD more generally. Our consideration of prospective studies in TRD is also restricted to those that utilize pharmacotherapy, repetitive trans-cranial magnetic stimulation (rTMS) or electroconvulsive therapy (ECT). We do not consider studies of deep brain stimulation due to the highly specialized nature of the intervention and the extreme phenotypes of the samples. This narrative review is necessarily selective, wherein we focus on studies that utilize MRI (rather than other imaging modalities), define TRD as a failure of at least 2 trials of antidepressant med-ications, and highlight studies that exhibit relatively more rigorous design characteris-tics and larger sample sizes, where available. The review is organized such that we begin with findings from structural MRI studies and then move to functional (specif-ically, RSFC) MRI studies. Within each of these categories, we present findings from retrospective study designs first, followed by those from prospective designs. When possible, we will point out significant areas of convergence on one hand, or lack of convergence or nonreplication of findings on the other hand.

STRUCTURAL ABNORMALITIES IN TREATMENT-RESISTANT DEPRESSION: RETROSPECTIVE STUDIES

Investigations of structural abnormalities in TRD have largely been conducted utilizing T1-weighted anatomic scans and subsequent GMV or cortical thickness analyses. DTI has also been used to examine integrity of white matter, estimated using fractional anisotropy (FA). Abnormalities in GMV that have been associated with TRD when compared to HCs and non-TRD patients include the anterior cingulate cortex (ACC), caudate nucleus, medial prefrontal cortex (mPFC), cerebellum, insula, and hippocampus.[5,6] Reduction in GMV in the ACC has been implicated across a variety of studies of individuals with TRD.[7–9] Serra-blasco and colleagues[7] compared individuals at different stages of depression (including 22 individuals each with first-episode, remitted-recurrent and TRD or chronic depression) with HCs and found that individuals with TRD had the largest reductions in GMV in fronto-limbic areas, including the ACC and insula. Moreover, when comparing the first-episode group to those with TRD, those with TRD had smaller insula and mPFC volumes, suggesting a specific relationship between these areas and resistance to treatment and/or maintenance of depressive symptoms.[7] In addition to changes in GMV, differences in cortical thickness have also been observed in patients with TRD. In a longitudinal study conducted during 1 year, thicker right caudal ACC at baseline was associated with greater symptom improvement among those with TRD.[8] When comparing those with TRD to those with non-TRD and HCs, individuals with TRD had significantly reduced right frontal and striatal GMV loss.[9] Similarly, Ma and colleagues[10] found that when both patients with non-TRD and patients with TRD were compared with HCs, only those with TRD exhibited GMV reduction in the bilateral caudate. Thus, severe and/or nonremitting subtypes of MDD may be characterized by caudate GM atrophy, a finding that has been posited by others.[11]

The literature on changes in white matter volume, integrity, and microstructure associated with TRD is quite variable. Some studies have found reduced FA values in the anterior limb of the internal capsule, body of the corpus callosum, and bilateral external capsule,[12] and others in the left middle frontal gyrus, left limbic lobe uncus, and right cerebellum posterior lobe.[13] De Diego-Adelino and colleagues[14] investigated white matter microstructure in patients at various stages of illness (ie, TRD, remitted-recurrent, first-episode) and HCs, and defined TRD as those whose last episode lasted more than 2 years with no response to multiple antidepressant strategies. They found pervasive decreases of FA in the cingulum bundle, corpus callosum and superior and inferior longitudinal fascicule when those with TRD were compared with first episode MDD and HCs. Significant FA reductions in white matter within the ventral medial prefrontal cortex (vmPFC), a region that is thought to be particularly important to antidepressant treatment mechanisms, was also observed when patients with TRD were compared with those with remitted recurrent MDD. Finally, individuals with TRD also had significantly lower whole-brain mean FA values when compared with non-TRD individuals; when the FA reduction in the prefrontal white matter was further analyzed, it was found that increased depression severity and number of previous episodes accounted for 12% of the variance. Zhou and colleagues[15] conducted a whole-brain analysis of individuals with TRD versus MDD individuals who were responsive to treatment and did not find any significant differences in FA values or whole-brain mean FA value differences between groups. The authors did observe significantly reduced white matter FA values within the bilateral hippocampus in those with TRD. De Diego-adelino and colleagues[16] examined hippocampal volume and gray matter proportions in individuals at different stages of depression, and found no differences in volume. In that study, individuals with TRD had a higher proportion of white to gray matter volume within the left and right hippocampus than those with non-TRD. Considered together, this suggests that TRD may be characterized by reductions in FA, although there is a notable lack of convergence among anatomic regions.

STRUCTURAL ABNORMALITIES IN TREATMENT-RESISTANT DEPRESSION: PROSPECTIVE STUDIES

Neuromodulation Therapies

Structural predictors of treatment response in individuals with TRD have primarily been studied with neuromodulation therapies, such as ECT and rTMS. Volumetric differences in the hippocampus have been suggested to be key baseline predictors of subsequent response to neuromodulation therapies. Patients with TRD have been found to have smaller hippocampal volumes compared with healthy volunteers at baseline before ECT treatment, and smaller hippocampal volume at baseline in individuals with TRD can be predictive of clinical improvement.[17] Similarly, Furtado and colleagues[18] found that smaller pretreatment left hippocampal volume showed a trend toward predicting subjective improvement in MDD symptoms after a course of an rTMS.

A few studies have also implicated the ACC, and in particular subgenual ACC (sgACC), as an important predictor of response to ECT. Schmitgen and colleagues[19] found that increased rostral ACC (rACC) thickness at baseline, in contrast to cortical complexity or cortical gyrification, had the greatest predictive power for clinical response to ECT. Additionally, lower pretreatment sgACC-mPFC structural connectivity has also been associated with response (>50% symptom improvement) to ECT.[20] Although limited, current research suggests that the structural brain feature that is most commonly predictive of response to neuromodulation therapies are changes in the hippocampus, with some studies also highlighting the ACC and sgACC.

Antidepressant Pharmacotherapy

To our knowledge, no studies have prospectively examined baseline brain features of those with TRD that are predictive of response to conventional oral pharmacotherapy; however, a few studies highlight potential structural biomarkers of response to ketamine treatment. In contrast to typical pharmacotherapy for MDD, which largely targets monoamine systems in the brain, ketamine is a glutamate N-methyl-D-aspartate (NMDA) receptor antagonist and is observed to lead to rapid treatment effects in individuals with TRD. In a pilot study of 13 individuals with TRD who received a single ketamine infusion, Sydnor and colleagues[21] demonstrated that higher preinfusion FA in the left cingulum bundle and the left superior longitudinal fasciculus was associated with greater depression symptom improvement 24 hours later. Abdallah and colleagues[22] found that change in depression scores after treatment with ketamine was significantly correlated with the pretreatment volumes of the left hippocampus, but not the right hippocampus, further highlighting the hippocampus as an important potential biomarker of response in TRD. Finally, Siegel and colleagues[23] explored the association between limbic structural volumes and clinical response to ketamine and found that smaller pretreatment right hippocampal volume predicted greater response to ketamine. Further studies in these areas are needed to better understand the nature of these relationships and their potential as biomarkers.

FUNCTIONAL ABNORMALITIES IN TREATMENT-RESISTANT DEPRESSION: RETROSPECTIVE STUDIES

Functional abnormalities in TRD have primarily been investigated via resting-state fMRI (rs-fMRI) in order to compute RSFC and will therefore be the focus of this review. Such studies in TRD individuals largely point toward altered RSFC and activity within the default mode network (DMN), and between the DMN and other brain regions and networks.[5,10,24,25] De Kwaasteniet and colleagues[26] conducted a cross-sectional seed-based rs-fMRI analysis comparing patients with TRD to those with non-TRD and HCs to investigate salience network, cognitive control nework, and DMN dysfunction among those with TRD. They found decreased RSFC in TRD relative to non-TRD and HC between the (1) anterior and posterior parts of the DMN, (2) cognitive control network and the posterior DMN, and the (3) motor cortex and superior temporal gyrus. He and colleagues[25] investigated large-scale functional connectivity differences using whole-brain rs-fMRI and found that individuals with non-TRD (ie, first-episode and treatment naïve) were characterized by disconnection in the fronto-parietal top–down control network, whereas those with TRD exhibited more extensive disconnection within the DMN and between the DMN and other networks. Notably, other studies have found altered DMN connectivity in both individuals with TRD and individuals with non-TRD; thus, specific nodes within this network may be critical in differentiating those who are resistant versus responsive to treatment. For example, when examining FC of the middle temporal cortex, Ma and colleagues[10] found that individuals with non-TRD, whose current episode was less than 6 months, exhibited abnormal RSFC in the supramarginal gyrus, parahippocampus gyrus, precuneus and angular gyrus while patients with TRD exhibited abnormal RSFC in the precuneus, cuneus, middle frontal gyrus, middle temporal gyrus and superior frontal gyrus. Moreover, Guo and colleagues[24] found that significantly decreased interhemispheric coordination in the middle cingulum and hippocampus, a white matter tract that links various DMN regions, in individuals with TRD compared with those with first-episode, treatment naïve MDD. Interestingly, a recent study comparing differences in habenular RSFC among individuals with TRD, symptom-remitted MDD individuals and HCS found that those with TRD exhibited hyperconnectivity of the left habenula to the left precuneus cortex and right precentral gyrus, when compared with the remitted group, and to the right precuneus cortex, when compared with the remitted and HC groups.[27] Thus, studies examining functional connectivity in individuals with TRD compared with those with treatment sensitive depression (TSD) seem to largely implicate hypoconnectivity between the DMN and other neural regions/networks, with some studies suggesting hyperconnectivity between the habenula and regions within the DMN. This perhaps suggests a unique relationship between hyperconnectivity of the habenula, a critical node of the reward-circuit, and the precuneus cortex, a region implicated in difficulties with positive future scene simulation for those experiencing anhedonia, in patients with TRD.[27,28]

It has also been suggested that TRD may be specifically associated with functional connectivity abnormalities in the thalamo-cortical circuits, whereas those that are responsive to treatment may have more widespread decreased connectivity in the limbic-striatal-pallidal-thalamic circuit.[29] In a cross-sectional study of those with TRD, treatment-responsive MDD and HCs, those that responded to antidepressants were found to have distributed decreases in RSFC, especially in the ACC and the left and right prefrontal cortex, hippocampus, insula and amygdala while patients with TRD were found to primarily have decreased connectivity in prefrontal areas and the thalamus, bilaterally.[29] Thus, altered connectivity within the DMN, between the DMN and other regions (eg, habenula) and within the thalamo-cortical circuit may uniquely characterize those with TRD.

FUNCTIONAL ABNORMALITIES IN TREATMENT-RESISTANT DEPRESSION: PROSPECTIVE STUDIES
Neuromodulation

Studies of baseline functional brain features predictive of response to neuromodulation therapies, including ECT and rTMS, in TRD have primarily been investigated using rs-fMRI. Such studies largely implicate the PFC, ACC, and sgACC dysfunction as brain features that associate with treatment outcome in TRD. For example, Van Waarde and colleagues[30,] collected fMRI scans before ECT treatment and utilized multivariate pattern analysis to discover networks that predicted recovery from depression. They found 2 resting-state networks, one centered in the dorsomedial PFC and another in the ACC, that showed relatively high sensitivity and specificity for the classification of treatment outcome. Argyelan and colleagues[31] demonstrated that those with TRD had higher baseline levels of fractional amplitude of low-frequency fluctuation (fALff) in the sgACC than HCs, and that higher baseline sgACC fALff values predicted better clinical response to ECT. Studies of functional biomarkers of treatment response to rTMS have been more widely studied than ECT and highlight similar abnormalities. Ge and colleagues[32] found that weaker baseline RSFC between the sgACC and right dorsolateral prefrontal cortex (dlPFC) and stronger rACC RSFC to left lateral parietal cortex was associated with more clinical improvement after 6 weeks of rTMS and that these brain signatures were also predictive of eventual response and/or remission at the 3-month follow-up visit. Avissar and colleagues[34] found that higher baseline functional connectivity of the left dlPFC to the executive division of the striatum correlated with treatment response to rTMS over the left dlPFC, suggesting that an intact pathway from frontal regions toward deeper regions may be responsible for treatment response to rTMS in those with TRD. Interestingly, Weigand and colleagues[33] used neuronavigation to prospectively determine patient-specific locations of rTMS stimulation within the dlPFC, with the hypothesis that stimulation sites that were more anterior-lateral and functionally connected to the sgACC (at baseline) would result in better response. They found that baseline RSFC between the targeted cortical site and sgACC prospectively predicted antidepressant response, and in particular, cognitive and affective symptoms (but not somatic). Considered together, the literature on functional biomarkers of response to ECT and rTMS suggest that functional connectivity within the PRC and between the PFC and subcortical limbic regions is critical to response to neuromodulation therapies in TRD.

Antidepressant Pharmacotherapy

Functional neuroimaging markers of clinical response to traditional antidepressant pharmacotherapy has largely been studied in the context of MDD more generally, rather that TRD specifically. Most prospective pharmacotherapy MRI studies have been conducted using ketamine, which is generally administered for the treatment of TRD (rather than non-TRD forms of MDD). Overall, studies show that brain features predictive of ketamine response include the PFC, DMN, and the sgACC. Siegel and colleagues[23] demonstrated that individuals with TRD exhibited baseline hyperconnectivity within mesiotemporal regions, within the DMN, and between the DMN and sgACC, when compared with HCs. Interestingly, no RSFC differences were found between individuals with HCs and those with postketamine TRD. This "normalizing" effect, from brain signatures unique to TRD to those more similar to HCs, has also been observed in other studies. Abdallah and colleagues[22] found that those with TRD had reduced global brain connectivity with global signal regression (GBCr) in the PFC but increased GBCr in the posterior cingulate, precuneus, lingual gyrus, and cerebellum at baseline. Posttreatment, they found that GBCr was significantly increased in the PFC and significantly reduced in the cerebellum and that only 310 voxels were significantly different from HCs (as compared with the 2174 voxels at baseline). Considered together, the literature on baseline predictors of response to ketamine is limited but highlight connectivity within DMN, between the DMN and other regions, and the sgACC, as biomarkers of treatment response.

DISCUSSION

Herein we provide a selective, narrative review of the available literature concerning both retrospective and prospective MRI studies of structural and RSFC brain features that associated with TRD. First, we find that there is marked heterogeneity in both the design of the studies reviewed, as well as in the findings. Some common limitations in the design of studies include variable or lack of specificity regarding enrollment criteria or the definition of TRD used, and relatively small samples sizes. In the case of most studies, it is also generally not possible to separate the effects of illness duration or illness severity from treatment-resistance *per se*. Although we restricted our review scope to MRI studies to increase the homogeneity of the literature under consideration, we found widespread variability in the MRI acquisition, preprocessing, and analytical approaches. We also found ambiguity or lack of specificity in neuroanatomical delineations and nomenclature used across studies, further confounding a clear integration of study results to date.

The preceding points notwithstanding, we do note a few areas of potentially important convergence across studies. Regarding structural brain features, lower GMV across cortical and subcortical areas in TRD samples emerges as a relatively consistent theme. Among brain regions, the PFC, ACC, hippocampus, and caudate seem to be most significantly involved. Available findings suggest that GMV loss may track with illness duration, particularly within the PFC. In another point of tentative convergence, multiple studies indicate loss of white matter integrity in TRD as indexed by reduced FA. Major white matter tracts are implicated, including the cingulum bundle, corpus callosum, and the superior longitudinal fascicule; however, the disparate nature of the tracts and brain regions across studies precludes clear anatomic localization.

Regarding functional brain features, aberrant connectivity both within subregions of the DMN as well as between regions of the DMN and other brain regions and networks in TRD is a modestly consistent find, although a few caveats are noted below. It should be noted at the outset that there is a lack of convergence in the field regarding the precise definition of the DMN, which likely contributes to discrepancies observed in the current literature. The DMN is generally considered to encompass regions of the vmPFC, together with dorsal regions of the PFC and the posterior cingulate cortex. Various authors also consider areas of parietal cortex, the precuneus, medial temporal cortex, parahippocampus, and other limbic regions within the definition of the DMN. Conceptualized as supporting internally directed and self-referential processing, the regions identified as comprising the DMN are observed to show relative coherence with each other, and to show enhanced activity during task-free or resting-state periods in individuals during functional imaging. Studies have found both increased and decreased RSFC within the DMN in individuals with TRD compared with non-TRD; the preponderance of evidence currently suggests overall a decrease in intrinsic DMN connectivity in TRD. Aberrant connectivity between regions of the DMN and other brain regions outside the DMN is also consistently reported in TRD but, similarly, the directionally of the findings are mixed.

Among the prospective treatment studies in TRD samples reviewed, the majority of studies have examined brain features at baseline that associate with treatment response to ECT or rTMS. The few studies done of structural MRI treatment predictors to ECT implicate the hippocampus as well as the ACC, although the studies are small and lack a control group, thereby limiting the conclusions that can be drawn. A somewhat larger literature addresses the question of RSFC predictive markers of treatment response to ECT or rTMS and the findings do partially converge on the PFC and ACC (particularly the sgACC) as important predictive regions. In terms of treatment studies utilizing pharmacotherapy, the majority feature the use of ketamine, whereas there is a notable dearth of prospective pharmacotherapy MRI studies otherwise. The studies of ketamine, limited by small samples sizes and other design limitations such as lack of a control group, preliminarily suggest that baseline hippocampal volume associates with treatment response and implicate the PFC and sgACC in the antidepressant mechanism of action of ketamine.

Considered together, we find substantial heterogeneity in the current literature regarding MRI studies of TRD. Given this, the field will need to wait for additional larger, high-quality MRI studies to inform an understanding of the brain mechanisms of TRD. Retrospective and case-control study designs in TRD are limited by risk of confounding and in difficulty decerning the relative contribution of illness duration, illness severity, and other clinical and demographic features known to be associated with TRD. Prospective neuroimaging studies that follow treatment-seeking individuals with MDD over time may be costly and complex but will likely be required in order to provide reliable and ultimately clinically actionable information regarding neurobiology features that predict or associate with treatment-resistance.

CLINICS CARE POINTS

- Given the great societal burden of TRD, it is critical that we increase our understanding of the neurobiological mechanisms underlying TRD.
- Continued advances in—and standardization of—structural and functional imaging techniques will be important to identify reliable, actionable brain features of TRD.
- Studies of structural abnormalities in TRD implicate reduction of FA and GMV across various regions. Notable regions in studies investigating GMV include the ACC, caudate, mPFC, cerebellum, insula, corpus callosum, and hippocampus. Investigations of WM are more heterogenous.
- Studies of functional abnormalities in TRD implicate altered connectivity and activity in the DMN and between the DMN and other cognitive networks/brain regions.
- Longitudinal investigations of individuals with MDD across stages of treatment will be critical to our furthered understanding of TRD.

FUNDING

This work was supported in part by the Ehrenkranz Laboratory for Human Resilience, a component of the Depression and Anxiety Center for Discovery and Treatment at the Icahn School of Medicine at Mount Sinai, and by the Gottesman Foundation.

DECLARATION OF INTERESTS

In the past 5 years, Dr J.W. Murrough has provided consultation services and/or served on advisory boards for Compass Pathfinder, Boehreinger Ingelheim, Clexio Biosciences, Engrail Therapeutics, FSV7, Otsuka, and Sage Therapeutics. Dr J.W. Murrough is named on a patent pending for neuropeptide Y as a treatment for mood and anxiety disorders and on a patent pending for the use of KCNQ channel openers to treat depression and related conditions. The Icahn School of Medicine (employer of Dr J.W. Murrough) is named on a patent and has entered into a licensing agreement and will receive payments related to the use of ketamine or esketamine for the treatment of depression. The Icahn School of Medicine is also named on a patent related to the use of ketamine for the treatment of PTSD. Dr J.W. Murrough is not named on these patents and will not receive any payments. All other authors declare no conflicts. None of the authors received any support or payments for this study.

REFERENCES

1. American Psychiatric Association. *Diagnostic and Statistical Manual of Mental Disorders*. 5th edition. Arlington, VA: American Psychiatric Association; 2013.
2. Ferrari AJ, Charlson FJ, Norman RE, et al. Burden of depressive disorders by country, sex, age, and year: findings from the global burden of disease study 2010. Plos Med 2013;10(11):e1001547.
3. Rush AJ, Trivedi MH, Wisniewski SR, et al. Acute and longer-term outcomes in depressed outpatients requiring one or several treatment steps: a STAR*D report. Am J Psychiatry 2006;163(11):1905–17.
4. Fonseka TM, MacQueen GM, Kennedy SH. Neuroimaging biomarkers as predictors of treatment outcome in Major Depressive Disorder. J Affect Disord 2018; 233:21–35.
5. Runia N, Yücel DE, Lok A, et al. The neurobiology of treatment-resistant depression: A systematic review of neuroimaging studies. Neurosci Biobehav Rev 2022; 132:433–48.
6. Klok MPC, van Eijndhoven PF, Argyelan M, et al. Structural brain characteristics in treatment-resistant depression: review of magnetic resonance imaging studies. BJPsych Open 2019;5(5):e76.
7. Serra-Blasco M, Portella MJ, Gómez-Ansón B, et al. Effects of illness duration and treatment resistance on grey matter abnormalities in major depression. Br J Psychiatry 2013;202:434–40.
8. Phillips JL, Batten LA, Tremblay P, et al. A Prospective, Longitudinal Study of the Effect of Remission on Cortical Thickness and Hippocampal Volume in Patients with Treatment-Resistant Depression. Int J Neuropsychopharmacol 2015;18(8): pyv037.
9. Shah PJ, Glabus MF, Goodwin GM, et al. Chronic, treatment-resistant depression and right fronto-striatal atrophy. Br J Psychiatry 2002;180:434–40.
10. Ma C, Ding J, Li J, et al. Resting-state functional connectivity bias of middle temporal gyrus and caudate with altered gray matter volume in major depression. PLoS One 2012;7.
11. Lorenzetti V, Allen NB, Fornito A, et al. Structural brain abnormalities in major depressive disorder: a selective review of recent MRI studies. J Affect Disord 2009;117(1–2):1–17.
12. Guo WB, Liu F, Xue ZM, et al. Altered white matter integrity in young adults with first-episode, treatment-naive, and treatment-responsive depression. Neurosci Lett 2012;522(2):139–44.
13. Peng HJ, Zheng HR, Ning YP, et al. Abnormalities of cortical-limbic-cerebellar white matter networks may contribute to treatment-resistant depression: a diffusion tensor imaging study. BMC Psychiatry 2013;13:72. https://doi.org/10.1186/1471-244X-13-72.
14. de Diego-Adeliño J, Pires P, Gómez-Ansón B, et al. Microstructural white-matter abnormalities associated with treatment resistance, severity and duration of illness in major depression. Psychol Med 2014;44(6):1171–82.
15. Zhou Y, Qin LD, Chen J, et al. Brain microstructural abnormalities revealed by diffusion tensor images in patients with treatment-resistant depression compared with major depressive disorder before treatment. Eur J Radiol 2011;80(2):450–4.

16. de Diego-Adeliño J, Portella MJ, Gómez-Ansón B, et al. Hippocampal abnormalities of glutamate/glutamine, N-acetylaspartate and choline in patients with depression are related to past illness burden. J Psychiatry Neurosci 2013; 38(2):107–16.

17. Joshi SH, Espinoza RT, Pirnia T, et al. Structural Plasticity of the Hippocampus and Amygdala Induced by Electroconvulsive Therapy in Major Depression. Biol Psychiatry 2016;79(4):282–92.

18. Furtado CP, Hoy KE, Maller JJ, et al. Cognitive and volumetric predictors of response to repetitive transcranial magnetic stimulation (rTMS) - a prospective follow-up study. Psychiatry Res 2012;202(1):12–9.

19. Schmitgen MM, Kubera KM, Depping MS, et al. Exploring cortical predictors of clinical response to electroconvulsive therapy in major depression. Eur Arch Psychiatry Clin Neurosci 2020;270(2):253–61.

20. Tsolaki E, Narr KL, Espinoza R, et al. Subcallosal Cingulate Structural Connectivity Differs in Responders and Nonresponders to Electroconvulsive Therapy. Biol Psychiatry Cogn Neurosci Neuroimaging 2021;6(1):10–9.

21. Sydnor VJ, Lyall AE, Cetin-Karayumak S, et al. Studying pre-treatment and ketamine-induced changes in white matter microstructure in the context of ketamine's antidepressant effects. Transl Psychiatry 2020;10(1):432.

22. Abdallah CG, Salas R, Jackowski A, et al. Hippocampal volume and the rapid antidepressant effect of ketamine. J Psychopharmacol 2015;29(5):591–5.

23. Siegel JS, Palanca BJA, Ances BM, et al. Prolonged ketamine infusion modulates limbic connectivity and induces sustained remission of treatment-resistant depression. Psychopharmacology (Berl) 2021;238(4):1157–69.

24. Guo W, Liu F, Xue Z, et al. Decreased interhemispheric coordination in treatment-resistant depression: a resting-state fMRI study. PLoS One 2013b;8.

25. He Z, Cui Q, Zheng J, et al. Frequency-specific alterations in functional connectivity in treatment-resistant and -sensitive major depressive disorder. J Psychiatr Res 2016;82:30–9.

26. de Kwaasteniet BP, Rive MM, Ruhé HG, et al. Decreased Resting-State Connectivity between Neurocognitive Networks in Treatment Resistant Depression. Front Psychiatry 2015;6:28.

27. Barreiros AR, Breukelaar I, Mayur P, et al. Abnormal habenula functional connectivity characterizes treatment-resistant depression. Neuroimage Clin 2022;34: 102990.

28. Yang ZY, Zhang RT, Wang YM, et al. Altered activation and functional connectivity in individuals with social anhedonia when envisioning positive future episodes [published online ahead of print, 2021 Mar 29]. Psychol Med 2021;1–9. https://doi.org/10.1017/S0033291721000970.

29. Lui S, Wu Q, Qiu L, et al. Resting-state functional connectivity in treatment-resistant depression. Am J Psychiatry 2011;168(6):642–8.

30. van Waarde JA, Scholte HS, van Oudheusden LJ, et al. A functional MRI marker may predict the outcome of electroconvulsive therapy in severe and treatment-resistant depression. Mol Psychiatry 2015;20(5):609–14.

31. Argyelan M, Lencz T, Kaliora S, et al. Subgenual cingulate cortical activity predicts the efficacy of electroconvulsive therapy. Transl Psychiatry 2016;6(4):e789.

32. Ge R, Downar J, Blumberger DM, et al. Functional connectivity of the anterior cingulate cortex predicts treatment outcome for rTMS in treatment-resistant depression at 3-month follow-up. Brain Stimul 2020;13(1):206–14.

33. Weigand A, Horn A, Caballero R, et al. Prospective Validation That Subgenual Connectivity Predicts Antidepressant Efficacy of Transcranial Magnetic Stimulation Sites. Biol Psychiatry 2018;84(1):28–37.
34. Avissar M, Powell F, Ilieva I, et al. Functional connectivity of the left DLPFC to striatum predicts treatment response of depression to TMS. Brain Stimul 2017;10(5):919–25.

Immune Dysregulation in Treatment-Resistant Depression

Precision Approaches to Treatment Selection and Development of Novel Treatments

Cherise R. Chin Fatt, PhD, Taryn L. Mayes, MSc,
Madhukar H. Trivedi, MD*

KEYWORDS

- Immune function • Precision medicine • Treatment-resistant depression

KEY POINTS

- Major depressive disorder has been shown to be associated with increased inflammation.
- One main step toward reducing the burden of treatment-resistant depression, and more generally major depressive disorder is immune-targeted precision medicine.
- There are multiple tools available to understand the complexity of the immune system, ranging from genetic composition to protein breakdown.

INTRODUCTION

Major depressive disorder (MDD) affects one in six adults in the United States during their lifetime and is one of the biggest causes of disability worldwide.[1] Owing to the heterogeneity of MDD, the symptom profile is quite different from person to person, and although it is a single disorder, it may be more appropriate to view MDD as composed of multiple subtypes.[2] According to the Diagnostic and Statistical Manual of Mental Disorders - Fifth Edition (DSM-5), five out of nine symptoms (low mood, anhedonia, weight loss or gain, insomnia or hypersomnia, psychomotor agitation, fatigue, feeling worthless or excessive/inappropriate guilt, decreased concentration, and thoughts of death/suicide) need to be met for the diagnosis of MDD. If we consider the compounding criteria separately (such as weight loss or gain) this may result in over 900 unique symptom profiles.[2] In fact, a study by Fried and Nesse[3] of 3703

Center for Depression Research and Clinical Care, UT Southwestern Medical Center, 5323 Harry Hines Boulevard, Dallas, TX 75235-9086, USA
* Corresponding author.
E-mail address: madhukar.trivedi@utsouthwestern.edu

Psychiatr Clin N Am 46 (2023) 403–413
https://doi.org/10.1016/j.psc.2023.02.010
0193-953X/23/

depressed outpatients identified 1030 unique symptom profiles underscoring the heterogeneous nature of MDD.

Findings from the landmark Sequenced Treatment Alternatives to Relieve Depression (STAR*D) study showed that one in three adults with MDD did not attain remission even after four consecutive trials of antidepressant treatment.[4] Although these findings informed the field on conceptualizing the definition of treatment-resistant depression (TRD) as inadequate improvement with two or more antidepressants in the current episode, a key confounding factor could be that patients may not have received the treatment that is matched to their biological and clinical profiles.[5] For example, we have previously found that patients with MDD who have elevated markers of systemic inflammation (such as c-reactive protein [CRP]) respond poorly to predominantly serotonergic antidepressant (such as selective serotonin reuptake inhibitors [SSRIs]) but have higher chances of improvement with a noradrenergic/dopaminergic antidepressant such as bupropion. Therefore, it may result in apparent TRD if a patient with MDD with elevated CRP receives two or more courses of SSRIs without ever being prescribed to the biomarker-matched antidepressant, such as bupropion. Based on this and other recent research, it is possible that a dysregulated inflammatory profile is a distinguishing factor between TRD and non-TRD.[6,7] This dysregulated inflammatory profile in TRD has been shown to be linked to some core symptoms of TRD such as physical illness or poor physical health,[8] recurrence of depressive illness,[9] cognitive impairments,[10] or early life trauma.[11,12]

Owing to the link between immune dysfunction and TRD and overwhelming evidence that immune dysregulation and MDD are associated with each other,[13–15] use of immune profiles to identify biologically distinct subgroups may be a step forward in understanding MDD and TRD. This report aims to briefly review (1) the role of inflammation in the pathophysiology of MDD, (2) the role of immune dysfunction to guide precision medicine, (3) tools used to understand immune function, and (4) novel statistical techniques that may allow for the use of immunological data to usher an era of precision medicine for psychiatry.

ROLE OF INFLAMMATION IN THE PATHOPHYSIOLOGY OF MAJOR DEPRESSIVE DISORDER

MDD has been shown to be associated with increased inflammation and this relationship has been extensively summarized in numerous review articles.[12,16–19] Multiple hypotheses have been developed to unravel the pathophysiology of MDD. One such theory is the cytokine theory which was originally developed by Smith[20] as the "The Macrophage Theory of Depression," and later expanded by Ur and colleagues.[21] This theory suggests that psychological stress together with genetic factors increases cytokine production and thus leads to depressive symptoms. Others have shown that MDD is associated with elevated levels of pro-inflammatory cytokines, acute phase proteins in blood and cerebrospinal fluid (CSF), decreased adaptive immune response, differences in the relative abundance of specific immune cells types, increased activation of microglia, and other immune changes.[13] There are a number of factors that are associated with inflammation such as obesity, childhood trauma, bacterial or viral infections, and medical illness such as diabetes and autoimmune and inflammatory disorders.[22] This suggests that it is possible that not every patient with MDD or TRD has increased inflammation and not every patient with increased inflammation has MDD or TRD. By characterizing the subtypes of MDD, it may be possible to determine which MDD subgroup is associated with increased inflammation or with other biological factors.

Immune Dysregulation and Specific Aspects of Depression

Owing to the large number of possible symptoms associated with MDD, it is important to explore the link between immune dysregulation and individual MDD symptoms. In a pooled analysis of 15 population-based cohorts of over 50,000 individuals over the age of 18, CRP, interleukin (IL)-6, and 24 depressive symptoms assessed with self-report measures were measured at baseline.[23] Frank and colleagues[23] found that higher CRP concentrations were strongly associated with increased risk of four physical symptoms (namely, changes in appetite, felt everything was an effort, loss of energy, and sleep problems) and one cognitive symptom (little interest in doing things). Interestingly, four symptoms that were strictly related to emotion (namely, bothered by things, hopelessness about the future, felt fearful, and life had been a failure) were not associated with inflammation. These results align with the findings of previous cross-sectional studies that showed differential associations between systemic inflammation and changes in appetite,[24–26] lower energy levels,[24,25,27] and sleep problems.[24,25,27]

Immune dysregulation specific to patients with treatment-resistant depression

In the first meta-analysis that examined the relationship between inflammation and TRD, it was found that elevated levels of inflammation contribute to MDD being treatment-resistant.[28] More specifically, Strawbridge and colleagues[28] showed that over time, there is a decrease in tumor necrosis factor α (TNFα) levels in patients who respond to treatment compared with those who are treatment-resistant. In addition, greater treatment resistance has been shown to be associated with higher levels of inflammatory markers, namely TNF, soluble TNF receptor 2, and IL-6.[29] These findings align with preliminary findings from Raison and colleagues[30] who showed that "TNFα antagonist, infliximab, can improve depression in some treatment-resistant patients." Patients with TRD have also been shown to have elevated CRP. In a study comparing 48 MDD patients responding to treatment, 102 treatment-resistant patients, 48 MDD patients not on medication, and 54 healthy controls, the TRD group had significantly elevated CRP compared with the healthy controls, whereas the other two MDD groups did not.[31] Thus, although inflammation is linked to depression in general, there may be even greater association between inflammation and treatment nonresponsiveness.

ROLE OF IMMUNE DYSFUNCTION TO GUIDE PRECISION MEDICINE

The role of inflammation as a marker of clinical response to treatment in TRD has been extensively detailed.[32] A review by Yang and colleagues[33] of 10 studies, showed that in 5 of the studies, "higher baseline IL-6 or CRP/high-sensitivity-CRP in blood predicted better response to medication with anti-inflammatory characteristics, such as ketamine and infliximab. Yet, markers such as TNFα and interferon-y did not show any predictive value in predicting response." However, many studies that seek to demonstrate the interaction between inflammatory factors and treatment outcomes only focus on a small subset of inflammatory markers. These findings need to be replicated so that a more definitive conclusion regarding the role of inflammation on treatment response and TRD can be reached.

Immune Mechanisms to Guide Precision Medicine

One potnetial avenue for reducing the burden of MDD is precision medicine. The National Research Council has pointed out that precision medicine does not mean creating a drug or medical device that is unique to each patient, but rather classifying individuals into subgroups that differ in their disposition to a particular disease or treatment response.

Immune dysfunction could contribute to depression that is associated with clinical inflammation as well as those with MDD who have low-grade inflammation. In addition, heterogeneity also exists within these groups of patients. As previously mentioned, when considering DSM-5 criteria, there are over 900 unique symptom profiles.[2] Therefore, there is a critical need to develop subtypes for MDD and TRD patients based on their clinical and biological profiles. A comprehensive definition of these subtypes and then identification of targets to treat these subtypes may get us closer to the goal of immune-targeted precision medicine.

Drevets and colleagues[13] proposed the 4-step criteria for immune-targeted precision medicine in MDD, namely (1) causality, (2) targetability, (3) diagnosability, and (4) unmet need (**Fig. 1**). Briefly, for causality, the authors suggest that for immune-targeted precision medicine, there must be a causal link between immune dysfunction and MDD.

Causality: As previously shown, there is compelling evidence that immune dysregulation and depression are correlated with each other.[14,15] However, these studies do not infer that there is a causal link between inflammation and MDD. The preclinical evidence has pointed to this causal relationship, where immune mechanisms can have "adverse effects on neuronal function and thus cause anhedonia, and other depressive-live behavior."[34–37] Longitudinal human studies have begun testing the hypothesis that inflammation precedes MDD.[38–40] For example, using data from the Netherlands Study of Depression and Anxiety (NESDA), Lamers and colleagues[40] showed that among women with depression, higher levels of IL-6 predicted a chronic course of MDD. Another example is the Texas Resilience Against Depression Study (T-RAD).[41]

The T-RAD study is composed of two inter-linked studies—D2K and RAD—which are designed to be natural history, longitudinal studies that follow participants with current or past diagnosis of a unipolar or bipolar depressive disorder or are at risk for depression but not yet suffering from the disease. The D2K study follows participants (ages 10 years and older) who have a current or past diagnosis of depression or bipolar disorder. The RAD study follows participants aged 10–24 years who are at risk for depression but not yet suffering from the disease. The assessments collected as part of T-RAD are similar between the two studies, thus the individuals with depression as well as those at risk can be compared in future analyses. This is an example of one study that may allow us to identify MDD subtypes and to determine the causal link between immune dysfunction and MDD as well as other biological and clinical factors that are related to the subtypes.

Targetability: The cause of the biological change must be targetable using either peripheral or centrally acting drugs. Several immune-targeted compounds have been evaluated for potential antidepressant effects. The studies assessing these effects have used three approaches: (1) meta-analyses of changes in depressive symptoms within aggregate data from clinical trials of primary immunological disorders, (2) analyses of mood effects in immunology clinical trials for which patient-level data were available, and (3) randomized-controlled trials in patients with MDD. Drevets and

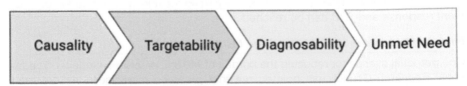

Fig. 1. The 4-step criteria for immune-targeted precision medicine defined by Drevets and colleagues.[13] For successful drug development of an immune-related marker in MDD, researchers need to establish causality, targetability, diagnosability, and unmet need.

colleagues[13] have provided a comprehensive review of immune targets for therapeutic development.

Diagnosability: An approach to selecting patients based on the biological model and matching to a treatment needs to be identified. This approach needs to be scalable, affordable, and accessible to all. Although subtyping the population based on immune dysregulation would be a major step forward, understanding the mechanisms in the immune system and the brain which mediate the depressive symptoms will drastically advance the field. Neuroimaging biomarkers assessed using MRI, PET, and magnetic resonance spectroscopy (MRS) have given us insight into the link between MDD and the brain. Each of these neuroimaging modalities has a different set of trade-offs between immune specificity of the imaging signal, spatial resolution, cost, and accessibility. Therefore, we need to work toward taking a holistic view that uses the strengths of different measurement tools, so that we can better subtype and get to the point of precision medicine.[13]

Unmet clinical need: For an immune-targeted precision medicine in MDD to be a viable step in drug discovery, the introduction of a treatment should substantially reduce the burden of depression. MDD affects one in six adults in the United States during their lifetime and is one of the biggest causes of disability worldwide.[1] Owing to the high prevalence of MDD as well as its chronicity, there is a heavy burden on the economy, health care systems, insurance systems, and most importantly the patients themselves.

The National Institute of Mental Health took a major step toward precision medicine, by launching the Research Domain Criteria Project (RDoC) in 2009.[42] RDoC was launched after a growing awareness that in order to better understand the development and treatment of mental health disorders, there is a need to increase knowledge of biological, physiological, and behavioral components and mechanisms, how these factors interact with each other, and which are of these factors actually serve as protective factors against mental health disorders. This framework is already being explored in various studies where investigators are moving beyond symptom-based research or limiting investigation to a subset of constructs. Two such examples are the Bipolar-Schizophrenia Network on Intermediate Phenotypes studies[43] and T-RAD.[41] For the later, T-RAD, the goal is to integrate variability in multiple aspects (neuroimaging, electroencephalography, mobile health, behavioral phenotype, biospecimens, and clinical phenotypes) to offer a comprehensive approach to understanding MDD to aid in novel drug development, optimal treatment assignment, and precision medicine.

TOOLS USED TO UNDERSTAND IMMUNE DYSREGULATION

There are multiple tools available to understand the complexity of the immune system, ranging from genetic composition to protein breakdown. A review by Gadad and colleagues[44] provides a comprehensive overview of these tools. Briefly, these tools can be broken down into three main categories, namely (1) gene transcription through pharmacogenomics, epigenomics, and transcriptomics, (2) proteomics, and (3) metabolomics. See **Table 1** for a brief overview of the technologies for development of peripheral blood-based biomarkers of MDD.

NOVEL STATISTICAL ANALYSIS OF IMMUNOLOGICAL DATA

There are multiple points to consider when analyzing immunological data. See Genser and colleagues[45] for a guide to statistical analysis for immunological data. Briefly, before reviewing the statistical techniques used to analyze immunological data, it is

Table 1
Technologies for development of peripheral blood-based biomarkers of major depressive disorder

	Example of Possible Technologies	Application of Technology in MDD or TRD
Gene transcription	• Single-nucleotide polymorphism identification • Epigenetic modification • Whole-gene/exome sequencing • Transcriptomics	Garriock et al,[48] 2010 Uher et al,[49] 2010
Proteomics	• Enzyme-linked immunosorbent assays (ELISA) • Multiplex	Köhler et al,[50] 2017
Metabolomics	• Mass spectrometry • Multiplex-based metabolites	Martins-de-Souza,[51] 2022 Paige et al,[52] 2007

important to review the structure of the data. Immunological data often does not meet the common data assumptions such as normality and is often highly correlated (ie, multicollinear). As such, for these types of data, a data transformation (eg, logarithmic transformation to make skewed data approximately normally distributed) is applied, or a statistical technique that has less stringent data assumptions (eg, nonparametric statistical techniques) is used. As for multicollinearity, the statistical techniques that assume independence between observations should not be used, but rather techniques that take these situations into account are more applicable.

As for the statistical techniques used to analyze immunological data, it strongly depends on the research question, the type of data collected, the size of the sample, and statistical distribution of the data (eg, normally distributed or skewed). Before applying the statistical techniques, it is important to first explore the data by reviewing summary statistics such as mean, standard deviation, and range, as well as visualizing the data (eg, heatmaps, scatter plots, boxplots). This will help to determine the structure of the data, identify possible outliers, and identify possible issues with the data set (such as batch effects). The next main issue to consider is sample size. Immunological data sets commonly have a large number of variables and a relatively small number of participants; thus, the dimension reduction techniques can be useful. Techniques, such as elastic net, can help to identify the variables that are related to the outcome of interest (eg, remission).

As for the statistical techniques, it can be divided into two groups, namely univariate and multivariate techniques. The examples of univariate techniques include the analysis of variance, T-test, Mann–Whitney U-test, and linear regression. As for multivariate techniques, examples of this include, principal component analysis, clustering techniques such as k-means, and logistic regression.

DISCUSSION

There is a significant burden associated with TRD-medical costs, patient health-related quality of life, and health status decreased by severity of disease.[46] As such there is an urgent need to work toward identifying MDD subgroups and immune-targeted precision treatments related to each subgroup. To get to this point of immune-targeted precision medicine, it is important to consider (1) the pathophysiology of TRD, (2) the role of immune dysfunction to guide precision medicine, (3) the

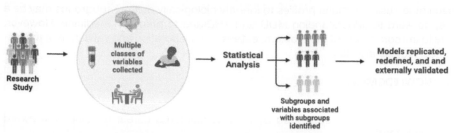

Fig. 2. The path toward precision medicine involves (1) recruiting a diverse group of participants, (2) collecting information from multiple units of data (biospecimens, brain-based markers, clinical assessments, and self-report assessments), (3) having a sound analytical plan that involves ensuring the data are carefully reviewed and cleaned, (4) identifying subgroups and markers associated with the subgroups, and (5) validation and replication of the model. With internal validation, these models can be improved and thus replicated in external data sets.

tools used to understand immune function, and (4) design of a statistical plan for quality control and answering the immune-related scientific questions.

One main step toward reducing the burden of TRD, and more generally MDD is immune-targeted precision medicine. Although precision medicine is the path forward, there are multiple challenges. It is a key to incorporate not only immune markers and clinical measures, but as suggested by the RDoC framework, to also include cells, circuits, physiology, behavior, and self-report paradigms. Several studies such as NESDA and T-RAD have been designed to address these questions. However, the models that are then built would need to be replicated and validated (**Fig. 2**). This venture would thus require extensive collaboration across not only personnel, such as psychiatrists, immunologists, neuroscientists, and data scientists, but also academic institutions and industry. As for the model building, the data sets involve a very large number of variables, and statistical models that are built are usually complex and difficult to interpret. Therefore, there is need to ensure that the data are clean, dimension-reduction methods are implemented, analytical plans are detailed, results are clearly explained, and results are replicated (or plans are clearly stated on how the findings will be replicated/validated).[47]

CLINICS CARE POINTS

- Symptom profiles of those with MDD are extremely heterogenous.
- Immune dysfunction is linked to MDD and TRD.
- Immune profiles may be useful for identifying biologically distinct subgroups in those with MDD.
- Precision medicine initiatives that utilize immunological data to guide treatment are currently under development and are not yet clinically actionable; once further developed immunological data may guide treatment selection to reduce incidence rates of TRD.

SUMMARY

In sum, due to the link between immune dysfunction and TRD as well as overwhelming evidence that the immune dysregulation and MDD are associated or correlated with each other, using immune profiles to identify biologically distinct subgroups may be a step forward to understanding MDD and TRD and to precision medicine. However, due to the complexity of the problem, extensive collaboration and validation of the statistical models are vital.

ACKNOWLEDGMENT

This work was supported in part by the Center for Depression Research and Clinical Care. Dr. Chin Fatt is supported by an NIH mentored career development award (KL2TR003981).

DISCLOSURE

Dr. Trivedi has served as a consultant or advisor for Acadia Pharmaceuticals, Inc., Akili Interactive, Alkermes, Inc. (Pub Steering Comm-ALKS5461), Allergan Sales LLC, Alto Neuroscience, Inc., Applied Clinical Intelligence, LLC (ACI), Axome Therapeutics, Boehringer Ingelheim, Engage Health Media, Gh Research, GreenLight VitalSign6, Inc., Heading Health, Inc., Health Care Global Village, Janssen - Cilag.SA, Janssen Research and Development, LLC (Adv Committee Esketamine), Janssen Research and Development, LLC (panel for study design for MDD relapse), Janssen - ORBIT, Legion Health, Jazz Pharmaceuticals, Lundbeck Research U.S.A, Medscape, LLC, Merck Sharp & Dohme Corp., Mind Medicine (MindMed) Inc., Myriad Neuroscience, Neurocrine Biosciences Inc, Navitor, Pharmaceuticals, Inc., Noema Pharma AG, Orexo US Inc., Otsuka Pharmaceutical Development & Commercialization, Inc. (PsychU, MDD Section Advisor), Otsuka America Pharmaceutical, Inc. (MDD expert), Pax Neuroscience , Perception Neuroscience Holdings, Inc., Pharmerit International, LP, Policy Analysis Inc., Sage, Therapeutics, Rexahn Pharmaceuticals, Inc., Sage Therapeutics, Signant Health, SK Life Science, Inc., Takeda Development Center Americas, Inc., The Baldwin Group, Inc., and Titan Pharmaceuticals, Inc. Dr. Trivedi also received editorial compensation from Oxford University Press. Dr. Chin Fatt and Mrs. Mayes have no conflicts to report.

REFERENCES

1. Marcus M, Yasamy MT, van Ommeren MV, et al. Depression: A global public health concern. 2012.
2. Demyttenaere K, Van Duppen Z. The impact of (the concept of) treatment-resistant depression: an opinion review. Int J Neuropsychopharmacol 2019; 22(2):85–92.
3. Fried EI, Nesse RM. Depression is not a consistent syndrome: an investigation of unique symptom patterns in the STAR* D study. J Affect Disord 2015;172:96–102.
4. Rush AJ, Trivedi MH, Wisniewski SR, et al. Acute and longer-term outcomes in depressed outpatients requiring one or several treatment steps: a STAR* D report. American Journal of Psychiatry 2006;163(11):1905–17.
5. Ionescu DF, Rosenbaum JF, Alpert JE. Pharmacological approaches to the challenge of treatment-resistant depression. Dialogues Clin Neurosci 2015;17(2): 111–26.
6. Strawbridge R, Young AH, Cleare AJ. Biomarkers for depression: recent insights, current challenges and future prospects. Neuropsychiatric Dis Treat 2017;13: 1245–62.
7. Raison CL, Felger JC, Miller AH. Inflammation and treatment resistance in major depression: the perfect storm. Psychiatr Times 2013;12.

8. Maes M, Kubera M, Obuchowiczwa E, et al. Depression's multiple comorbidities explained by (neuro) inflammatory and oxidative & nitrosative stress pathways. Neuroendocrinol Lett 2011;32(1):7–24.

9. Anisman H, Ravindran A, Griffiths J, et al. Endocrine and cytokine correlates of major depression and dysthymia with typical or atypical features. Mol Psychiatry 1999;4(2):182–8.

10. Li H, Sagar AP, Kéri S. Microglial markers in the frontal cortex are related to cognitive dysfunctions in major depressive disorder. J Affect Disord 2018;241:305–10.

11. Grosse L, Ambrée O, Jörgens S, et al. Cytokine levels in major depression are related to childhood trauma but not to recent stressors. Psychoneuroendocrinology 2016;73:24–31.

12. Strawbridge R, Hodsoll J, Powell TR, et al. Inflammatory profiles of severe treatment-resistant depression. J Affect Disord 2019;246:42–51.

13. Drevets WC, Wittenberg GM, Bullmore ET, et al. Immune targets for therapeutic development in depression: towards precision medicine. Nat Rev Drug Discov 2022;21(3):224–44.

14. Miller AH, Raison CL. The role of inflammation in depression: from evolutionary imperative to modern treatment target. Nat Rev Immunol 2016;16(1):22–34.

15. Branchi I, Poggini S, Capuron L, et al. Brain-immune crosstalk in the treatment of major depressive disorder. Eur Neuropsychopharmacol 2021;45:89–107.

16. Dowlati Y, Herrmann N, Swardfager W, et al. A meta-analysis of cytokines in major depression. Biol Psychiatry 2010;67(5):446–57.

17. Hannestad J, DellaGioia N, Bloch M. The effect of antidepressant medication treatment on serum levels of inflammatory cytokines: a meta-analysis. Neuropsychopharmacology 2011;36(12):2452–9.

18. Hiles S, Baker A, de Malmanche T, et al. Interleukin-6, C-reactive protein and interleukin-10 after antidepressant treatment in people with depression: a meta-analysis. Psychol Med 2012;42(10):2015–26.

19. Miller AH, Maletic V, Raison CL. Inflammation and its discontents: the role of cytokines in the pathophysiology of major depression. Biol Psychiatry 2009;65(9):732–41.

20. Smith RS. The macrophage theory of depression. Med Hypotheses 1991;35(4):298–306.

21. Ur E, White PD, Grossman A. Hypothesis: cytokines may be activated to cause depressive illness and chronic fatigue syndrome. Eur Arch Psychiatry Clin Neurosci 1992;241(5):317–22.

22. Miller AH. Five things to know about inflammation and depression. Psychiatr Times 2018;35(4):2018.

23. Frank P, Jokela M, Batty GD, et al. Association between systemic inflammation and individual symptoms of depression: a pooled analysis of 15 population-based cohort studies. Am J Psychiatr 2021;178(12):1107–18.

24. Fried EI, Von Stockert S, Haslbeck J, et al. Using network analysis to examine links between individual depressive symptoms, inflammatory markers, and covariates. Psychol Med 2020;50(16):2682–90.

25. Jokela M, Virtanen M, Batty GD, et al. Inflammation and specific symptoms of depression. JAMA Psychiatr 2016;73(1):87–8.

26. Lamers F, Milaneschi Y, De Jonge P, et al. Metabolic and inflammatory markers: associations with individual depressive symptoms. Psychol Med 2018;48(7):1102–10.

27. White J, Kivimäki M, Jokela M, et al. Association of inflammation with specific symptoms of depression in a general population of older people: The English Longitudinal Study of Ageing. Brain Behav Immun 2017;61:27–30.

28. Strawbridge R, Arnone D, Danese A, et al. Inflammation and clinical response to treatment in depression: a meta-analysis. Eur Neuropsychopharmacol 2015; 25(10):1532–43.

29. Haroon E, Daguanno AW, Woolwine BJ, et al. Antidepressant treatment resistance is associated with increased inflammatory markers in patients with major depressive disorder. Psychoneuroendocrinology 2018;95:43–9.

30. Raison CL, Rutherford RE, Woolwine BJ, et al. A randomized controlled trial of the tumor necrosis factor antagonist infliximab for treatment-resistant depression: the role of baseline inflammatory biomarkers. JAMA Psychiatr 2013;70(1):31–41.

31. Chamberlain SR, Cavanagh J, De Boer P, et al. Treatment-resistant depression and peripheral C-reactive protein. Br J Psychiatry 2019;214(1):11–9.

32. Strawbridge R, Young AH, Cleare AJ. Inflammation as a marker of clinical response to treatment: a focus on treatment-resistant depression. In: Inflammation and immunity in depression. London, England: Academic Press; 2018. p. 473–87.

33. Yang C, Wardenaar KJ, Bosker FJ, et al. Inflammatory markers and treatment outcome in treatment resistant depression: a systematic review. J Affect Disord 2019;257:640–9.

34. Dantzer R, O'connor JC, Freund GG, et al. From inflammation to sickness and depression: when the immune system subjugates the brain. Nat Rev Neurosci 2008;9(1):46–56.

35. Bhattacharya A, Derecki NC, Lovenberg TW, et al. Role of neuro-immunological factors in the pathophysiology of mood disorders. Psychopharmacology 2016; 233(9):1623–36.

36. Felger JC. Role of inflammation in depression and treatment implications. In: Antidepressants. Cham, Switzerland: Springer; 2018. p. 255–86.

37. Hodes GE, Pfau ML, Leboeuf M, et al. Individual differences in the peripheral immune system promote resilience versus susceptibility to social stress. Proc Natl Acad Sci U S A 2014;111(45):16136–41.

38. Khandaker GM, Pearson RM, Zammit S, et al. Association of serum interleukin 6 and C-reactive protein in childhood with depression and psychosis in young adult life: a population-based longitudinal study. JAMA Psychiatr 2014;71(10):1121–8.

39. Bell J, Kivimäki M, Bullmore E, et al. Repeated exposure to systemic inflammation and risk of new depressive symptoms among older adults. Transl Psychiatry 2017;7(8):e1208.

40. Lamers F, Milaneschi Y, Smit JH, et al. Longitudinal association between depression and inflammatory markers: results from the Netherlands study of depression and anxiety. Biol Psychiatry 2019;85(10):829–37.

41. Trivedi MH, Chin Fatt CR, Jha MK, et al. Comprehensive phenotyping of depression disease trajectory and risk: rationale and design of Texas Resilience Against Depression study (T-RAD). J Psychiatr Res 2020;122:22–32.

42. Insel TR. The NIMH research domain criteria (RDoC) project: precision medicine for psychiatry. Am J Psychiatr 2014;171(4):395–7.

43. Tamminga CA, Ivleva EI, Keshavan MS, et al. Clinical phenotypes of psychosis in the Bipolar-Schizophrenia Network on Intermediate Phenotypes (B-SNIP). Am J Psychiatr 2013;170(11):1263–74.

44. Gadad BS, Jha MK, Czysz A, et al. Peripheral biomarkers of major depression and antidepressant treatment response: current knowledge and future outlooks. J Affect Disord 2018;233:3–14.

45. Genser B, Cooper PJ, Yazdanbakhsh M, et al. A guide to modern statistical analysis of immunological data. BMC Immunol 2007;8(1):1–15.

46. Johnston KM, Powell LC, Anderson IM, et al. The burden of treatment-resistant depression: a systematic review of the economic and quality of life literature. J Affect Disord 2019;242:195–210.

47. Roche D, Russell V. Can precision medicine advance psychiatry? Ir J Psychol Med 2021;38(3):163–8.

48. Garriock HA, Kraft JB, Shyn SI, et al. A genomewide association study of citalopram response in major depressive disorder. Biological psychiatry 2010;67(2):133–8.

49. Uher R, Perroud N, Ng MY, et al. Genome-wide pharmacogenetics of antidepressant response in the GENDEP project. The American Journal of Psychiatry 2010;167(5):555–64.

50. Köhler CA, Freitas TH, Maes M, et al. Peripheral cytokine and chemokine alterations in depression: a meta-analysis of 82 studies. Acta Psychiatrica Scandinavica 2017;135(5):373–87.

51. Martins-de-Souza D. Proteomics, metabolomics, and protein interactomics in the characterization of the molecular features of major depressive disorder. Dialogues in Clinical Neuroscience 2014;16:63–73.

52. Paige LA, Mitchell MW, Krishnan KRR, Kaddurah-Daouk R, Steffens DC. A preliminary metabolomic analysis of older adults with and without depression. International Journal of Geriatric Psychiatry 2007;22(5):418–23.

Moving?

Make sure your subscription moves with you!

To notify us of your new address, find your **Clinics Account Number** (located on your mailing label above your name), and contact customer service at:

Email: **journalscustomerservice-usa@elsevier.com**

800-654-2452 (subscribers in the U.S. & Canada)
314-447-8871 (subscribers outside of the U.S. & Canada)

Fax number: 314-447-8029

Elsevier Health Sciences Division
Subscription Customer Service
3251 Riverport Lane
Maryland Heights, MO 63043

*To ensure uninterrupted delivery of your subscription, please notify us at least 4 weeks in advance of move.

Printed and bound by CPI Group (UK) Ltd, Croydon, CR0 4YY